National Healing, Integration and Reconciliation in Zimbabwe

This book brings together scholars from diverse backgrounds to provide interdisciplinary perspectives on national healing, integration, and reconciliation in Zimbabwe.

Taking into account the complex nature of healing across moral, political, economic, cultural, psychological, and spiritual dimensions of communities and the nation, the chapters discuss approaches, disparities, tensions, and solutions to healing and reconciliation within a multidisciplinary framework. Arguing that Zimbabwe's development agenda is severely compromised by the dominance of violence and militancy, the contributors analyse the challenges, possibilities and opportunities for national healing.

This book will be of interest to scholars of African studies, conflict and reconciliation, and development studies.

Ezra Chitando serves as a professor in the Department of Religious Studies, Classics, and Philosophy at the University of Zimbabwe and a theology consultant on HIV and AIDS for the World Council of Churches. He has published extensively on religion and HIV, gender, masculinity, politics, and methodology.

Kelvin Chikonzo is a senior lecturer who has researched intensively on protest theatre in Zimbabwe. He is interested in studying various aspects of democracy protest theatre as a way of ensuring that protest theatre does not replicate the oppression that it purports to fight against in terms of multi-vocalism, mediation of agency and liberating the spectator.

Nehemiah Chivandikwa is an Associate Professor at the University of Zimbabwe. He teaches theatre and development communication and applied media technologies. His research interests are in performance and body politics, gender, disability, applied theatre performances and media. He has published several articles in both regional and international journals in these areas. Prof Chivandikwa has been involved in several projects in applied theatre on gender, political violence, disability and rural and urban development. His latest 2017 publications are: 'Subverting Ableist Discourse as an Exercise in Precarity' in the Journal of Applied Theatre and Performance, 35(3):pp.61–75 and 'Political-Ethical Approach to Disability in Theatre for Development Context' in Applied Theatre Research, 5(2):83–97.

Routledge Contemporary Africa Series

For more information about this series, please visit: www.routledge.com/series/RCAFR

National Healing, Integration and Reconciliation in Zimbabwe

Edited by
Ezra Chitando, Kelvin Chikonzo
and Nehemiah Chivandikwa

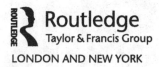

Routledge
Taylor & Francis Group

LONDON AND NEW YORK

First published 2020 by Routledge

2 Park Square, Milton Park, Abingdon, Oxon OX14 4RN
605 Third Avenue, New York, NY 10017

Routledge is an imprint of the Taylor & Francis Group, an informa business

First issued in paperback 2021

Publisher's Note

The publisher has gone to great lengths to ensure the quality of this reprint but points out that some imperfections in the original copies may be apparent.

British Library Cataloguing-in-Publication Data
A catalogue record for this book is available from the British Library

Library of Congress Cataloging-in-Publication Data
A catalog record for this book has been requested

ISBN: 978-0-367-34246-3 (hbk)
ISBN: 978-1-03-217617-8 (pbk)
DOI: 10.4324/9780429327049

Typeset in Bembo
by Apex CoVantage, LLC

Contents

Author biographies

Everisto Benyera is an Associate professor of African Politics in the Department of Political Sciences at the University of South Africa in Pretoria, South Africa. He holds a PhD in African Politics from the same university. He is a decolonial scholar and researches on transitional justice focusing on traditional and non-state reconciliation, peacebuilding and healing process. He is the author of 21 peer reviewed journal articles and book chapters. His two edited books are: *Indigenous, Traditional, and Non-State Transitional Justice in Southern Africa: Namibia and Zimbabwe* (Rowman and Littlefield: New York) and *Reimagining Justice, Human Rights and Leadership in Africa Challenging Discourse and Searching for Alternative Paths* (Springer: Cham).

Kudzai Biri is Associate Professor in the Department of Religious Studies, Classics and Philosophy at the University of Zimbabwe. She has published widely in the areas of Pentecostalism, African Traditional Religions, gender, politics and disability. In 2018 she was awarded the Alexander von Humboldt Research Fellowship, University of Bamberg, Germany.

Kelvin Chikonzo is a senior lecturer who has researched intensively on protest theatre in Zimbabwe. He is interested in studying various aspects of democracy protest theatre as a way of ensuring that protest theatre does not replicate the oppression that it purports to fight against in terms of multivocalism, mediation of agency and liberating the spectator.

Patrick Chiroro is a Professor in Cognitive Psychology supervising Post-Graduate Students in the Department of Psychology at the University of Zimbabwe. His research and publication interests include cognitive psychology, gender and psychology and youths employability.

Nehemiah Chivandikwa is an Associate Professor at the University of Zimbabwe. He teaches theatre and development communication and applied media technologies. His research interests are in performance and body politics, gender, disability, applied theatre performances and media. He has published several articles in both regional and international journals in these areas. Prof Chivandikwa has been involved in several projects in applied theatre on gender, political violence, disability and rural and urban development. His latest 2017 publications are: 'Subverting Ableist Discourse as an Exercise in Precarity' in the Journal of Applied Theatre and Performance, 35(3):pp.61–75 and 'Political- Ethical Approach to Disability in Theatre for Development Context' in Applied Theatre Research, 5(2):83–97.

Wellington Gadzikwa is a senior lecturer of Journalism and Media Studies at the University of Zimbabwe. His research interests are in journalism standards and practice, media framing, tabloids and tabloidization.

Mediel Hove is a professor of International and local conflicts, peacebuilding and Security in the War and Strategic Studies Section-History Department at the University of Zimbabwe and a Research Associate at the Durban University of Technology-South Africa. His research interests include conflict studies, peacebuilding, nonviolence, human and state security and strategic studies.

Diana Jeater is Emeritus Professor of African History at UWE, Bristol, and currently Associate Dean (Education) in the School of Histories, Languages and Cultures at the University of Liverpool. Her research and publication interests focus on diverse cultural and social aspects of Zimbabwean history, including gender and sexuality, law, language, knowledge construction, religion, witchcraft and healing, and spirits and reconciliation.

David Kaulemu is the Acting Dean of the School of Philosophy and Humanities and the Director of the Center for Ethics at Arrupe Jesuit University. He teaches social, economic and environmental philosophy. His research and publication interests include social justice, transitional justice, leadership and social transformation, global citizenship and Christian social teaching.

Ruby Magosvongwe is an Associate Professor in the Department of English, Faculty of Arts, University of Zimbabwe, for which she is currently Chairperson. Ruby is also a Research Fellow with the Department of English Studies in the Faculty of Humanities at UINSA. She joined the Department of English at University of Zimbabwe in 2001. She holds a Doctor of Philosophy Degree from the University of Cape Town. She has been the Acting Editor-in-Chief of *Zambezia*, University of Zimbabwe's Humanities Journal since April 2017. Her research thrusts are on development issues, focussing primarily on Comparative Literature; Literature and Gender, Land and Sustainable Livelihoods, and Cultural Studies.

Ruth Makumbirofa is a lecturer in the Theatre Arts Department at the University of Zimbabwe, where she teaches Applied Drama and Performance studies. Her research interests and publications include drama and life-skills development, African performance studies, drama and bereavement therapy as well as drama in peace building.

Tobias Marevesa is a New Testament Lecturer in the Department of Philosophy and Religious Studies, under the Joshua Nkomo School of Arts and Humanities at the Great Zimbabwe University where he teaches New Testament Studies and New Testament Greek. He is pursuing doctoral studies at the University of Pretoria in South Africa. His areas of interest are New Testament studies and politics, Pentecostal expressions in Zimbabwean Christianity, culture, human rights, and gender-based violence. He has also published in the area of New Testament studies and conflict-resolution in the Zimbabwean political landscape. He has attended and presented a number of papers in both regional and international conferences and has published articles in reputable international journals. He is a member of the New Testament Society of Southern Africa (NTSSA), Reading Association of Nigeria (RAN), Association for the Study of Religion in Southern Africa (ASRSA), African Consortium for Law and Religion Studies (ACLARS), and the International Consortium for Law and Religion Studies (ICLARS).

Francis Matambirofa is an Associate Professor of African languages and Literature at the University of Zimbabwe who teaches Comparative Bantu Linguistics and Shona language structure. His research interests are in the areas of theoretical linguistics, culture, lexicography and African politics at a general and/or observational level.

Samson Mhizha is a Lecturer of Developmental, Social and Cross-Cultural Psychology in the Department of Psychology at the University of Zimbabwe. His research and publication interests include developmental psychology, resiliency, the psychology of nationhood and psychological citizenship.

Tafadzwa Mlenga is currently pursuing a DPhil in film studies at the University of Zimbabwe. Her research interests are in theatre design, community theatre, and film studies.

Josephine Muganiwa is a Senior Lecturer in the Department of English of the University of Zimbabwe specialising in aspects of African and European literatures. Her research and publication interests include literature and: genres, gender, religion and culture.

Teddy Mungwari holds a Doctor of Literature and Philosophy in Communication Sciences and is a senior lecturer at Chinhoyi University of Technology. His research and publications are in political conflict and gender studies.

Tinashe Muromo is a Senior Lecturer of Research Methodology and Health Psychology in the Department of Psychology at the University of Zimbabwe. His research and publication interests include developmental psychology and health psychology.

Darlington Mutanda is currently a full-time lecturer at the University of Zimbabwe in the History Department (War and Strategic Studies unit) and a PhD student in the Department of Politics and International Relations at the University of Johannesburg, South Africa. His research interests include strategic studies and peacebuilding as it relates to: reconciliation, peace journalism, African security and conflict transformation, among others.

Enock Ndawana is a PhD candidate in the Department of Politics and International Relations, University of Johannesburg, South Africa and a full time lecturer in the War and Strategic Studies Section of the History Department, University of Zimbabwe, Zimbabwe. His research interests include: human security, African peace and politics, gender and conflict, conflict resolution and transformation.

Nisbert Taisekwa Taringa is an Associate Professor of Religious Studies at the University of Zimbabwe, Department of Religious Studies, Classics and Philosophy. He has published a book, *Towards an African-Christian Environmental Ethic* (University of Bamberg Press, 2014) and many book chapters and journal articles on religions and contemporary issues such as ecology, development, gender, HIV and AIDS, sexuality, animals in religions, religions and reconciliation, peace and conflict resolution, and human rights.

Joram Tarusarira (PhD) is currently serving as an Assistant Professor of Religion, Conflict and Peacebuilding in the Faculty of Theology and Religious Studies and as the Director, Centre for Religion, Conflict and Globalisation, University of Groningen, the Netherlands. He has expertise in Religion, Conflict, Peacebuilding and Reconciliation; Religion and Politics; Community Development; Civil Society and Social Movements. He has published widely in these areas. One of his latest publications (co-edited with E. Chitando) is *Religion and Human Security in Africa*. London: Routledge, 2019.

Liveson Tatira is a senior lecturer at the University of Zimbabwe, where he has been teaching in the Department of Curriculum and Arts Education for more than two decades. He holds a PhD in Shona Literature and another PhD in Arts (Onomastics). He has published in Folklore, Literature, Education and Indigenous Knowledge Systems. He is also a published Shona poet. He is married to Shamiso and they are blessed with two adult children, Herbert and Cephas.

Stanley Tsarwe is a senior lecturer of Journalism and Media Studies at the University of Zimbabwe. His research interests include media, conflict and peace; African radio and democracy; Mobile phones and emerging mobilities. He is an alumnus of the African Peacebuilding Network (APN).

Ephraim Vhutuza is currently a senior Lecturer and the founding chairperson of the Department of Film and Theatre Arts Studies, Midlands State University, Zimbabwe. He holds a Doctor of Literature and Philosophy in Zimbabwean drama written in English. His research interests and publications are in African literature, nationalism and written drama in Zimbabwe and theatre and in 2018, he published a book titled *Emerging Perspectives on Drama and Social Change in Zimbabwe*.

Introduction

National healing, integration and reconciliation in Zimbabwe

*Ezra Chitando, Kelvin Chikonzo, and
Nehemiah Chivandikwa*

Zimbabwe aspires to be an upper-middle income country by 2030. It seeks to embark on this trajectory and overcome the many years of economic turmoil. Under the late Robert Mugabe, who was removed from the office of president in November 2017 in a "military-assisted transition," Zimbabwe recorded high levels of inflation and unemployment. To achieve this goal of becoming an upper-middle income country by 2030, it is vital to achieve peace, healing, and integration too in the country. In order to move the country forward, all stakeholders must be able to address the past with honesty, justice, and creativity. This is because, "[T]he past is always present in Zimbabwe" (Peace Direct, Circa, 2017: 22).

The presence of the past in the present in Zimbabwe calls for patient reflection and interrogation. It implies that in the arena of conflict transformation, the past is not history. In everyday language, history belongs to the past, that is, what is now "gone." Yet, the past resists erasure. The past is stubborn. The past is persistent. The past does evolve into the present and affects it. Further, engaging with the past is not merely an intellectual exercise predicated on "facts." No. Deep feelings and emotions are involved. The past is not available for rewriting. It stares at us; confronting us with unpleasant events. The saving grace is that it can be redeemed (Lapsley, 2012). John Paul Lederach, a leading practitioner of conflict transformation, proposes that "[T]o rebuild relationships, we must develop innovative ways of providing space within which the emotional and psychological aspects of the conflict can be addressed" (Lederach, 1997: 152).

The desire by Zimbabwe to achieve socio-economic progress is salutary. However, it must be anchored on a very dynamic and creative approach to national healing. The concept of healing is unsettling to some scholars and activists. They regard it as being too tied to emotional and religious dimensions. However, healing entails contending with, and mending, the memories of trauma. It is informed by the understanding that, "[I]f left unaddressed, trauma leaves behind corrosive narratives that further erode the foundations of social harmony and peaceful coexistence" (Girma, 2018: xii). Focusing on healing emerges from appreciating the sobering reality that there can be no future without forgiveness (Tutu, 1999). According to Machinga (2012: 4), "For healing and restoration of broken relationships to take place, the feelings, emotions, and thoughts of survivors need to be acknowledged and validated."

Zimbabwe is, indeed, an intriguing case study on cycles of violence. After the removal of Mugabe and the heavily contested elections of 2018, serious violence broke out in the urban areas in January 2019. It is clear that addressing violence and facilitating healing is not only about looking back: It is also about the present and the future! Zimbabwe has continually hit the global news headlines as the place where violence is endemic. This volume seeks to contribute to the healing of the nation and offer possible insights into how future generations can live together in peace and harmony. Further, Zimbabwe's quest for healing offers valuable lessons to other countries in Africa (Uwazie, 2018; Mawere and Marongwe, 2018) and throughout the world.

No development for a divided and bleeding nation

Healing, integration, forgiveness, and reconciliation have different nuances, but they refer to the desire to inculcate and nurture cultures of peace. They speak to the desire to realistically and courageously confront pain, denial, injustice, and exclusion. They propose healing, acknowledgement, justice, and inclusion. Zimbabwe's history of violence (Schmidt, 2013; Kaulemu, 2011; Sachikonye, 2011; Human Rights Watch, 2011; Mukonori, 2012) makes the call for healing a compelling one. In particular, the Gukurahundi (Shona for "the rains that wash away the dirt") of the early 1980s heads the country's "unfinished business." This was when thousands of civilians in the Matabeleland and Midlands provinces of Zimbabwe were killed by the state's Fifth Brigade. Among others, Eppel (2004), Muzondidya and Ndlovu-Gatsheni (2007), Ndlovu-Gatsheni (2012), and others have sought to examine the implications of Gukurahundi on the national question. Ngwenya (2018, 2016) interrogates the urgency of holistic healing when addressing Gukurahundi. Ndlovu-Gatsheni and Benyera (2015) have explored the challenges that have characterized efforts to tackle healing and reconciliation in Zimbabwe, while Ndlovu and Harris (2015) lay bare the consequences of not healing.

It is clear that Zimbabwe is in dire need of healing. Mugabe's successor, Emmerson D. Mnangagwa, who finished Mugabe's term (November 2017–July 2018) and was inaugurated president of Zimbabwe in August 2018 after fractious elections (he was pronounced the winner over Nelson Chamisa), has popularised two sayings. One of them has been that, "Zimbabwe is open for business." This is a bold statement designed to appeal particularly to foreign investors. The other one is that, "the voice of the people is the voice of God." This declaration seeks to present the post–Mugabe era as democratic and guided by the will of the people. A massive investment in the project of national healing is needed urgently if both statements are to get traction. It is envisaged that the National Peace and Reconciliation Commission (NPRC) will contribute towards national healing and reconciliation (Heal Zimbabwe, 2018: ix).

Peace is the sine qua non for holistic and sustainable development. It is not possible to be open for business without having attended to "unfinished business."Without national healing and integration, scarce resources will be devoted towards identifying and neutralising "enemies and upstarts" at the expense of development.Tschirgi (2003: 2) maintains that peacebuilding is intricately tied to security and development. One of the critical investments the Zimbabwean government in particular and society in general can make is in the area of healing. A nation that is cohesive and shares a common vision is more attractive to investors than one that is characterised by strife. Mnangagwa's rhetoric has been designed to promote healing and reconciliation.At his inauguration, he reached out to different players, declaring that "What unites us is far greater than what divides us" (Ndlovu, 2018: 198). However, the declaration needs to be followed by practical and concrete actions that lead to conflict transformation in Zimbabwe. Unfortunately, violence appears to be the default mode of engagement in the country.

Healing is not a luxury. It is not an exercise of political brinkmanship. Healing is central to the progress of Zimbabwe. It is healing that will provide the platform for national development.A divided nation will not fly.The wrongs of the past must be righted.There must be truth telling and justice if Zimbabwe is to achieve its developmental goals. Here, it is important to cite the Zimbabwean philosopher and educationist, Hapanyengwi-Chemhuru, at length when he reflects on the meaning of reconciliation.Thus:

> It has to be a product of genuine realisation and acknowledgement by all that continued conflict is detrimental to the well-being of all the parties involved in the conflict, and that in the end no one will profit from the continuation of the conflict. As a process, reconciliation is sustained through the renewal of effort to promote justice, peace and national healing. When genuine reconciliation takes place, the parties come together to agree that there is need to work together, to admit guilt for crimes, to cease hostilities, and to forge or chart the way forward. It does not involve glossing over the causes of the conflict, but it does involve honest and sincere commitment to the attainment of peace. It, of necessity, involves the acknowledgement of the wrongs of the past, preparedness to forgive, and the expression of a desire to forge new relations and a new direction for the interest of all. But the wrongs of the past can only be forgiven if the truth of the past has been revealed or is known.
>
> (Hapanyengwi-Chemhuru, 2013: 83)

Zimbabwe needs to adopt a creative response to Gukurahundi. While the state has tried a number of initiatives, there must be a major investment in an effort to address this highly emotive issue.We believe that truth-telling, confession, and justice are central to processes that can contribute towards healing (Tshuma, 2018). Further, there must be radical vulnerability where those who were involved in Gukurahundi will apologise for errors of commission and omission. Although it is often accepted that no amount of cash can replace the lives of loved ones, there must be an accompanying process of reparation for survivors. No government will become bankrupt (financially) because it has sought to address an urgent national issue. Also, apart from the top-down initiatives by government, there must be more community-based healing initiatives. Traditional leaders, church leaders, non-governmental organisations (NGOs), and other players must build on indigenous healing mechanisms in order to facilitate the healing of memories. According to Villa-Vicencio:

> Indigenous African healing and reconciliation practices provide both *pre-verbal* and *nonverbal* spaces as a pretext for rational debate and conversation to take place as a way of dealing with the violence and trauma of the past. Through ceremony and ritual, perpetrators and victims are encouraged to make an attitudinal and behavioral shift from a prelinguistic state to the point where they can begin to articulate their experiences in words and ritual. Perpetrators can begin to acknowledge how they violated human rights and victims can begin to deal with their suffering. When effective, it can provide solace for individuals and groups sharing in these practices – drawing adversaries into an experiential bond that provides a basis from which to make reparations and promote community reconciliation and healing.
>
> (Villa-Vicencio, 2009: 134)

Additional challenges to be negotiated

There are a number of other issues that Zimbabwe needs to address in order to achieve healing. Kaulemu submits that there are inequalities that "threaten to destroy our nation which is deeply wounded and in need of healing" (2010: 1). We have already highlighted the challenges associated with the issue of Gukurahundi. In this section, we draw attention to some of the key challenges that Zimbabwe must negotiate if it is to make progress on the path to national healing, reconciliation, and integration. Although we concentrate on national conflicts or factors that have a bearing on peace (in both this section and the book more generally), it is vital to acknowledge that conflicts are found at different levels. Thus, there are conflicts at the family, community, provincial, and national levels (CCSF, 2014).

A poisoned approach to politics

Alongside the challenge relating to ethnicity, the nation will need to address the issue of aggressive political contestation. From the nationalist tensions in the 1960s, different political parties have been involved in intense rivalry, often involving violence. The struggle for independence and contestation for power also generated a culture of violence. Munemo (2016) has highlighted the political history of Zimbabwe, tracing how the various agreements between and amongst political parties have struggled to deliver peace, reconciliation, and unity.

The government of national unity (GNU), emerging out of the 2008 political and economic crisis, can be rightly viewed as a conflict transformation mechanism (Mutambudzi, 2015; Mapuva, 2010; Mukuhlani, 2014). While it is possible to critique challenges that characterised the GNU, it is clear that the collaboration amongst the different political parties enabled citizens to get some respite in the face of a debilitating socio-economic and political context. The GNU facilitated a rapid recovery of the economy. Although there were challenges, the reality of politicians from different political parties working together to promote the well-being of Zimbabweans left a lasting impression for many. It also proved that when politicians invest their energies towards the national cause, citizens benefit immensely.

Given the national benefits of harnessing talent from across the political divide, it is important for political actors to invest in dialogue and healing. The tension created by campaigns must not be allowed to cloud the national vision. Dialogue is not a sign of weakness. If anything, it is a mark of maturity and commitment to the national cause. Tendai Biti, one of the GNU actors, articulates the call for unity of purpose well when writing:

> The Zimbabwean example highlights the importance of forging a consensus around a common national strategy or vision. Without a fundamental agreement over the country's developmental trajectory, effective policy-making and reform cannot take root. Much has to do with leadership. A strong, focused and transformational leadership that puts the national interest above all else can drive an effective economic reform agenda at a sustained pace, as evidenced in Rwanda, Ghana and Botswana.
>
> (Biti, 2014: 22)

The 2018 elections delivered yet another contested result. This has exacerbated division along political lines, with voters being split between Mnangagwa and Chamisa (Bratton and Masunungure, 2018). A new approach to politics must be adopted in Zimbabwe. The preoccupation with the winner takes all overlooks the value of harnessing talent from across the political divide. Instead of slavishly following a model of politics that has stalled development, Zimbabweans must create a new electoral system that minimises tension and generates optimum returns for the country. Further, active citizen participation must be prioritised if the country is to engender democracy and national ownership of processes (ZCC, 2018: 36).

The mobilisation of ethnicity

The quest for and retention of political power has authored a related challenge of divisive ethnicity in Zimbabwe. While a few scholars have invested in elaborating on the creation of ethnicity in Zimbabwe (Ranger, 1985; Chimhundu,

1992; Sithole, 1999), there have been limited reflections on the extent to which many citizens overcome ethnicity in their day to day interactions. Thus, street vendors in the city of Masvingo, for example, flee municipal police together, irrespective of their ethnic identities. Love defies ethnic constructions and there are countless marriages across the ethnic groups. Many deep and lasting friendships at workplaces, in religious groups and within the communities have been formed across ethnic affiliation. The idea that there must be a socially engineered process to form friendship between the Shona and the Ndebele, for example (Muchemwa, 2015), is tenuous. It is politicians who mostly exaggerate ethnic differences and use these to generate loyalty. In contexts characterised by resource constraints, ethnicity is used as a tool to access resources. Thus, politicians mobilise ethnic sentiments to build a power base.

One of the most effective healing strategies when addressing the question of ethnicity is to acknowledge and celebrate ethnic differences. Efforts to address the challenges of ethnicity by placing a prefix, for example, "negative ethnicity" or "positive ethnicity," do not resolve them. The starting point must be to accept the reality of ethnicity and to acknowledge that both in the past and in the present, ethnicity has been appropriated and deployed to achieve definite political goals. Further, the project of state/nation building must not be done at the expense of celebrating ethnic diversity. The Nation building in Africa has tended to both suppress and minimise ethnic identities.

It is important to acknowledge the consequences of some ethnic groups being convinced that they do not belong. This generates resentment, withdrawal, or active resistance. The emergence of social media enables the expression of deeply held sentiments of exclusion. In Zimbabwe, social media has given some individuals ("nationalist" or "ethnic extremists") an opportunity to put across their views in very strong language (Mpofu, 2013). Addressing the reality of the cleavage brought about by ethnicity remains critical in Zimbabwe. It is vital to acknowledge that, "If we cannot live together, we surely will be buried here together. We must choose life rather than death" (Bhebhe, 2013: 23).

The challenge of ethnicity can be addressed by emphasising the capabilities that people from diverse groups bring to the national developmental agenda. By running a meritocracy, where anyone who is qualified for a position stands an equal chance to access it, Zimbabwe can overcome problematic appropriations of ethnicity. No ethnic group should ever feel that the best they can be is to deputise those from another ethnic group. Further, languages such as Chishona, isiNdebele, and other indigenous languages, should be taught from primary school, across the nation. The excitement around and popularity of isiNdebele at Umvukwesi Primary School in Mvurwi (Mashonaland Central) confirms the possibility of teaching indigenous languages across the different regions of the country (Mwase, 2011).

Trauma of lost savings

It is unfortunate that most of the scholars writing on healing and reconciliation in Zimbabwe have completely overlooked the trauma that many citizens have from the loss of savings when the Zimbabwe dollar was retired in favour of the multi-currency regime in 2009. No in-depth study has been undertaken to examine the extent to which many citizens are hurting from the loss of savings, pensions, and insurance policies. The personal experiences of the authors, who had their own savings wiped out, indicate that the pain is real and deep. The sense of powerlessness and feelings of vulnerability and having been taken for granted require urgent attention. The government adopted a unilateral policy when introducing the multi-currency system, resulting in massive losses. Thus:

> Firstly, there was no agreed exchange rate to use when converting debts and savings. Secondly, government did not require banks to convert money held in savings accounts and other investment portfolios, allowing banks to use the zero balance system, erasing the savings of millions of Zimbabweans. Finally the government authorised local authorities, the power utility and telecommunication companies to convert debts accrued prior to the transition to USD. Many people ended up with huge debts that to this day they cannot pay whilst at the same time their savings were wiped out and their salaries were not backdated.
>
> (PBNZ, n.d.: 15–16)

Mental illnesses such as anxiety, depression, and loneliness have become more widespread as Zimbabwe's economy has taken a plunge. Although it is helpful to investigate the resilience that citizens continue to demonstrate in the face of serious socio-economic and political challenges, there is need to acknowledge the need for healing from trauma induced by a collapsed economy. The respite that had been induced by the GNU has dissipated and renewed suffering had set in at the time of writing. The impact on health and well-being has not received adequate scholarly attention.

To his credit, in 2015 former President Mugabe established a Commission of Enquiry into the Conversion of Insurance and Pension Values from the Zimbabwe Dollar to the United States Dollar. The Commission presented its report in 2018 and made some valuable proposals. However, poor economic performance has meant that direct victims/survivors of dollarization have not been compensated. Worse still, it would appear that the issue of compensation is not on the agenda of the government. We are convinced that the government must address the question of compensation in order to bring healing. The feelings of having been fleeced of hard-earned savings elicit resentment, alienation, and resistance to the project of nation building.

Generational conflict

Adolescents and youth now constitute the majority of Zimbabwe's population. However, the dominant ideology in the country relates to celebrating the past and keeping the memory of the liberation struggle alive. In many senses, the generational conflict is also expressed in the political conflict. Although it would be misleading to suggest that there are no young people who support

Mnangagwa and his party, it is probably correct to observe that many young people are in Chamisa's corner (Bratton and Masunungure, 2018: 2). Outside politics, many young people are frustrated by the lack of employment or upward social mobility.

The generational conflict has generated tension between older people and youth in Zimbabwe. Young people feel that their futures have been stolen by older people. Consequently, they challenge narratives of sacrifice and commitment to the nation by their elders. Although young people have been deployed to perpetrate violence by the different political parties (Mude, 2014), it is important to view them more positively. Young people have creativity, talent, resilience, and skills that must be mobilised for national development. Unfortunately, most young in Zimbabwe feel left out of the national project. They have seen their future disappear in front of them, while adults continue to pontificate and reminisce about the struggle for liberation. Ironically, Mugabe, who insisted in his landmark 1980 independence and reconciliation "sermon" that it was vital to be forward-looking, spent the larger part of his leadership looking backwards! In this scheme, young people felt marginalised. It is, therefore, vital to initiate processes to bring the different generations into dialogue and effect healing.

Addressing sexual and gender-based violence

It requires a separate project to seek to do justice to the extent to which sexual and gender-based violence is rampant in Zimbabwe. As is the case in many conflicts, women have borne the brunt of election-related violence. Unfortunately, efforts to bring healing have not been gendered and Hunhu /Ubuntu has not taken women's experiences seriously (Manyonganise, 2017, 2015). Women have suffered horrendous abuse, with society appearing to accept the violation of women as an integral part of life. Although the 16 Days Against Gender-based Violence campaign (25 November – 10 December) has gained momentum, many people have not undergone personal transformation to internalise resistance to violence against women.

Violence against women is rampant in homes and institutions. Women who seek political office are routinely attacked as "prostitutes," and there are no consequences for the men who use violent language. Across the political parties, religious organisations, and in everyday language, women endure physical, psychological, spiritual, and other forms of violence. While this is a global phenomenon, Zimbabwe must demonstrate greater commitment towards addressing sexual gender-based violence. After all, it boasts of having a highly educated populace!

Multiple approaches to healing

One of the major challenges characterising the quest for healing in Zimbabwe has been the dominance of government-led, top-down, formal processes. While it remains important for the government to demonstrate commitment to healing, reconciliation, and integration, it is vital to embrace diverse approaches. Thus, indigenous approaches of conflict transformation and healing, such as understanding *ngozi* (justice-seeking spirit), *nhimbe* (traditional communal way of working together), *usahwira* (covenant friendships), proverbs, and others must be explored in creative ways.

The arts must be employed fully in the quest for the healing of individuals, communities, and the nation. Music, dance, and drama are powerful resources that can be harnessed to bring healing. What is critical is for politicians, and religious, and community leaders to recognise the urgency of the task at hand. The current approach that regards healing as a footnote is not sustainable. Zimbabweans must have the courage to face the (our) past with courage in order to shape the future together. The words of Kgalema Monthlante, who led the Commission of Enquiry into the 1 August 2018 post-election violence are helpful in this regard: "The past we inherit, the future we create" (Ncube, 2018).

Chapters in this volume

The chapters in this volume interact with most of the issues that we have outlined in the foregoing sections. The chapters are organised thematically. Chapters that have a historical (and political) outlook in terms of engaging with the quest for healing constitute the first set. In Chapter One, Teddy Mungwari and Ephraim Vhutuza provide an overview of the episodes of violence in independent Zimbabwe. The chapter is an overview of key issues and challenges around the question of national healing and reconciliation in Zimbabwe. David Kaulemu doubts the capacity of the post-colonial state to deliver healing and reconciliation due to its faulty foundations in Chapter Two, while in Chapter Three Mediel Hove and Darlington Mutanda revisits the multiple challenges that Zimbabwe must address. In Chapter Four, Tobias Marevesa examines one attempt at conflict transformation, namely, the Global Political Agreement. In Chapter Five, Evaristo Benyera critiques the use of Commissions of Inquiry as a transitional justice mechanism in Zimbabwe. He is convinced that sincerity has not been a defining feature in the setting up of Commissions of Inquiry in the country, as the results have remained opaque and there has not been any political will to ensure that the recommendations are implemented. In Chapter Six, Joram Tarusarira theorises on national healing and reconciliation in Zimbabwe. He brings fresh theoretical perspectives to this discourse and offers new ways of thinking about healing and reconciliation in the nation.

The role of language in facilitating national healing is the theme of Chapter Seven. In it, Francis Matambirofa contends that new terms must characterise political discourse in order to inculcate a more tolerant culture. Liveson Tatira reflects on the potential of proverbs to promote peace, healing, and reconciliation in Chapter Eight. One indigenous cultural institution, namely that of the *sahwira* (intimate friend), has a lot of potential to facilitate healing in families and communities. In Chapter Nine, Ruth Makumbirofa, Kelvin Chikonzo, and

Nehemiah Chivandikwa explore the role of the *sahwira* and the potential of this institution to contribution to national healing and reconciliation. Theatre has been one avenue for exploring the tension around national healing and reconciliation. In Chapter Ten, Nehemiah Chivandikwa, Kelvin Chikonzo, and Tafadzwa Mlenga critique the play, "Heal the Wounds" in its efforts to promote reconciliation in Zimbabwe. This is followed by an examination of the *ngozi* (justice-seeking spirit) in Chapter Twelve by Diana Jeater. She reflects on the politics of translation and minimisation of indigenous concepts in the quest for justice, healing, and integration in Zimbabwe.

From here, the volume shifts to the role of the written word in promoting national healing. In Chapter Twelve, Stanley Tsarwe and Wellington Gadzikwa focus on the media and healing, while in Chapter Thirteen, Josephine Muganiwa analyses the book, *Running with Mother*, and its engagement with Gukurahundi. Recognising the value of literary works from other parts of the continent, in Chapter Fourteen, Ruby Magosvongwe reflects on the selected works of Nigeria's Chimamanda Ngozi Adichie and their implications for Zimbabwe. The role of peace education is the focus of the chapter that follows. In Chapter Fifteen, Hove Enock Ndawana discuss the importance of peace education and argue that it should be at the heart of post-conflict restructuring in Zimbabwe.

Religion plays a major role in conflict transformation. In Chapter Sixteen, Kudzai Biri reflects on Pentecostal discourses on nation building, while in Chapter Seventeen Ezra Chitando and Nisbert T. Taringa propose the transformation of theology and religious studies in order to ensure that graduates are better equipped to promote national healing. In Chapter Eighteen, Samson Mhizha, Tinashe Muromo, and Patrick Chiroro, and Tinashe Muromo remind readers of a constituency that is often neglected in national healing discourses, namely, children on the streets. They reflect on the need to promote healing among children on the streets in Zimbabwe. The closing chapter in this volume, namely, Chapter Nineteen, reminds the reader of the urgency of addressing environmental degradation in Zimbabwe. Taringa argues that the healing of the land provides a platform where all other forms of healing can be accomplished.

Overall, we are encouraged by the fact that scholars from diverse disciplines answered our call to reflect on the key issues relating to national healing in Zimbabwe. The regular outbreaks of violence and strong language that flares up frequently on social media are indicative of a body politic that is in dire need of healing. More work needs to be done to ensure more voices of women and that women's issues are addressed. Further, there is need to accord more space to scholars from excluded ethnic, racial, and other social groups. Thus, other forms of exclusion based on geographical location, social status, political party affiliation, the extent of rootedness in Zimbabwe (e.g. having a totem), race, disability status, living with albinism, sexual orientation and gender identity, and others, will require another volume. This volume, however, refocuses the debate on national healing and confirms the urgency of multidisciplinary perspectives in the quest for healing, integration, reconciliation, and national cohesion. It is envisaged that the volume will inspire reflections in other African contexts.

References

Bhebhe, P. 2013. "Zimbabwe: Integration, Reconciliation and Rehabilitation Processes," *Journal of Emerging Trends in Educational Research and Policy Studies* 4(1), 17–24.

Biti, T. 2014. *Rebuilding Zimbabwe: Lessons from a Coalition Government.* Washington, DC: Centre for Global Development.

Bratton, M. and E. V. Masunungure. 2018. *Heal the Beloved Country: Zimbabwe's Polarized Electorate.* Afrobarometer Policy Paper No. 49.

CCSF (Church and Civil Society Forum). 2014. *Local Conflict Resolution Mechanisms Mapping Report.* Harare: CCSF.

Chimhundu, H. 1992. "Early Missionaries and the Ethnolinguistic Factor During the 'Invention of Tribalism' in Zimbabwe," *The Journal of African History* 33(1), 87–109.

Eppel, S. 2004. "'Gukurahundi': The Need for Truth and Reparation," in Brian Raftopoulos and Tyrone Savage (eds.), *Zimbabwe: Injustice and Political Reconciliation.* Cape Town: Institute for Justice and Reconciliation.

Girma, M. 2018. "Introduction," in M. Girma (ed.), *The Healing of Memories: African Christian Responses to Politically Induced Trauma.* Lanham: Lexington Books.

Hapanyengwi-Chemhuru, O. 2013. "Reconciliation, Conciliation, Integration and National Healing," *African Journal of Conflict Resolution* 13(1), 79–99.

Heal Zimbabwe. 2018. *A Baseline Study Report on the Peace and Reconciliation Process in Zimbabwe.* Harare: Heal Zimbabwe Trust.

Human Rights Watch. 2011. *Perpetual Fear: Impunity and Cycles of Violence in Zimbabwe.* New York: Human Rights Watch.

Kaulemu, D. 2010. *Zimbabwe: Promotion of Equality, National Healing, Cohesion and Unity.* Harare: Konrad Adenauer Stiftung.

Kaulemu, D. 2011. *Ending Violence in Zimbabwe.* Harare: Konrad Adenauer Stiftung.

Lapsley, M. 2012. *Redeeming the Past: My Journey from Freedom Fighter to Healer.* Maryknoll, NY: Orbis Books.

Lederach, J. P. 1997. *Building Peace: Sustainable Reconciliation in Divided Societies.* Washington, DC: United States Institute of Peace Press.

Machinga, M. M. 2012. "Grassroots Healing and Reconciliation in Zimbabwe: Introducing the RECORE Process," *Practical Matters* 5, 1–11.

Manyonganise, M. 2015. "Oppressive and Liberative: A Zimbabwean Woman's Reflections on *Ubuntu*," *Verbum et Ecclesia* 36(2), Art. #1438, 7 pages.

Manyonganise, M. 2017. "Invisibilising the Victimised: Churches in Manicaland and Women's Experiences of Political Violence in National Healing and Reconciliation in Zimbabwe," *Journal for the Study of Religion* 30(1), 110–136.

Mapuva, J. 2010. "Government of National Unity (GNU) as a Conflict Prevention Strategy: The Case of Zimbabwe and Kenya," *Journal of Sustainable Development in Africa* 12, 247–263.

Mawere, M. and N. Marongwe (Eds.) 2018. *Violence, Politics and Conflict Management in Africa: Envisioning Transformation, Peace and Unity in the Twenty-First Century.* Mankon, Bamenda: Langaa Research & Publishing CIG.

Mpofu, S. 2013. "Social Media and the Politics of Ethnicity in Zimbabwe," *Ecquid Novi: African Journalism Studies* 34(1), 115–122.

Muchemwa, C. 2015. "Building Friendships Between Shona and Ndebele Ethnic Groups in Zimbabwe," A Thesis Submitted in Fulfilment of the Requirements of the Degree of Doctor of Philosophy in the Faculty of Management Sciences Public Management (Peacebuilding), Durban University of Technology.

Mude, T. 2014. "Political Violence: Major Socio-Political Consequences of Urban Youth Unemployment in Zimbabwe," *Review of History and Political Science* 2(1), 107–139.

Mukonori, F. 2012. *The Genesis of Violence in Zimbabwe*. Harare: Centre for Peace Initiatives in Africa.

Mukuhlani, T. 2014. "Zimbabwe's Government of National Unity: Successes and Challenges in Restoring Peace and Order," *Journal of Power, Politics & Government* 2(2), 169–180.

Munemo, D. 2016. "The Search for Peace, Reconciliation and Unity in Zimbabwe: From the 1978 Internal Settlement to the 2008 Global Political Agreement," A Doctoral Thesis in Development Studies, University of South Africa, Pretoria.

Mutambudzi, A. 2015. "Conflict and the Resolution Process in Zimbabwe from 2000 to 2013," A Thesis Submitted to the Faculty of Commerce, Law and Management, University of the Witwatersrand, in Fulfilment of the Requirements for the Degree of Doctor of Philosophy.

Muzondidya, J. and S. J. Ndlovu-Gatsheni. 2007. "'Echoing Silences': Ethnicity in Post-Colonial Zimbabwe, 1980–2007," *African Journal of Conflict Resolution* 7(2), 275–297.

Mwase, E. 2011. "Ndebele gains popularity in Mashonaland," *The Sunday Mail*, Harare, 31 October.

Ncube, X. 2018. "Motlanthe Speaks on His Zim Connection: The Big Interview," *The Standard*, 2–8 December.

Ndlovu, R. 2018. *In the Jaws of the Crocodile: Emmerson Mnangagwa's Rise to Power in Zimbabwe*. Cape Town: Penguin Books.

Ndlovu-Gatsheni, S. J. 2012. "Rethinking Chimurenga and Gukurahundi in Zimbabwe: A Critique of Partisan National History," *African Studies Review* 55(3), 1–26.

Ndlovu-Gatsheni, S. and E. Benyera. 2015. "Towards a Framework for Addressing the Justice and Reconciliation Question in Zimbabwe," *African Journal of Conflict Resolution* 15(2), 9–33.

Ngwenya, D. 2016. "'Our Branches Are Broken': Using the Tree of Life Healing Methodology with Victims of Gukurahundi in Matabeleland, Zimbabwe," *Peace and Conflict Studies* 23(1), Article 2.

Ngwenya, D. 2018. *Healing the Wounds of Gukurahundi in Zimbabwe: A Participatory Action Research Project*. New York: Springer.

Ngwenya, D. and G. Harris. 2015. "The Consequences of not Healing: Evidence from the Gukurahundi Violence in Zimbabwe," *African Journal of Conflict Resolution* 15(2), 35–55.

PBNZ (Peace Building Network of Zimbabwe). n.d. *The Role of the Business Sector in National Healing in Zimbabwe*. Harare: PBNZ.

Peace Direct. Circa. 2017. *Local Voices for Peace in Zimbabwe: Civil Society Perspectives on Peace and Conflict Issues in Zimbabwe*. London: Peace Direct. www.peacedirect.org/wp-content/uploads/2017/06/P661-PD-LVP-Zimbabwe-Report_LR.pdf (accessed on 23 November 2018).

Ranger, T. 1985. *The Invention of Tribalism in Zimbabwe*. Gweru: Mambo Press.

Sachikonye, L. 2011. *When a State Turns on its Citizens: 60 years of Institutionalised Violence in Zimbabwe*. Johannesburg: Jacana Media.

Schmidt, H. I. 2013. *Colonialism and Violence in Zimbabwe: A History of Suffering*. Woodbridge: Currey.

Sithole, M. 1999. *Zimbabwe: Struggles Within the Struggle*. Harare: Rujeko Publishers.

Tshirgi, N. 2003. *Peacebuilding as the Link Between Security and Development: Is the Window of Opportunity Closing?* New York: International Peace Academy Studies in Security and Development.

Tshuma, D. 2018. "Reconciliation, Integration and Healing Efforts in Zimbabwe," *Conflict Trends* 2, 19–26.

Tutu, D. 1999. *No Future Without Forgiveness*. New York: Doubleday.

Uwazie, E. E. (Ed.) 2018. *Peace and Conflict Resolution in Africa: Lessons and Opportunities*. Newcastle upon Tyne: Cambridge Scholars Press.

Villa-Vicencio, Charles. 2009. *Walk with Us and Listen: Political Reconciliation in Africa*. Washington, D. C.: Georgetown University Press.

ZCC (Zimbabwe Council of Churches). 2018. *2018 Harmonized Elections: Prospects for Democratic Transition in Zimbabwe*. Harare: ZCC.

1 The elusive search for national healing and reconciliation in Zimbabwe

Teddy Mungwari and Ephraim Vhutuza

Introduction

The chapter is an overview of key issues and challenges around the question of national healing and reconciliation in Zimbabwe. The search for national peace, reconciliation, and justice has a long history that can be traced back to the pre-colonial and colonial eras. However, this chapter mainly focuses on Zimbabwe after independence. We argue that the 1983–1987 infamous Gukurahundi massacres, the excesses of the land reform programme in 2000 and after, Operation Murambatsvina in 2005 and the violent June 2008 presidential re-run election have made Zimbabwe a candidate for serious dialogue around national healing, reconciliation, and justice mechanisms. The chapter argues that Zimbabwe has never comprehensively attempted to prosecute and/or compel perpetrators or instigators of mainly political violence to publicly acknowledge their transgressions. The policy of amnesia has always outweighed the imperatives of victim-sensitive national healing and reconciliation processes. We argue in this chapter that the major deficiency in Zimbabwe has been lack of clear and binding instruments and political will for achieving national healing and reconciliation. Individuals and institutions that foment violence and cause trauma to sections of the society have not been held accountable and subsequently this has had the negative effect of foreclosing any meaningful national healing, reconciliation, and inevitably any form of justice. The chapter concludes by reiterating that reconciliation and national healing are demanding responsibilities that call for greater commitment, dedication, and acknowledgement, and that there is need for the national political leadership to support processes already happening in various communities at the local level. Thus, a more holistic approach is needed to resolve the politics of reconciliation and national healing in Zimbabwe.

Background

Zimbabwe has been experiencing bloody conflicts dating back to the colonial and indeed, pre-colonial eras. At independence in 1980, then President Robert

Mugabe (now late), who was then the new Prime Minister, proclaimed a policy of national reconciliation between former belligerents that included the former white coloniser. The liberation struggle had been traumatic to all and the Prime Minister concluded that the country would need to move forward by proclaiming and promoting the policy of reconciliation without perpetrators of violence and murders acknowledging their past. Even after he announced that policy, many racist white Rhodesians could not believe his word. As a result, many left the country for fear of retribution from the new black leadership that had assumed political power notwithstanding certain privileges guaranteed by the 1979 Lancaster House Constitution. What this clearly demonstrates is that the policy of reconciliation in 1980 on its own, minus public acknowledgment of the past by the perpetrators, was not enough, hence the flight by some of the white people. However, this does not imply that only white people were perpetrators of violence and needless killings. On all sides, including among the black nationalists, there were perpetrators who should have been given the opportunity to confess their past during the years leading to independence in 1980.

Because individuals and institutions were not asked to acknowledge their past, mistrust and fear became the order of the day. It did not take more than two years before the Gukurahundi era started. Gukurahundi, easily the bloodiest civil conflict to-date, was mainly confined to the Matabeleland and Midlands provinces and saw thousands of civilians being maimed and killed by the North Korean-trained 5th Brigade; a now disbanded division of the Zimbabwe National Army. The Army was unleashed to crush rebellion among dissident elements who were black Zimbabweans perceived to be fighting state interests. According to the Catholic Commission for Justice and Peace (CCJP) report of 1997, over 20,000 people were massacred between 1983 and 1987 before the signing of the Unity Accord between Mugabe's Zimbabwe African National Union (ZANU), and the Zimbabwe African People's Union (ZAPU), then led by the late Vice President Joshua Nkomo. That 1987 Unity Accord brought the two warring parties together to form the Zimbabwe African National Union Patriotic Front (ZANU PF).

According to the Zimbabwe Catholic Bishops' Conference *et.al* report (2006), the conflicts which render national healing and reconciliation imperative in Zimbabwe can be traced back to the pre-colonial times. Cases in point are the ethnic conflicts between the Shona and Ndebele and later the racial tension and violence, mainly between black and white during the colonial period. In post-colonial times, apart from the Gukurahundi era, there has been recurrent state and inter-party sponsored violence unleashed on unarmed civilians. After the formation of a strong and formidable party in the Movement for Democratic Change (MDC) in 1999, some war veterans and ZANU PF youth militias in rural and farming areas have been implicated in violence against perceived political opponents (Primorac, 2007). Political violence continuously reared its ugly head at election times and as a result it is not surprising that the word "election" has become synonymous with violence in the general tapestry of an otherwise peace-loving nation. The June 2008 Presidential Re-run election easily emerges as one of the bloodiest since independence. Also, around 2000, a number of victims, mainly composed of white farmers, were maimed and killed during the land reform programme. All these violent episodes in the history of Zimbabwe beg for clearly thought-out and meaningful national healing and reconciliation mechanisms. Unfortunately, these have not been forthcoming to date despite some attempts such as the creation of the Organ on National Healing and Reconciliation during the life of the Inclusive Government from 2009–2013.

The Organ on National Healing and Reconciliation (ONHR) formed during the life of the Inclusive Government, also known as the Government of National Unity, was an attempt to promote national healing and reconciliation in Zimbabwe following years of conflicts and violence among Zimbabwe after independence. However, according to Goredema et al. (2014), the continued mistrust and inter-party violence among the two formations of the Movement for Democratic Change (MDC), one led by the then Prime Minister, Morgan Tsvangirai and the other by the Industry and Commerce Minister, Welshman Ncube and President Robert Mugabe's ZANU PF, did not bring any meaningful national healing and reconciliation to the nation. Thus, the formation of the ONHR did not yield the intended result.

Savage (2003) argues that violence and conflicts in independent Zimbabwe are products of an incomplete and corrupted transition from colonial rule. To buttress Savage's (2003) observation, Paul Juru, co-chair of the Church and Civil Society Forum (CCSF), a non-governmental organisation (NGO) that has attempted to help with the promotion of national healing, was quoted in the *News Day* of 25 March 2015 arguing that Zimbabwe's predicament was that, for years, it has not attempted to heal its past wounds. He further argued that the only way the country could break from its sad past is through a comprehensive national healing and reconciliation programme that is capable of uniting both the victims and the perpetrators of past violations. We argue that this is yet to happen at the time of writing.

Will a Zimbabwean version of the South African Truth and Reconciliation Commission (TRC) be the answer to the trauma that has been suffered by some sections of the population since independence? According to South Africa's Nobel Prize laureate and human rights activist, Archbishop Desmond Tutu, who was also the chairperson of the TRC, "peace without justice is an impossibility" (*Financial Gazette*, 20 July 2017). He further argues that:

> I hope that the work of the Commission, by opening wounds to cleanse them, will thereby stop them from festering. We cannot be facile and say bygones will be bygones, because they will not be bygones and will return to haunt us. True reconciliation is never cheap, for it is based on forgiveness,

which has to be based on an acknowledgement of what was done wrong and therefore on disclosure of the truth.

You cannot forgive what you do not know.

(Tutu, on his appointment as chairperson of the TRC on 30 November 1995 as cited in *Financial Gazette* of 20 July 2017)

Tutu is a strong advocate of forgiveness and the Ubuntu way of finding justice. We agree with his observation in the previous quote that reconciliation should be encouraged, but that it should be predicated on the acknowledgement of what was done wrong by perpetrators of the trauma. Tutu was further quoted in the *New Yorker* of November 1996 (cited in *Financial Gazette*, ibid.) saying that there are two kinds of justice, the retributive, which is largely Western, and the African understanding of justice, which he argues is far more restorative and not meant to punish as an end in itself. Although we agree with Tutu on restorative justice, we argue that in the Zimbabwean context, perpetrators have not been forthcoming in acknowledging their hand in the trauma that was played on innocent victims, especially if the perpetrators are highly placed in society. Thus, to ensure national reconciliation and healing in Zimbabwe, we argue that the state and/ or political parties must be willing to openly admit their role as individuals and collectively in the violence and massacres that have happened in Zimbabwe since independence. Only if this is done can national healing and reconciliation be complete and acceptable in our view.

Healing will only come if the truth is told. We argue in this chapter that the right to truth is both in individual and the collective. Each survivor has the right to know the truth and how violations affect(ed) them. In this regard, informing broader society about fundamental freedoms and how they have been violated is a vital safeguard against the occurrence of abuses. We also note that despite government's unwillingness to promote debate and initiate programmes on national healing and reconciliation, non-governmental organisations seem to be making more inroads towards this. The Zimbabwe Human Rights Non-Governmental Forum (ZHR NGO Forum), a consortium of over 20 peace and pro-democracy civil organisations, has been holding meetings across the country urging people to demand clear mechanisms and implementation of statues on national healing and reconciliation in Zimbabwe.

Against this background, the Human Rights Bill which sailed through Parliament in July 2017 limits the scope of the Zimbabwe Human Rights Commission to the period after the 2008 political violence. This is despite the fact that the Organ on National Healing and Reconciliation has not meaningfully addressed the traumatic events that happened before 2008. We argue in this chapter that despite ZANU PF's advantage of a two-thirds majority in Parliament to pass through bills, Zimbabweans should continue to debate and push for programmes that promote national healing and reconciliation at local level. However, uncertainty is forever haunting Zimbabweans as Mugabe would sometimes remind citizens of old wounds from past massacres such as the Gukurahundi. For example, in 2016, when a section of the war veterans expressed their succession preference of then Vice President Emmerson Mnangagwa, it provoked then President Robert Mugabe into saying: "Zimbabwe National Liberation War Veterans Association (ZNLWVA) was formed to cater for the welfare of our veterans and not to champion the struggle for political change . . . Do we see another rise of dissident activity? . . . It's not your business to talk a lot on who shall be the president" (*Daily News* of 10 June 2016).

The reference to dissident activity easily reminds Zimbabweans of the Gukurahundi era and this sends chills down the spines of many Zimbabweans. It is worsened by the fact that a lot of secrecy and denial still surrounds the Gukurahundi era a thing that does not augur well for national healing and reconciliation let alone issues of justice.

In pursuit of national healing and reconciliation in Zimbabwe

The pre-colonial era, colonial era, and the post-colonial era serve as identifiable historical periods in which our conflicts have taken place. Each era has its own sources of conflict that can be seen as political, economic, and cultural. However, the different eras have deeply influenced each other. What has made the situation complex is the fact that conflicts that existed before colonisation were used by the colonial system's divide and rule strategies for the purposes of maintaining power and control, only to have some of the same modes of thinking, strategies, and institutions inherited and perpetuated in the post-colonial period (CCJP, 1997). This makes the challenges of healing, reconciliation, justice, and peace in Zimbabwe very complex, as it becomes necessary to deal with the present hurts and wounds, as well as trace the wounds of the past. We argue in this chapter that historical wounds have been carried to the present through memories, oral traditions, and recorded reports. Members of one group that were victims to violence in one era have sometimes turned out to be the perpetrators in another.

Murambadoro (2014) discusses critical insights around issues surrounding national healing and reconciliation efforts in the country and suggests that the government of Zimbabwe has undermined the reconciliation process in the country by failing on several occasions to implement measures to address and prevent the occurrence of social injustices. Murambadoro (2014), posits that the government repeatedly ignored the demands of victims of the Gukurahundi massacres in 1983–1987, the land invasions of 2000–2001, and Operation *Murambatsvina* in 2005, with perpetrators protected from accountability by amnesty provisions, the Clemency Orders of 1980, 1988, and 2000, as well as government security agents (Benyera, 2014; Mashingaidze, 2010; Ndlovu-Gatsheni and Benyera, 2015).

Instead of acknowledging state and in some cases individual and party violence on innocent civilians, the national leadership has mostly attempted to reconcile the population at the political level by signing agreements with its rival parties (Sachikonye, 1996). This may have been the case with the Gukurahundi massacres. Other reconciliation efforts arguably have become ceremonial projects that serve to silence any claims that the government is unwilling to account for past injustices (Mlambo, 2009). This chapter posits that there is need for deeper and more lasting national healing and reconciliation efforts in Zimbabwe and this can be a reality if the magnitude of the happenings in the affected areas is more widely understood and acknowledged by all those concerned. Only when those who inflicted untold hardships are prepared to acknowledge what they did, can lasting reconciliation take place between all who live in Zimbabwe. And only then can the bitterness and fear of the past be eased although not necessarily forgotten. The CCJP (ibid.) posits that unless past atrocities are sincerely acknowledged, fear among victims and survivors will not recede and that they will themselves not feel able to speak out about their experiences without dreading retribution. This applies to a wide range of victims and survivors of the 1983–1987 Gukurahundi, 2000 land invasions, the 2005 Operation Murambatsvina, and the 2008 presidential election re-run.

Ndlovu-Gatsheni and Benyera (2015) argue that there have been numerous amnesties and pardons in Zimbabwe. These amnesties gave blanket immunity, thereby stifling the processes of truth telling, truth recovery, healing, and reconciliation. The Inclusive Government's Organ on National Healing and Reconciliation's effectiveness in national healing and reconciliation efforts has been largely dismissed by Goredema et al. (2014). The capacity of the National Peace and Reconciliation Commission (NPRC) to remedy these historical shortcomings remains to be seen. The state's track record at healing and reconciliation which, besides being littered with amnesties and pardons, is heavily punctuated characterised by an amnesia that has become its official position regarding past human rights abuses thereby limiting effectiveness of commissions. Ndlovu-Gatsheni and Benyera (2015) posit that the National Reconciliation Policy of 1980 and the Unity Accord of 1987 are the cornerstone of this amnesia policy. Amnesia is a policy which entails a conscious decision by the government not to investigate past atrocities on the grounds that such investigations will jeopardise precarious peace-building efforts (Tendi, 2010). This happened after the unity between ZANU and ZAPU and thereafter all attempts to dialogue around the Gukurahundi era have been seen as debilitative to Zimbabwe's peace-building efforts.

In 1980, reconciliation efforts were reduced to the prescription of amnesia (Mungwini, 2013; Ndlovu-Gatsheni and Benyera, 2015) by Mugabe through his 1980 inaugural speech, in which he proclaimed that all parties should "let bygones be bygones" (Nyarota, 2006: 145). But Tutu (cited in *Financial Gazette*, 20 July 2017) argues that such mere pronouncements will return to haunt people if no truth telling, acknowledgements, and forgiveness are done in an open manner. Murambadoro (ibid.) observes that this expectation that the violence-stricken communities would forget the past without recourse was dispelled in the 1983–1987 period with the outbreak of a conflict between ZAPU and ZANU.

Following Gukurahundi massacres, a Unity Accord of 1987 was an attempt for the second reconciliation project. There was no further effort by government to address the social injustices that occurred during the atrocities, instead; it issued an amnesty proclamation pardoning all crimes committed and forcing the population to move on (Murambadoro, ibid.). The implication was that the more than 20,000 victims of the massacres were part of collateral damage that occurs in any conflict situation, which is why, in a public speech at Nkomo's burial in 1999, Mugabe referred to the Gukurahundi massacres as a "moment of madness." This is the closest that the former president came to openly acknowledging wrongdoing during the Gukurahundi era. Other than that, the state has not tolerated any dialogue around the massacres.

Former President Mugabe's admission that it was "a moment of madness" has prompted Muzondidya and Ndlovu-Gatsheni (2007) into challenging the government to explain who was mad at the time of the massacres, and whether the madness has been treated. These concerns arise from the view that subsequent actions of the government – such as the land invasions in 2000–2001, Operation Murambatsvina in 2005, and the post-electoral violence in 2008 – seem to indicate the "madness" has continued. Sadomba (2011) also writes about election-related violence, code-named Operation *Mavhoterapapi* [where did you place your vote?] of 2008 power struggles pitting the ruling ZANU PF against the opposition MDC formations.

Election times have rarely been peaceful in Zimbabwe since 1980 (Mungwari, 2016). Belonging to a different ideological persuasion provokes hatred and violence in a country where constitutional provisions such as freedom of political affiliation are sometimes not respected. As a result of these realities, conflict and violence have continued to be a major challenge in Zimbabwe (Mashingaidze, 2010). Ironically, there has never been any serious national commitment to finding truth, establishing justice, and forging durable reconciliation in Zimbabwe.

According to Murambadoro (2014), government made efforts at a formal reconciliation process as the third project in which it adopted the Organ for National Healing and Reconciliation. She argues that a third attempt at reconciliation emerged in 2008 from a mandated transitional Inclusive Government (IG), comprising ZANU PF, led by President Robert Mugabe and the two MDC formations, namely, MDC-T, led by the then Prime Minister Morgan Tsvangirai and MDC-N, led by Welshman Ncube. The IG resulted from a Global Political Agreement (GPA) signed in September 2008 following a mediation process initiated by the Sothern African Development Community (SADC) led by former President of South Africa Thabo Mbeki, to resolve the polarised June 2008 elections.

The ONHRI did not achieve its intended goal mainly because of its top-down approach which failed to cater to the demands of the grassroots. ONHRI might also have failed because, although it was expected to run as an independent body, the authority to exercise its mandate remained in the hands of government. The conflict of interests among parties could not be resolved because the ruling party, ZANU PF, had been implicated in many of the violent incidents whose perpetrators ONHRI was supposed to bring to account. Deliberations concerning the reconciliation process that might have exposed the actions of the ruling party pushed the organ to a deadlock (Mashingaidze, 2010).

Thus, in the interest of preserving the power-sharing agreement, opposition parties apparently calculated that the coalition would most likely collapse if the demands for truth and reconciliation remained a top priority on the unity government's agenda. ONHRI's mandate ended in 2013 when the IG was dissolved, having made little progress in addressing the social injustices of the past and promoting social cohesion, integration, and reconciliation in Zimbabwe. It should be pointed out that the IG was characterised by antagonism, contestations, and animosity throughout its tenure because ZANU PF was fighting to regain its lost hegemony (Mungwari, 2016).

Murambadoro (2014) posits that the fourth reconciliation project pertains to Chapter 12 on Commissions. She argues that reconciliation remains a work in progress for the government of Zimbabwe. Chapter 12 of the country's 2013 amended constitution prescribes that the government sets up independent commissions to promote democracy, harmony, and social cohesion in the country. Among the commissions are the Zimbabwe Human Rights Commission (ZHRC) and the National Peace and Reconciliation Commission (NPRC). The ZHR NGO Forum (2013) argues that the effectiveness of these commissions and their ability to work independently remains questionable. It points out that, given the past record of the government of Zimbabwe; it is unlikely the provisions in section 235 of the new Constitution (which postulates the commissions' independence) can be satisfied by the current ruling party and government. We concur and add that ZANU PF is not likely to implement policies that are unfavourable to its power and control. Therefore, the ruling party and government cannot reform itself given the circumstances at hand. It is envisaged that the proclamations by the new president, Emmerson Mnangagwa, promising a new era of engagement will yield favourable results.

Given this state of affairs, Zimbabwe does not seem to present an enabling environment in which to engage in national healing and reconciliation processes. The government's persistent inaction since independence concerning perpetrators of social injustices suggests a lack of political will. Another explanation for Zimbabwe's failure in terms of reconciliation is that the country has not yet undergone full transition. ZANU PF has been in power since independence in 1980. It has been using its dominance to ensure the political and personal interests of individuals in the party are not threatened by calls to address the past. Murambadoro (2014) further argues that consequently, when representatives of the ruling party engage in deliberations about reconciliation, they tend to focus on the party's familiar redistributive demands such as the land reform programme, compensation of war veterans, and the indigenisation programme to justify the recurrence of violence.

The question to ask is; when is the appropriate time to address past injustices and how should they be addressed in Zimbabwe? That largely remains unclear and unanswered, but we argue that ignoring the past will only perpetuate the cycles of violence in Zimbabwe, particularly during election periods. Violence in Zimbabwe over the past three decades has dehumanised victims and perpe- trators, families and the nation's integrity and willingness to engage in genuine national healing and reconciliation processes.

Conclusion

With past traumas unresolved and/or glossed over by politicians, Zimbabwe remains a politically volatile country. Political differences continue to be settled through the use of violence or the threat of its use and political intolerance has remained the cornerstone of Zimbabwe's political contests. Ndlovu- Gatsheni and Benyera (2015) argue that whatever mechanisms and methodolo- gies employed to achieve justice and reconciliation must, therefore, be capable of engaging with the historical legacies of conflict and violence, and this engagement should not be seen as hindering efforts at nation-building. In this chapter, we conclude by saying that there has to be political will to implement government decisions and allow commissions to fully operate as independent organs without interference.

The role of civil society should be seen by the state as complementing and completing the efforts of the state towards national healing and reconciliation. This could take various forms such as raising awareness, disseminating infor- mation, establishing education programmes around the work of commissions, producing and distributing information, funding radio and television pro- grammes, and advertisements that focus on publicising the work of the com- mission (Ndlovu-Gatsheni and Benyera, 2015). It is important to point out that the role of Zimbabwean media, which currently and unfortunately is polarised, should be to encourage peace resolutions rather than exacerbate or foment conflict which is already fragile and precarious (See the chapter by Tsarwe and Gadzikwa in this volume). The media should adopt Galtung's (2000) peaceful resolution strategies in reporting conflict issues. It is interesting that in South Africa, the media was an integral part of the work of the Truth and Rec- onciliation Commission, broadcasting the location of future hearing venues and raising public awareness (Shea, 2000: 4). The media also facilitated the live broadcast of the hearings, thereby helping to bring the work of the TRC to the nation (Cole, 2010). This generated public interest enhanced participation and indeed in our view played a huge part in bringing national healing and reconciliation in post-apartheid South Africa.

We also conclude that national healing and reconciliation efforts should be holistic to embrace the role of faith-based organisations such as the involve- ment of the church and other religious faiths (See also the chapters by Biri, and, Chitando and Taringa in this volume). Concepts used in justice and reconcilia- tion such as confession and forgiveness also have their basis in religion and faith.

This symbiotic relationship between faith-based organisations and the NPRC becomes a sine qua non for the effective delivery of justice and reconciliation in Zimbabwe (Benyera, 2014). Non- governmental organisations working on healing and reconciliation in Zimbabwe can support the process with the provision of technical support, expertise, and even personnel in support areas such as communication, logistics, advertising, and data analysis. Their visibility and participation in various ways will have the ability to bring international credibility to the whole process, as was the case in South Africa.

In pursuit of this goal, the NPRC needs to work with faith-based organisations such as the Zimbabwe Catholic Bishops Conference, Zimbabwe Christian Alliance, and Evangelical Fellowship of Zimbabwe among others (Chitando and Manyonganise, 2011). It should be pointed out that NPRC is a temporary mechanism, hence the need for permanent grassroots-based structures such as the church to partner with the NPRC in the implementation of its mandate. According to Machakanja (2010), African traditional leaders play a central role in Zimbabwe's customary law and we concur with her observation that these can be used to create cultural spaces needed for the facilitation of the victims-perpetrator acknowledgment. At a spiritual level, they are expected to lead their various constituencies in performing certain rites, rituals, and ceremonies in cleansing the land. We therefore, conclude that a holistic and comprehensive approach will be ideal in Zimbabwe's national healing and reconciliation efforts.

References

Benyera, E. 2014. "Debating the Efficacy of Transitional Justice Mechanisms: The Case of National Healing in Zimbabwe, 1980–2011," Unpublished PhD Thesis, University of South Africa, Pretoria.

Catholic Commission for Justice and Peace (CCJP). 1997. *Breaking the Silence, Building True Peace: Report on the 1980s Disturbances in Matabeleland and the Midlands.* www.rhodesia.nl/Matebeleland%20Report.pdf.

Chitando, E. and Manyonganise, M. 2011. "Voices from Faith Based Communities," in Tim Murithi and Aquilina Mawadza (eds.), *Zimbabwe in Transition: A View from Within.* Sunnyside: Jacana Media, 77–111.

Cole, C. M. 2010. *Performing South Africa's Truth Commission: Stages of Transition.* Bloomington: Indiana University Press.

Galtung, J. 2000. *Conflict Transformation by Peaceful Means (the Transcend Method): Participants' Manual, Trainers' Manual.* Geneva: The United Nations, Module 111.

Goredema, D., P. Chigora and Q. P. Bhebe. 2014. "Reconciliation in Zimbabwe: Where, When and How?" *Journal of Global Peace & Conflict* 2(1), 207–223.

Machakanja, P. 2010. *National Healing and Reconciliation in Zimbabwe: Challenges and Opportunities.* Zimbabwe Monograph Series. (No. 1). Cape Town: Institute for Justice and Reconciliation.

Mashingaidze, T. M. 2010. "Zimbabwe's Illusive National Healing and Reconciliation Processes: From Independence to the Inclusive Government 1980–2009," *Conflicts Trends* (1), 19–27.

Mlambo, A. S. 2009. "From the Second World War to UDI, 1940–1963," in B. Raftopoulos and A. S. Mlambo (eds.), *Becoming Zimbabwe: A History from the Pre-Colonial Period to 2008*. Harare: Weaver Press.

Mungwari, T. 2016. "Representation of Political Conflict in Zimbabwean Press: The Case of *The Herald, The Sunday Mail, Daily News* & *The Standard*, 1999–2016," Unpublished PhD Thesis, University of South Africa, Pretoria.

Mungwini, P. 2013. "Conscripts and Not Volunteers: Indigenous Peoples, Transition & the Post-Colonial Question of Reconciliation in Zimbabwe," *Journal on African Philosophy* 7, 19–31.

Murambadoro, R. 2014. *The Politics of Reconciliation in Zimbabwe: Three Times Failure – Will the Fourth Time Count?* 17 December 2014. Mediation and Reconciliation. Centre for the Study of Governance Innovation. Pretoria: University of Pretoria.

Muzondidya, J. and S. J. Ndlovu-Gatsheni. 2007. "Echoing Silences: Ethnicity in Postcolonial Zimbabwe 1980–2007," *African Journal on Conflict Resolution* 7(2), 275–297.

Ndlovu-Gatsheni, S. and E. Benyera. 2015. "Towards a Framework for Resolving the Justice and Reconciliation Question in Zimbabwe," *African Journal on Conflict Resolution* 15(2), 9–33.

Nyarota, G. 2006. *Against the Grain: Memoirs of a Zimbabwean Newsman*. Cape Town: Zebra Press.

Primorac, R. 2007. "The Poetics of State: Terror in Twenty-First Century Zimbabwe," *Interventions* 9(3), 434–450.

Sachikonye, L. M. 1996. "The Nation-State Project and Conflict in Zimbabwe," in Adebayo O. Olukoshi and Liisa Laakso (eds.), *Challenges to the Nation-State in Africa*. Uppsala: Nordic African Institute, 136–153.

Sadomba, Z. W. 2011. *War Veterans in Zimbabwe's Revolution: Challenging Neo-Colonialism, Settler and International Capital*. Harare: Weaver Press.

Savage, T. 2003. *Zimbabwe: A Hundred Year War*. Trenton, NJ: Africa World Press.

Shea, D. 2000. *The South African Truth Commission: The Politics of Reconciliation*. Washington, DC: United Nations Institute of Peace Press.

Tendi, B. M. 2010. *Making History in Mugabe's Zimbabwe: Politics, Intellectuals and the Media*, Vol. 4. New York: Peter Lang.

The Zimbabwe Catholic Bishops Conference, The Evangelical Fellowship of Zimbabwe and The Zimbabwe Council of Churches. 2006. *The Zimbabwe We Want: Towards a National Vision for Zimbabwe*. Harare: ZCC, EFZ and ZCBC.

Zimbabwe Human Rights NGO Forum. 2013. *The Transitional Justice Second International Conference Report*. www.hrforumzim.org/wp-content/uploads/2014/o7/ICTJ-11Conference-Report.pdf

2 The social imaginary for healing and reconciliation

David Kaulemu

Introduction

We have reached a stage through globalization, when we can no longer talk about a nation-state without making reference to the global economic and political architecture. Oswald de Rivero has convincingly demonstrated that globalization has made sure that third-world countries become "non-viable economies" which are "quasi nation-states" with "perforated sovereignties" (Rivero, 2001: 13–41). With the consolidation of global capitalism all nation-states have become surrogates for the "new global aristocracy" (Rivero, 2001: 45) emanating from transnational corporations. This position is further developed by David Korten (2015). It is the same with talking about the prospects for national healing and reconciliation in Zimbabwe. Nothing can any longer escape the gaze and interests of global capitalism. National healing must necessarily be placed in the context of the agenda of global capitalism.

Many Zimbabweans have expressed the need for national healing and reconciliation to facilitate nation building that will bring prosperity to Zimbabwe as a nation-state and individuals and families of Zimbabweans. This belief in national healing and reconciliation is based on an unwavering faith in the nation-state and an optimistic belief that post-colonial Zimbabwe is or can become a viable nation-state whose citizens are not only prosperous and happy, but also healed and reconciled. The healing and reconciliation are understood to be processes that will address the various historical wounds, memories of social hurting, and conflicts that date back from pre-colonial ethnic encounters. The hurts and conflicts are understood to range from the pre-colonial encounters between indigenous communo-cultural groups to confrontational colonial encounters and oppressions as well as post-colonial abuses and political confrontations.

This is too much hope invested in a European social artifact – the nation-state. Africans had limited choice in constructing the character of the nation-state which is expected to solve social, political, and economic challenges that have accumulated since time immemorial. To begin with, the nation-state was never constructed for this purpose. The Europeans who proposed these nation-states aimed at maximum exploitation of the natural and human resources of the regions they demarcated and controlled. They hoped they would continue this exploitation even after these regions had fought for and gained their political independence. Africans continue to play this role given to them by the global economic powers. Those who have attempted to reconceptualize this role, have been brutally eliminated. These include Kwame Nkrumah, Thomas Sankara, Patrice Lumumba, and many others.

There are indeed too many wounds, memories, and conflicts expected to be dealt with within a time period that is shorter than the time taken in accumulating these historical wounds. It is, therefore, legitimate to ask whether the current expectations for success are realistic. This essay raises these questions and provides grounds for their legitimacy.

I argue that issues of social cohesion in Africa must rely essentially on African local moral and spiritual resources and authentic appropriation of other relevant resources emanating from global solidarities. We need the solidarity of global social and political movements that share similar values with us. But these should not include the dominant political and economic forces. They also should not include enlisting the help of the nation-state. A world ruled by corporations and their surrogate nation-states will not help Africa achieve the goals of social cohesion. We need a different paradigm. We need more than having just a few wonderful leaders that can inspire us into building a better world. This leader-inspired paradigm failed. Nkrumah, Nyerere, Kaunda, Mandela, Mugabe, etc. led failed experiments because they worked within the dominant economic and political systems and in many ways they appropriated these systems. More importantly, they failed because their ideas never developed into a social imaginary, which we need to transform society. This chapter calls for our withdrawal from a phantom system that is based on the worship of money (Korten, 2010), to reconnect to a real economy that is based on efforts to respond to fundamental human needs (Max-Neef, 1992). It also interrogates the relevance and usefulness of European social and political constructs such as the nation-state and the corporate dominated market.

Interrogating the nation-state

For the majority of analysts, the responsibilities attributed to the nation-state to deliver on these expectations are based on the confidence that the largely colonially constructed nation-state is desirable and realizable. This is the prescription pill that Europe gave us. The one silver bullet! The majority of us have swallowed it, as it were, hook, line, and sinker. There is, therefore, a strong belief that Rhodesia, a colonial artifact that was renamed Zimbabwe, is worth appropriating and building as an African social, political, and economic entity that can respond to the basic needs of Africans.

African leaders of the (then) Organization of African Unity (OAU) (later to become the African Union) cursorily considered alternatives and decided to keep the European-drawn boundaries as a European gift which they renamed as the African nation-state. It was never meant by the Europeans to be an independent and viable nation-state. Yet our African leaders felt that to change the boundaries would cause even more problems among Africans. The OAU had no confidence in the African leadership and African peoples' capacity to chart a new dispensation less influenced by Europe. In fact, by taking up the responsibilities of the nation-state, African leaders took up moral responsibility of social, economic, and political issues they had no capacity to resolve.

In the context of Zimbabwe, most analysts have focused on healing and reconciliation emanating from issues of local conflicts and confrontations. Colleagues have legitimately raised issues of the need for healing from the experiences of Gukurahundi, Murambatsvina, and political violence. I have confidence that my colleagues can deal with these issues. This chapter, on the other hand, places these issues in a wide global context. Gukurahundi happened when there was already a great need for healing and reconciliation. It is also interesting to note that it happened when the British Army was officially in the country training the new integrated Zimbabwean army. Also, even if Robert Mugabe and Zanu PF were to offer genuine apologies for their sins, we are still left with unfulfilled human needs and other reasons for further conflict. We are still left with poverty created by global corporations, disruptions and atrocities of the European political powers, and the restrictions effected by the imposed nation-state. At independence, when African political leaders agreed to raise the flag of political independence, they took the European political and corporate powers off the hook. After years of slavery, colonial oppression, and post-colonial exploitation, European and American corporations and states still find themselves free of any responsibility for the poverty, conflicts, and environmental damage they caused – no apology, no compensation, no retribution, no restitution!

No one seems to be talking about the need for healing and reconciliation between Africans and Europeans. Why is that? While we hear a lot about the genocide in Rwanda, we do not hear much about the German genocide against the Herero, Nama, and San people in what is now Namibia (Sarkin 2009). The history of atrocities by Belgians in the Congo and many other European countries in other parts of Africa has been sanitized and deodorized without any attempt to propose healing and reconciliation as a solution. American political interference and assassinations of African leaders is recorded in history and yet no talk of reconciliation and healing is put on the agenda. European countries are still reluctant to return to Africa many artifacts, trophies, and cultural wealth plundered from the continent. Many European museums, gardens, and art galleries would be impoverished if they would return what was plundered from Africa alone and not considering those from other parts of the developing world. Some of the plundered include tombs, skulls, and skeletons of slain Africans who resisted the colonial abuses.

This is what is called having your cake and eating it. The conclusion we might make from this is that when you are in power, or when you benefit from global power, you do not need healing and reconciliation. Why, in the context of Zimbabwe, is it easier to talk about the need for healing between the Ndebele and the Shona and not between the blacks and the whites? When it comes to the latter, it is the issue of property – the land – that needs to be resolved and not the issue of relationships and healing. I am yet to see any proposal for healing and reconciliation that involves white people in Africa. Yet we have seen many cases where white people make claims for property. Property rights are their healing magic box. Uganda is an interesting case where the issue was settled, not so much with healing, but with the return of properties confiscated from Asians by Idi Dada Amin. Don't white people also need healing and reconciliation? Yet when Africans make claims for property – especially land – they are encouraged to go for healing and reconciliation. The issue becomes not so much of property and rights, but of good governance, morality, and conciliation. Who is setting the agenda?

It seems to me that Africans need to deal with issues of property, economy, and the ecological system before they focus on healing and reconciliation. The latter without the former seems a waste of energy and time. It may be that Maslow's hierarchy of needs (Maslow, 1954) is correct. Maslow argued that people always want to address basic physical needs before attending to issues of safety and security, love and belonging, self-respect and personal growth. It may be that issues of healing and reconciliation in Zimbabwe will only be relevant when issues of physical needs have been addressed. By basic physical needs is meant issues of subsistence and fulfillment of the needs for food, clothing, shelter, water, health, and so on. These are the basic issues of the living economy. Not until people's subsistence needs are settled will they be ready for healing and reconciliation. Yet, today, in Zimbabwe, healing and reconciliation is being shoved down the throats of African people whose subsistence has not been guaranteed. For whites, however, it is their property they need to get back. Healing and reconciliation, they do not need.

We need new ways of thinking

In spite of the comments made earlier, I have hope for global healing and reconciliation, but harbour serious doubts about the capacity of the African nation-state to deliver on the promises of economic, political, and social prosperity under the present global economic and political architecture. While I have hope in social healing and reconciliation, I do not claim to be optimistic about it. I think that Africans should work hard to bring about social harmony between different peoples on the continent and in the world and especially to bring themselves in harmony with the ecological system. To do so requires fundamental changes in the global and local social, political, and economic arrangements. It also requires fundamental changes in the kinds of beliefs we have about ourselves, our neighbours, and the ecological system that we are a part of. I do not think that we should invest much of our efforts, resources, and planning in maintaining, monitoring, and effecting the separating boundaries drawn by the colonial powers. I also believe that we should interrogate some of the invented traditions, ethnicities, gender roles, and racial identities that have supported the hegemony of colonialism and capitalism (Vail, 1996). Part of what reconciliation and healing in Africa should mean is the healing of the wounds that were created by the European-drawn boundaries and separations. A lot of the African ethnicities and their "traditional cultures" are largely colonial inventions (Ranger, 1985).

Reflection on Zimbabwean nationhood

Krejci and Velimsky argue that, "there are five objective factors which can contribute to the identification of a group as a nation" (1996: 2). For them, the five objective factors are territory, state, language, culture, and history. They add a sixth subjective factor of national consciousness (1996: 2). They add a critical point which says that, "The subjective factor of consciousness is the ultimate factor which eventually decides the issue of national identity" (1996: 2). For Zimbabwe, divisions and conflicts have characterized the five objective factors as follows:

1   Territory: Modern Zimbabwe relies on imposed country boundaries and invented Tribal Trust Lands which are now being called rural areas and were used by the colonial system and are still being used by the post-colonial leaders to divide people in ways that undermine national consciousness. What Fanon (1963: 148) called "the pitfalls of national consciousness" are still evident in post-colonial Zimbabwe.
2   State or political formation: It is clear that the colonial powers, in forming the colonies, had no plans of making them viable political formations. They used divide-and-rule tactics, inventing and playing different ethnic groups against one another. The legacy of this still exists in post-colonial countries. In most African countries political loyalty is more towards ethnic groups and regional groups than to the nation-state (Fanon, 1963: 3). As Fanon has demonstrated, the former colonial states cultivated a local ruling elite through which they continue to maintain a neocolonial hegemony. He says that "By its very structure, colonialism is separatist and regionalist. Colonialism does not simply state the existence of tribes; it also reinforces it and separates them. The colonial system encourages chieftaincies and keeps alive the old Marabout confraternities" (Fanon, 1963: 3).
3   Language: Many of the dominant languages in modern African states are codified by colonial powers and imposed on the population in ways that were convenient to the colonial administrative requirements and not to the development of local national consciousness. Hence many African disputes are centered around the issues of language imposition. The official status of the English, French, and Portuguese and their exaltation over local languages resulted in the non-development of local languages. The difficulties in investing in local languages at this stage is seen in the predicaments of countries like Tanzania who seem to be pulled more and more by the

forces of globalization towards abandoning using Kiswahili Swahili as an official language. The mammoth task that African states face in trying to honour the numerous languages that are part of the nation-state is almost insurmountable. South Africa, for example, has declared 11 languages as official languages. It would be interesting to find out how many languages would be spoken today in the United Kingdom if the English had followed this language policy.

4   Culture: Our sense of culture as Africans is cultivated within the European intellectual and administrative traditions. The role of European missionaries, anthropologists, administrators, and academics in contributing to the "invention" of African traditions should never be underestimated. Placide Tempels's (1959) *Bantu Philosophy* is very clear on its role in the administration of Africans.

5   History: African history still needs to be decolonised. The European gaze still dominates the African historical narrative. African historians respond to European questions, historical agendas, and conceptual frameworks.

It is a fact that the nation-state that is given the name Zimbabwe is not a natural entity. It is a fiction of European imperialism imposed on various ethno-cultural groups. It is also a fiction that many of these local groups simultaneously fight and yet also appropriate. On the whole, it is treated like some manna from heaven; like a felled elephant where all you need to do is "cut your piece and go." Very little effort is put into investing in the nation-state as a common good embedded in the local needs and aspirations. Most Africans, and especially the African leaders, expect the nation-state to fulfil their own private desires and appetites without them investing in building up the nation-state for the common good. This point has clearly been demonstrated in the case of many post-colonial countries, including Zimbabwe. Leaders who came into political power in Zimbabwe in 1980 went straight into looting, cannibalizing, and privatizing the nation-state without tangible investment in its institutional viability as an economic and political entity. Many post-colonial leaders and their governments expected to rely on financial and material support from their former colonizers in the running and maintenance of the new nation-state. Most of them depend on aid from Western countries. Apart from unsuccessful attempts by Patrice Lumumba in the DRC, Julius Nyerere in Tanzania, and Thomas Sankara in Burkina Faso, there has been very little attempt to develop serious and non-corrupt self-reliance efforts. It was not until Mugabe had lost popular support that he started thinking about his land reform programme. Before that, he had relied, like most African leaders, more on the generosity of Western powers than on his own people. Various groupings, defined by political affiliation, ethnicity, and regional location hover over the remnants of the cannibalized state like vultures ready to grab their pieces and go. Many government and state funds have been looted, including the War Veterans Compensation Fund and the National Youth Fund. In today's context, national unity, reconciliation, and solidarity seem far-fetched.

Re-imagining our reality

The challenge then is on how these groups could either ignore or heal the historical wounds and be ready to engage with others in a process of nation building. In order for such process to begin, there needs to be an admission of the fact that the nation state is a fiction. It has to be recognized that, despite all rhetoric, it is an invention. There needs to be a way of thinking, feeling, and behaving that could facilitate the whole process of healing, reconciliation, and nation building. There needs to be a common way of imagining the nation-state that will facilitate and make possible the desires of the Zimbabwean citizens. This social imaginary will inform the whole process. I argue that this social imaginary requires the following:

1   Recognition that Zimbabwe, as a nation–state, is a social and political experiment that is aimed at enhancing the dignity of all its people and searching for the common good.
2   A nuanced historical understanding of the present and inclusive narrative of the various histories, experiences, and contributions to the development of the nation–state as a deliberately chosen common good.
3   A recognition of the humanity and legitimacy of every participant individual and groups especially acknowledging their varied interests, anxieties, and visions without letting any of the individuals or groups count for more than others.
4   Humility of every group in recognizing and acknowledging its contribution to the creation of the obstacles to nation building.
5   A sense not only of optimism but that of hope.
6   A recognition and respect of the previous five points by the national political, social, and cultural leadership and especially and more importantly, also by the general population of the country. Charles Taylor (2004: 23) emphasizes that the difference between social imaginary and theory is that the former is possessed by the general population whereas the latter is only a property of the elite experts.
7   Recognition that Zimbabwe on its own could fail to realize the intended goals of the nation–state and that other means may need to be found to realize the goals. These could include regional political and economic integration or a complete redrawing of the country boundaries to cater for realistic economic and political prospects. As an economic entity, Zimbabwe has many disadvantages. I imagine that these disadvantages could be overturned by redrawing national boundaries. I imagine that if Zimbabwe were to coagulate with say, Mozambique, Zambia, and Malawi, we would have a much more economically viable entity with a respectable population, access to the ports and the sea, as well as a wider variety of natural resources. Such an entity would have greater chances of internal trade and investment to stimulate local industries capable of sustainable beneficiation than is possible today.

8   Recognition that under the present global economic and political architecture, the chances of realizing number 1 are very slim.

In order for all this to happen, there is need for political leadership that understands how to bring together a humanist, pan-Africanist national consciousness that recognizes the experiences of and expands the imagination of all who are to be part of the nation-state. To cut the story short, the post-colonial leadership have failed to play that role. Describing this failure, Fanon (1963: 147–148) observes that the post-colonial state has been built on shaky foundations.

Social imaginary

Charles Taylor defines 'social imaginary' as,

> the ways people imagine their social existence, how they fit together with others, how things go on between them and their fellows, the expectations that are normally met, and the deeper normative notions and images that underlie these expectations.
>
> (Taylor, 2004: 23)

Taylor is clear that the social imaginary is not the same as a social theory. A social theory is more or less an academic scheme used to understand social reality. However, a social imaginary is something that belongs to the ordinary people as they imagine their social reality. It includes what they think, how they feel, and what inspires them to act in certain ways rather than others. The social imaginary may not necessarily be self-conscious but it is expressed in the stories, images, and legends expressed by ordinary people (Taylor, 2004: 23).

The challenge for Zimbabwe has been the absence of the development of this kind of social imaginary. There is great need for a social imaginary that helps to create a sense of common understanding, recognition, and social solidarity. This will facilitate common national cultural practices that realize common norms and appropriate emotional responses to the environment, the economy, and life in general. The challenge has been about how to develop common understanding about who belongs; about legitimacy and mutual obligations and expectations; acceptance of historical responsibility to being complicit in the challenges facing the building of nation-state, especially being complicit to racism, tribalism, patriarchy, and provincialism. It has also been about the resolve to give hope to future generations, both human and non-human. This involves assessing our economic priorities. For example, it involves assessing and recognizing the difference between "real wealth and phantom wealth." David Korten explains real wealth in the following way:

> Real wealth includes land, fertile soils, clean air and water, our labor, ideas, Technology, physical infrastructure, tools, and all the essentials of human Living. The foundation of all real wealth is the living wealth of living

people, Communities, and Living Earth. A real-wealth living economy necessarily Begins with the health of Living Earth.

(Korten, 2015: 8)

The challenge today is how we can extricate ourselves from the phantom economy that we have been sucked into by global corporations. Pope Francis has called on the world to withdraw from this phantom economy when he warned that, "The worship of the ancient golden calf has returned in a new and ruthless guise in the idolatry of money and the dictatorship of an impersonal economy lacking a truly human purpose" (Pope Francis, 24 November 2013).

Our challenge today, as people living in Southern Africa, is how we can wake up from this corporate-induced dream about our reality. In order to continue feeding the capitalist growth of corporations, we are told and we have come to believe that we are naturally selfish individuals. The reality is that capitalism, and its surrogate European nation-states, created us as such when it uprooted us from our families and communities through slavery, wars, labour migration, education, religion, attack on our cultures, and participation in the phantom global economy. We must wake up from this corporate-induced dream that our ancestors do not live in the forest and that our air, water, land, trees, and the rest of creation are not sacred but simply natural resources that can be turned into commodities. Above all, we must wake up from the dream, rather, the nightmare of the nation-state and that of the so-called national economy. Given the power of corporations, the nation-state has lost its sovereignty. Oswaldo de Rivero convincingly argues this point when he calls the nation-state, "perforated sovereignties" and "powerless powers" (2010).

The idea that we are naturally Zimbabwean and naturally different from those who are naturally Zambian, Malawian, or Mozambican is a lie that runs into the face of history. It is a lie that is facilitating the continued rule of global corporations, consuming our wealth, draining our lives while creating human waste out of us and devastating our natural habitat – our physical and spiritual homes.

Our challenge today is to develop and cultivate the kind of social imaginary that will help us live authentic lives that address our fundamental human needs. Manfred Max-Neef calls this "barefoot economics" and his other colleagues call it "real-life economics." It is not just economics that knows facts about the economy, for example, what the gross national product is. It is an economics that "understands" what people are going through and aims to respond to their fundamental needs. (Ekins and Max-Neef, 1997). We need a social imaginary that will help us to disengage from the phantom economy and start responding to the needs of our families, communities, relationships, morality, and spirituality. When we do this, we will open up possibilities for authentic living with ourselves, with each other, and as part of our ecology. This new social imaginary will make many of our beliefs, ideas, and emotional responses redundant and self-defeating. This new social imaginary is capable of facilitating the development of enough social cohesion and positive attitudes to help the process of healing past wounds and move towards reconciliation at different levels of our societies. This is really a big challenge as it requires going beyond the borders of what is now the Zimbabwe nation-state. This is because some of the wounds that need to be healed include the ways in which communities were separated by the European-created country borders.

History of the idea of the nation-state and implications for Zimbabwe

The idea of a nation-state is originally a European idea that was used to resolve religious wars in Europe. It came out of a series of peace treaties signed between May and October 1648 in the Westphalian cities of Osnabrück and Münster. The Peace of Westphalia as it is known, ended the Thirty Years' War (1618–1648) in the Holy Roman Empire, and the Eighty Years' War (1568–1648) between Spain and the Dutch Republic, with Spain formally recognizing the independence of the Dutch Republic. It was based on the concept of coexisting sovereign states committed to non-interference in other states' domestic affairs and spheres of influence. These Westphalian principles, especially the concept of sovereign states, became central to international law.

European nations tried to extend the use of the Westphalia principles to the new "sovereign" states that emerged from their imperial territories after decolonization. They tried to promote the idea that these new states were as "sovereign" as the European states when they themselves knew that it could not be. As Fanon demonstrates, European powers clearly knew that de-colonization was a process of continuing colonialism in another form.

The whole notion of post-colonial nation-building makes a number of critical assumptions that may turn out to be chimera for Africa and Zimbabwe of today. First, it makes, for example, the assumption that Zimbabwe is potentially, at least, a viable political, economic, and cultural entity. There is a very serious question as to whether, on its own, this is true. The underlying reason is that, Zimbabwe, like all the other colonial entities created by European countries at the Berlin Conference of 1884, was never meant to be a viable independent political and economic entity. These African entities were carved out essentially as sources of raw materials and labour for the European countries that participated in the Berlin conference. Oswaldo de Rivero (2010), has argued convincingly that given this position allocated to former colonies like Zimbabwe in the global economic architecture, it is almost impossible that they can wriggle out of this position to develop into viable economic entities that can stand on their feet in the way in which European nations are generally understood to have done. It is true, as Rivero has argued that with the rule of corporations, even European nation-states have lost their sovereignty (2010: 25). The global economic powers, which today are led by global corporations, are constantly making sure that former colonial territories and others continue to play the roles they desire them to play (Korten, 2015). Hence Rivero calls them non-viable national economies that survive on "international aid, official loans and credits from private institutions, continually falling into insolvency and national bankruptcy" (Rivero, 2010: 81).

In any case the development theories used to encourage former colonies give the impression that these quasi-nation-states could take up the development trajectory that European countries took in the sixteenth century. It is clear from the history and conditions of the success of what Karl Marx (1928: 873) called "primitive accumulation" that was stimulated for the formation of European nation-states, that developing countries could never have access to such conditions. These conditions, which are the historical basis of the development of the economies of the European nation-states, included having the benefits of the system of slavery, colonialist exploitation, and piracy and plunder without international rules and regulations. David Harvey has pointed out that,

> The original accumulation of capital during late medieval times in Europe entailed violence, predation, thievery, fraud and robbery. Through these extra-legal means, pirates, priests and merchants, supplemented by the usurers, assembled enough initial 'money power' to begin to circulate money systematically as capital.
>
> (Harvey, 2009: 47)

Developing countries today have to face numerous international rules and regulations which European nation-state never had to face during their process of development. For example, developing countries cannot freely engage in piracy, slavery, and colonial expansion without consequences from global economic and political powers. Developing countries face many restrictions from global powers. They cannot develop nuclear power without supervision and approval from the global powers. They cannot own strategic minerals and resources and decide on their own how to use them. Experiences of DR Congo, Angola, Nigeria, Sudan, Iran, Iraq, and many others indicate that owning those resources has become more of a curse than it is a blessing for those countries.

Territory, nation, and state

This law of diminishing returns is the other side of the coin of the growth in the power of global corporations. When global corporations grow, they suck all life from our societies and environments. They are supported by a scientific and mechanistic view of the world which disenchants the world and presents it as lifeless and spiritless. They turn our natural living environments into commodities they exploit. They turn human beings into commodities they exploit for production. Because of advances in technology, production is more and more needing less and less labour power. Hence many human beings are being turned into redundant "human waste" not needed by the triumphant capitalist system (Bauman, 2007: 30). The move from production capitalism to finance capitalism means that we are now dominated more by money than inspired by production to feed human needs. Economic growth now means the accumulation of money and not the fulfilment of human needs. This financialized system makes humans not only massively unemployed but redundant. Unemployment suggests a temporary condition that can be corrected by job creation and improved economic conditions. Redundancy, on the other hand, is recognition of the permanency of the condition of unemployment. Millions of people all over the world have come to give up looking for employment as they have realized that capitalism has declared them irrelevant and permanently unemployable. This is what Bauman has called the production of human waste. As Zygmunt Bauman explains, "The volume of humans made redundant by capitalism's global triumph grows unstoppably and comes close now to exceeding the managerial capacity of the planet" (Bauman, 2007: 29).

It is important to the corporations and global political powers for us in developing countries to believe that in post-colonial society, we own territories and nation-states while they continue to extract wealth from those territories with our consent and at our expense. It is important for the corporate world that we continue to maintain a social imaginary created by the capitalist world. For as long as we continue to believe in the priority of the perforated nation-state, and believe that money is wealth, and allow our ecological system to be abused, privatized, and destroyed, we will continue to fight among ourselves in conditions of poverty, with no hope of healing and reconciling.

Towards the new economy

We need to find ways of escaping the clasp of the global corporations and their surrogate nation-states. In doing so, we must escape the money-centered economy and re-establish our close spiritual relations with the ecological system to build a new life-centered economy. It will also be helpful to connect with many peoples of the world who are trying to do the same. This new economy recognizes that water, air, land, trees, and animals are the true value. Their value is not counted in monetary terms and does not merely lie in their contribution to the gross national product. They are what life is about. A living economy – one that respects life – is one that focuses on people's well-being in terms of the fulfilment of their fundamental needs but fulfilled in the context of respecting other forms of life in the universe as well. This is not impossible. We need to learn from Bhutan, the first and so far the only country to have officially adopted gross national happiness instead of the gross national product as their main development indicator (World Happiness Report). What Bhutan teaches us is that there is an alternative to the way we construct our way of living and what things we can give priority to. For example, we could stop prioritizing growth and the gross national product and focus on people's welfare and the kinds of human and ecological relations that contribute to it. Instead of just focusing on development in the sense of the multiplication of the number of objects (food, water, houses, etc.), we can also assess what is happening to human beings and their relationships in terms of their physical, moral, and spiritual welfare. This approach will need to take seriously the Freirean (2000, 2005) approach which says that people must participate in their own development. This is the principle of subsidiarity. The principle says that decisions should be taken as much as possible at the points at which they are to be implemented. This means that as Africans, we must be skeptical of the global processes that are initiated on our behalf without our participation. It does not matter how much good intention there is in those initiatives. In fact, we must resist the tendency of development specialists to centralize the conceptualization of development and the attempt to standardize the decision-making and monitoring and evaluation of development. We must also resist the efforts to universalize models for healing, reconciliation, and transitional justice. The models tend to be rationalistic, mechanistic, and lifeless. They treat human beings like bricks to be moulded and joined into buildings.

True healing and reconciliation must be led and planned by those who are affected. Certainly not by consultants. It is interesting to note how transitional justice has become a business with so many experts, publications, and conferences being organized. The language, models, theories, and conceptual tools being invented for healing and reconciliation are complex and mostly irrelevant. Experts on these matters are meeting in seminars and conferences without and on behalf of the affected. Money is being exchanged in the name of transitional justice. This is another ideological smoke screen equivalent to the smoke screen of development – so much effort, no work done!

Neither should it be led by the nation-state, which is itself implicated as part of the root cause of the problem. The principle of subsidiarity emphasizes that the local people are the best people to assess the progress of their own development. This active transformative participation of people in their own development, healing, and reconciliation, will ensure that ordinary people develop the social imaginary necessary for the new economy which is inspired more by values than by the dominance of money. It is only then that people can consider seriously the prospects for genuine healing and reconciliation.

Conclusion

Albert Einstein once said, "No problem can be solved from the same level of consciousness that created it." Another way of saying the same thing is to say that problems cannot be solved without addressing their root causes. African countries, including Zimbabwe, are facing issues of social cohesion calling for healing and reconciliation. Most of these issues are a direct result of the global capitalist system that sequestrated us from the land and reorganized the world to feed the profit-seeking world corporations. I have argued that issues of healing and reconciliation in Zimbabwe cannot be resolved without interrogating the values, institutions, and practices that contributed to their formation. Healing and reconciliation cannot be achieved without responding to people's fundamental needs. Global capitalism makes this impossible and yet it creates smoke screens to make people believe they can use its surrogate institutions like the state, the market, and mechanistic science to resolve their social problems. Karl

Marx was right to recognize that capitalism cannot deliver on peace. Sustainable social cohesion in Southern Africa will need us to interrogate the role of capitalism, the nation-state, and mechanistic science in creating the challenges we face today. There will be need for a fundamentally different social imaginary to transform the historical wounds, social conflicts, political grudges, and economic hurts we carry today.

References

Bauman, Zygmunt. 2007. *Liquid Times in an Age of Uncertainty*. Cambridge UK: Polity Press.

Ekins, Paul and Max-Neef, Manfred (Eds.) 1997. *Real-Life Economics: Understanding Wealth Creation*. London and New York: Routledge.

Frantz, Fanon. 1963. *The Wretched of the Earth, Présence Africaine*. Broadway, New York: Grove Press, Inc.

Freire, Paulo. 2000. *Pedagogy of the Oppressed*. 30th Anniversary Edition. Translated by Myra Bergman Ramos with an Introduction by Donaldo Macedo. London and New York: Continuum.

Freire, Paulo. 2005. *Education for Critical Consciousness*. New York: Continuum. (First Published in 1974 by Sheed & Ward Ltd.)

Harvey, David. 2009. *The Enigma of Capital and the Crises of Capitalism*. London: Profile Books.

Herero and Namaqua genocide https://en.wikipedia.org/wiki/Herero_and_Namaqua_genocide.

Korten, David. C. 2010. *Agenda for a New Economy: From Phantom Wealth to Real Wealth*. San Francisco: Berrett-Koehler Publishers, Inc.

Korten, David C. 2015. *When Corporations Rule the World*. Oakland, CA: The Living Economies Forum, Berrett-Koehler Publishers Inc.

Krejci, Jaroslav and Velimsky, Vitezslav. 1996. "Ethnic and Political Nations in Europe," in John Hutchinson and Anthony D. Smith (eds.), *Ethnicity*. New York: Oxford University Press, Oxford Readers.

Marx, Karl. 1928. *Capital Volume 1*. Introduced by Ernest Mandel. Translated by Ben Fowkes. London: The Pelican Marx Library.

Maslow, Abraham. 1954. *Motivation and Personality*. New York: Harper and Row.

Max-Neef, Manfred. 1992. "Development and Human Needs," in Paul Ekins and Manfred Max-Neef (eds.), *Real Life Economics*. London and New York: Routledge.

Pope Francis. 2013. Apostolic Exhortation Evangelii Gaudium: To the Bishops, Clergy, Consecrated Persons and the Lay Faithful on the Proclamation of the Gospel in Today's World. 24 November 2013. Rome.

Ranger, O. Terence. 1985. *The Invention of Tribalism in Zimbabwe*. Gweru: Mambo Press.

Rivero, Oswaldo de. 2001. *The Myth of Development: The Non-Viable Economies of the 21st Century*. London and New York: Zed Books.

Rivero, Oswaldo de. 2010. *The Myth of Development: Non-Viable Economies and the Crisis of Civilization*. London and New York: Zed Books.

Sarkin, Jeremy. 2009. *Colonial Genocide and Reparations Claims in the 21st Century: The Socio-Legal Context of Claims Under International Law in Namibia, 1904-1908. Praeger Security International Reports*. Westport, Connecticut and London: Greenwood Publishing Group.

Taylor, Charles. 2004. *Modern Social Imaginaries*. Durham and London: Duke University Press.

Tempels, Placide. 1959. *Bantu Philosophy*. Paris: Présence Africaine. www.congoforum.be/ upldocs/Tempels%20BantuPhil%20English%201959.pdf.

Vail, Leroy. 1996. "The Creation of Ethnicity in South Africa," in John Hutchinson and Anthony D. Smith (eds.), *Ethnicity*. Oxford and New York: Oxford University Press.

World Happiness Report 2017 from Wikipedia. en.wikipedia.org/wiki/World_Happin ess_Report.

Yeros, Paris. 1999. *Ethnicity and Nationalism in Africa: Constructivist Reflections and Contemporary Politics*. London: MacMillan Press Ltd.

3 The significance of inclusivity

National healing and reconciliation in Zimbabwe

Mediel Hove and Darlington Mutanda

Introduction

This chapter identifies and explains the significance of inclusivity (involving all stakeholders) in the reconciliation process, an issue neglected by former President Robert Mugabe's government despite the fact that he had pronounced it in 1980. National healing and reconciliation in Zimbabwe can only be realised if the process values and takes into consideration the views and aspirations of different stakeholders. These include especially the church, civil society, civilians, government, academics, the media, traditional leaders, and the international community. As an important aspect of peacebuilding, reconciliation engages the deep-seated wounds of conflict that cannot be left unattended (Hutchison and Bleiker, 2013: 81). Reconciliation is considered essential in a drive to avert the desire for revenge (Fischer, 2011: 415). Bloomfield (2003: 12) refers to reconciliation as:

> an over-arching process which includes the search for truth, justice, forgiveness, healing and so on. . . . it means finding a way to live alongside former enemies . . . to coexist with them, to develop the degree of cooperation necessary to share our society with them, so that we all have better lives together than we have had separately.

Discussing the circumstances under which reconciliation must take place, Van Binsbergen noted that a necessary condition for reconciliation is "the express recognition by the parties concerned, that there is a specific, explicitly expressed conflict" (Van Binsbergen, 1999: 2).

Who is responsible for peacebuilding?

National healing, reconciliation, and integration require inclusivity in order to succeed. It should be a depoliticised process and be initiated from below. History has shown that where violations are experienced, the process does not accomplish its intended objectives. Muchemwa et al. (2013: 1) argue that state-centric approaches are problematic. Reconciliation can only succeed where it is treated as a multi-stakeholder process.

General citizens/civilians

The citizens play prominent roles in the reconciliation process in different environments where reconciliation is a necessity. Bottom-up approaches to peacebuilding yield durable peace because they involve people who experienced challenges as a result of particular decisions taken by the state. Lack of civilian input helps explain why reconciliation failed to take place in Zimbabwe. Civilians were victims of the Second Chimurenga (Hove, 2012b; Kriger, 1992: 27), the Gukurahundi massacres (Catholic Commission for Justice and Peace in Zimbabwe and Legal Resources Foundation, 1997), the Fast Track Land Reform Programme (Sachikonye, 2011), and the run up to the 27 June presidential run-off election when members of the security sector allegedly deployed violence (Hove, 2017). Their input to the process is invaluable. Civilian participation is integral in carrying out a locally initiated and durable reconciliation programme in Zimbabwe.

Civil society

For national healing and reconciliation to be achieved, there should be harmony between the government of the affected country and civil society. Where there is an acrimonious relationship, the prospects of peacebuilding are endangered. Colvin (2007) analysed how civil society organisations (CSOs) have been at the forefront of reconciliation in Southern Africa. He asserted that Southern African countries have put in place national reconciliation processes to deal with human rights abuses and address the deep ethnic, racial, political, and class-based divisions of the past (Colvin, 2007: 322). He further noted that CSOs have also been renowned for offering victim-support services such as legal-advice centres, skills training and economic empowerment, social-work services, mental and physical health care, and memorialisation (Colvin, 2007: 326). Civil society groups among other stakeholders such as human rights representatives, women, political party representatives, and religious leaders help to refine the terms of reference to respond to the challenges confronting societies (Hayner, 2011: 39). CSOs are important in Zimbabwe, especially in providing funding to projects that can help in transforming relationships, counselling, mediation and education.

For example, in Buhera West, villagers met regularly under Heal Zimbabwe's *Kugara Kunzwanana* (co-existence can happen when there is harmony) peacebuilding programme in 2011. Some of the activities included *Nhimbe* (community weeding and harvesting activities), sporting activities, burial societies, and face-the-communities interface meetings. Buhera was one of the areas worst affected by political violence in 2008 (The Legal Monitor, 2012a, 2012b, 2012c). Rights defenders such as Zimbabwe Peace Project director Jestina Mukoko were abducted by state security agents, held incommunicado, and tortured (The Legal Monitor, 2012a, 2012b, 2012c). Civil society organisations that were mostly vulnerable were those involved in monitoring the political environment in the country (*The Standard*, 2013: 10). There is consensus that governments and civil society should build national and local infrastructures for sustainable peacebuilding (SADC Gender Protocol Barometer, 2014: 277). To that end, Heal Zimbabwe Trust in September 2015 invited more than thirty survivors of political violence drawn from Masvingo and Manicaland to talk about their experiences with experts and moderators and this culminated in the discussions on how they could be assisted to deal with the after-effects of violence (Kandimire, 2015). Linked to this, commemorations were also done on the International Day of Peace.

The Zimbabwe Election Support Network (ZESN) encouraged peace prior to the 2013 harmonised elections. It posted adverts encouraging everyone to participate in the elections and to vote in peace. Some of its messages read in part: "Women you are the vote Zimbabwe needs. Register to vote now. The nation's future is in you! Vote in Peace" (*The Standard*, 2012: 7). These activities by ZESN demonstrate that political democratisation is an important component of peacebuilding. It is significant for people to be given a chance to vote for their leaders in a free and fair manner and this helps to diffuse tension.

Moreover, through the efforts of socialisation, democratization and the rebuilding of communities via the different bottom-up peacebuilding strategies under the Church and Civil Society Forum (CCSF), broken relationships were rebuilt, spaces were provided for interaction between perpetrators and victims, thereby rekindling the "values of mercy, justice, truth and peace in a context of deep political polarisation" (Ncube, 2014: 283).

The Church

The church undoubtedly plays an important role in peacebuilding. Summing up Mugabe's relationship with the church between 1980 and 2016, Hove and Chenzi (2017: 173) drew attention to the resurgence of the church in Zimbabwe. The significance of the church was apparent in 2013 when churches organised a peacebuilding event at Chinhoyi stadium. At the gathering politicians from different political parties such as Morgan Tsvangirai of MDC-T and Philip Chiyangwa of ZANU-PF denounced violence (Chibaya, 2013: 2). On separate occasions, the Apostolic Christian Council of Zimbabwe (AACZ) leader Johannes Ndanga pledged to assist in mediating the Gukurahundi conflict (Ndlovu, 2017: 7). This shows that the church is a critical institution in peacebuilding without withstanding the fact that at times the churches were in sharp conflict with the government and ruling party (Chitando and Togarasei, 2010: 157–59).

Besides, the church took part in developmental projects which benefited communities. For example, on 2 March 2012, the Apostolic Faith Mission (AFM) in Zimbabwe donated a classroom block at Chikanga Primary School in Chegutu (*The Sunday Mail*, 2013b: 3). Speaking at the ceremony, the then

Media, Information, and Publicity Minister Webster Shamu acknowledged the role of the church in peacebuilding when he said:

> AFM in Zimbabwe is one such big spiritual church which is not only contributing to national civilisation through education, but is also playing the pivotal role in moral shaping and maintenance of peace through the teaching of the Word and also spreading God's news from the Bible.
>
> (*The Sunday Mail*, 2013b: 3)

Also, the provision of humanitarian aid is an important peacebuilding measure in that it reduces the effects of economic structural violence. Speaking at one donation, the leader of Methodist congregation at All Souls Church, Reverend Sithole said they catered for many beneficiaries, including children's homes (Hudzerema, 2015: 5). Similarly, it was considered important to impart skills to the unemployed youths. In this regard, Caritas, a Roman Catholic affiliated organization, sponsored a skills training programme in 2015 for 80 youths at Nyahombe Primary School in Chivi South (Ward 27). The one-week courses included carpentry, building, hotel and catering.

However, some Apostolic churches patronised ZANU PF gatherings, with some of their leaders publicly aligning themselves with ZANU PF. This close alliance of some churches to the ruling party, exemplified in former Archbishop Nolbert Kunonga's openly pro-ZANU PF pronouncements and actions, tarnished the image of the church among many Zimbabweans (Chitando and Togarasei, 2010: 159). Addressing parishioners in Mhondoro in 2012, Kunonga pledged support for ZANU PF, saying the party's policies clearly demonstrated efforts to uplift the majority, "Indigenisation is a programme of God, it is initiated by agents such as Zanu-PF and its leaders for the benefit of the people . . . The President has been chosen by God as an agent" (*The Sunday Mail*, 2012: 4). Likewise, ZANU PF's national chairman, Simon Khaya Moyo, addressing thousands of congregants at the Johane Masowe Wechishanu church annual pilgrimage in Harare on 4 May 2013 urged members of the church to register as voters ahead of the July 2013 elections:

> We are saying we respect your church and its ideologies because you support the revolutionary party. Register to vote so that we do away with this animal called the inclusive Government.
>
> (*The Sunday Mail*, 2013a: 2)

The leader of the Johane Masowe Wechishanu Church, Madzibaba Edward Manyara, said they were fully behind the leadership of President Robert Mugabe because he was leading the country in fulfilment of prophecy and God's will: "The policies that President Mugabe and his party pursue are for the benefit of the majority and as a church we will continue to pray for him" (*The Sunday Mail*, 2013a: 2).

There, however, emerged a crop of church leaders who opposed state brutality and maladministration. Kariba-based pastor, Patrick Mugadza of the Remnant Church, staged a solo demonstration at the ZANU PF national conference in Victoria Falls in December 2015. He accused government of fueling poverty through misrule. The pastor marched through the resort town waving a placard which read, "Mr President, the people are suffering, Proverbs 21 verse 13" (Matenga, 2016: 1). He called on President Robert Mugabe to concede failure and step down immediately. The action resulted in his immediate arrest by the police. The pastor noted that elections had failed to solve the Zimbabwean crisis. He spent 18 days in remand prison after failing to raise the required US$500 bail (Matenga, 2016: 1). He was only released on New Year's Eve after the intervention of the Zimbabwe Lawyers for Human Rights (ZLHR) who also applied for a downward review of the bail to US$50 (Matenga, 2016: 1). From the forgoing, it is evident that the church can act as a mediator. Mediation comes as an important aspect in addressing the reconciliation elements raised by the citizens. This is where stakeholders such as the church, traditional leaders, government, artists and CSOs, to name a few, can play prominent roles in facilitating negotiations and stressing the need for forgiveness.

Artists

Artists have a huge a role to play in building peace in Zimbabwe. Musicians, for example, are influenced by what they see every day. This influences them to play major roles in encouraging and promoting peace in communities.

Banning Eyre (2015) captivatingly chronicled the contribution of Thomas Mapfumo, asserting that an assessment of his life and career simplifies and makes it easier for one to understand Zimbabwe (Hove, 2016: 190). The book covers colonial Rhodesia when Mapfumo was born in 1945, through the liberation struggle and post-independence euphoria epochs. It further stretches to the era when the musician challenged social injustices committed by the Mugabe regime, and this led to his eventual exile to the state of Oregon in the United States in 2000 (Hove, 2016: 190). Mapfumo's immense legacy is clear in his untiring struggle for social justice and African culture. Prior to Zimbabwe's independence, he was persistently and courageously outspoken and he became an enemy of the Smith regime. He criticised the corrupt presidency of Mugabe, although he had assisted him to rise to power and even sang praise songs for him during the euphoria for independence period (Hove, 2016: 190).

Takesure Zama's "*Kuregerera in advance*" (Forgiving in advance) song produced in 2015 preaches about the importance of forgiveness. Local gospel musicians sought to lift the fading spirits by promising that a new era was beckoning. One, Donna Chibaya, released an album *Zvichanaka* (It shall be well) in 2009 wherein she predicted that Zimbabwe would enjoy unparalleled prosperity in the near future. She proclaimed that in His own time, God would restore Zimbabwe's currency and its citizens would once again enjoy peace and prosperity. Another singer, Prince Mafukidze, stuck to the prosperity theme when he called upon the nation to persevere as salvation was around the corner. Various other gospel artists sought to promote healing and hope (Chitando and Togarasei, 2010: 154).

Before the harmonised elections of 31 July 2013, several musicians performed at the Book Café in Harare on 30 July 2013. The peace concert was organised by the Media Institute of Southern Africa (MISA) and the Book Café. Entrance was free. Musical groups such as Nehoreka, Aggabu Nyabinde, Joel Likembe, and Tinashe Mupambawashe performed. MISA spokesperson, Kholiwe Majama, highlighted the significance of the event when he said:

> We feel it is very necessary to help reinforce peace agenda messages being preached by most churches in Zimbabwe. Though we have not received many violence reports, we still feel it is very important to encourage people to observe peace during the July 31, 2013 elections.
>
> (Gumbo, 2013: 18)

Musician Leonard Zhakata at one time had some of his songs banned on national radio and television. However, he highlighted the important roles artists can play in national healing:

> Artists are popular and have fans from across the political divide. At times politicians tend to be biased and blinkered, they talk and address people with a certain bias . . . We want to be involved in national healing but we have a problem in that if you start acting on such issues you will be labeled politically.
>
> (Muguwu, 2012: 16)

The influence of artists can be demonstrated by their crowd pulling capabilities. During the Defence Forces Day commemorations held in Harare in August 2012, Alick Macheso's performance was brilliant to an extent that former President Mugabe had to ask Macheso for a face-to-face interaction. Then Vice-President Mujuru and then Prime Minister Tsvangirai could not also hide their joy at the performance (Chinowaita, 2012: 4). If musicians can unify politicians, they can also unify the nation through preaching and encouraging the practice of peace.

Actors have also proved central to peacebuilding efforts in the country. In peacebuilding the key thrust is to avoid a relapse to the hated past. Local Zimbabwean drama series called *Sabhuku Vharazipi* was popular not only because of the talent of its actors such as David Mubayiwa "Sabhuku Vharazipi" Kumbirai Chikonye "Mbuya Mai John" and Wellington Chindara "Svari/Chairman," but because of their creativity in revealing societal ills. The *Sabhuku Vharazipi* drama series unearthed perceived pressing social, economic, and political problems in Zimbabwe. These included gender-based violence manifesting itself in forms such as child marriages and labour, wife battering, and widow/bride inheritance, corruption, vote buying, and political violence. The popularity of the drama series made it a suitable platform for raising awareness and educating communities about what needs to be done to reduce violence and oppressive practices in communities.

Government

The government of Zimbabwe long undermined national healing and reconciliation processes and this was clear in the political leadership's lack of political will hence its failure to put in place strategies to redress and curtail social injustices (Murambadoro, 2014). It recurrently cast a cold shoulder on the calls by the victims of the Gukurahundi atrocities that took place between 1982 and 1987. Gukurahundi is a Shona term that refers to "the first rain that washes away chaff before the spring rains." It has been used to refer to the killings and torture of over 20,000 people by government security forces (the 5th Brigade and Police Intelligence) in the Midlands and Matabeleland regions of Zimbabwe between 1982 and 1987. This was a government campaign to eradicate the stronghold of the Zimbabwe People's Revolutionary Army (ZIPRA) ex-combatants in these regions (Catholic Commission for Justice and Peace in Zimbabwe and the Legal Resources Foundation, 1997). Again, there was violence during the Fast Track Land Reform Programme which began in 2000, Operation Murambatsvina in 2005 and the 27 June 2008 presidential run-off election among other incidences which demonstrate the role of violence in the survival of ZANU PF since 1980. Wrongdoers were not called to account as a result of government Clemency Orders of 1980, 1988, and 2000 which pardoned government security agents for almost all the atrocities they committed (Murambadoro, 2014).

The greatest contribution that the Zimbabwean government can do to facilitate reconciliation is to listen to the citizens, many of whom were victims of ZANU PF violence over the years. In addition, the government should be encouraged to create an environment that allows the church and civil society to carry out national healing and reconciliation activities. Zimbabwe was once seen as a model for reconciliation when Mugabe pronounced his intention to encourage the citizens to reconcile. In his Independence Day message delivered on 17 April 1980, Prime Minister, Mugabe, gave peace assurances to all Zimbabweans (Zimbabwe Press Statement 204/80/JEM). He called for reconciliation saying:

> Surely this is now the time to beat our swords into ploughshares so we can attend to the problems of developing our economy and our society . . . I urge you, whether you are black or white, to join me in a new pledge to forget our grim past, forgive others and forget, join hands in a new amity, and together, as Zimbabweans, trample upon racialism, tribalism and regionalism, and work hard to reconstruct and rehabilitate our society as we reinvigorate our economic machinery.
>
> (De Waal, 1990: 46)

Traditional leadership

Traditional leaders play a fundamental role in settling community differences throughout rural Zimbabwe. They are considered the custodians of traditional law and receive the majority of the cases relating to political and domestic violence, including antisocial behaviour. However, it appears that they have limited power and knowledge to curtail and sufficiently respond to violence. The regulatory objective of the traditional justice system headed by traditional leaders in Africa in general and Zimbabwe in particular seeks to restore peace and harmony in the community. This is accomplished through reconciling the disputants and their respective supporters.

Chiefs remain indispensable in encouraging peaceful societies. At the inauguration ceremony of Chief Samambwa in Zhombe in January 2018, president of Zimbabwe Council of Chiefs, Fortune Charumbira, encouraged villagers to live in peace and harmony despite one's political affiliation (Ndlovu, 2018). In this vein, community leaders such as kraalheads, headmen and chiefs have indispensable roles in safeguarding their communities from violence. These are important in influencing and preventing their subjects from resorting to violence by settling differences peacefully. In the process of conflict transformation, community leaders can take up the roles as mediators, advisors and mentors.

The media

The agenda-setting theory put forward by Maxwell McCombs and Donald Shaw (1972) posits that the mass media have the capacity to influence what people think about and how they think about certain issues because of their ability to identify, select, prioritise, include, and exclude issues. The theory is significant if one considers the stories that dominated the media during the Government of National Unity (GNU) era. The media focused on the issue of elections during the preparation of the 2013 harmonised elections. It was very rare to find a story which dealt with the economic issues of the inclusive government. There was political bickering as Patrick Chinamasa of ZANU PF and Tendai Biti of the MDC-T quarrelled over who introduced the multi-currency regime. On the other hand, Mugabe castigated the GNU as a "two headed creature." Headlines that appeared in the print and electronic media illustrated the role of the media in agenda setting. Examples were drawn from the GNU era. The headline of the *Herald*, 8 March 2013 was entitled, "Government drops poll funding request," while the *Patriot*, 3 to 9 August 2012 was headlined, "Black faces white minds at Book Fair." *The Sunday Mail*, 12 to 18 August, 2012 headline was "Ndabaningi Sithole was a sell-out," *Newsday* of 10 September 2012 was titled, "Mugabe 'plots' ambush," the *Standard*, 8 to 14 July 2012 it was "Mujuru flexes muscles," and the *Daily News on Sunday*, 30 September to 6 October 2012 had the headline, "Zanu PF will fail."

The media became more polarised following the establishment of the *Daily News* and the formation of the opposition. The state-owned newspapers rallied behind the ZANU PF-led government while the *Daily News* vigorously and unapologetically backed the MDC. Related to this, Patrick Chinamasa, ZANU PF justice minister at the time commented that: "I wonder why the MDC has Learnmore Jongwe as their spokesperson when they have the *Daily News* doing their job" (Chari, 2010: 133).

During the run up to elections the government-owned media was biased in favour of ZANU PF. To confirm this, Hove and Harris (2015: 157) wrote:

> the media and the Zimbabwe Electoral Commission acted in ways which strongly advantaged the Zimbabwe African National Union Patriotic Front to the detriment of the opposition political parties including the Movement for Democratic Change formations.

Furthermore, the media under Jonathan Moyo, then Minister of Information of Publicity was used as a tool of indoctrinating Zimbabweans in an effort to change their mind set in favour of ZANU PF. Moyo sought to introduce 100% local content in music by playing one revolutionary song out of every five songs on radio (Hove and Mukurunge, 2014).

Media reforms in Zimbabwe can lead to better prospects for good governance in the sense that bias would be minimised as issues affecting the nation would be fairly covered without considering the political affiliation of the persons involved. The national television was pro-ZANU PF and was willing to maintain the status quo as long as ZANU PF was in power. The electronic media produced and aired one-sided political content (The Legal Monitor, 2012a, 2012b, 2012c). Alternative sources of media such as short-wave radios were prohibited as shown by the confiscation of radios from civil society organisations which distributed them (The Legal Monitor, 2013a, 2013b).

The media is better positioned to build peaceful communities because it is close to the people. It reports stories as they happen, highlighting the nitty-gritties. The realities of xenophobic violence that gripped South Africa in 2015 were exposed by the media. On 19 April 2015, the *Sunday Times* produced horrible pictures showing the murder of a Mozambican man, Emmanuel Sithole, in Alexandra, Johannesburg (Tromp et al., 2015: 1). The pictures revealed the urgency required in order to thwart the recurrence of the murder of foreigners. The media also helped in building peace by publishing stories which slammed the behaviour of Zulu King Goodwill Zwelithini for his remarks which were believed to have sparked xenophobic attacks in Durban. Some of the attackers confessed to be following the King's call for foreigners to leave (Mashaba, 2015: 6). Overall, the media can be so influential in building peace in Zimbabwe through castigating the use of violence as a political tool.

Political parties

Global peacebuilding players have so far not been too excited about engagement with political parties. However, there is increasing appreciation of their significance since they play influential roles in castigating inter-party and intra-party violence, promoting healing and reducing politically-driven structural violence.

Former South African President Thabo Mbeki's mediation led to an almost-level political playing field due to the several amendments to some inflexible laws that stood in the way of democracy in Zimbabwe. Accordingly, during the run up to the March 29, 2008 harmonised elections, political parties urged their supporters to desist from violence. As a result these "were the most peaceful since the beginning of the Zimbabwean crisis in 2000 (Hove and Ndawana, 2016: 66). More so, the GNU provided for a democratic framework because it had executive power sharing (though top to bottom). The GNU principals were President Mugabe, Prime Minister Tsvangirai, Deputy Prime Ministers Thokozani Khupe (MDC-T), and Professor Arthur Mutambara (MDC).

The Constitution Parliamentary Select Committee (COPAC) was established to lead the constitution-making process in Zimbabwe. It was guided by the provisions of the Global Political Agreement whose Article VI noted that, "it is the fundamental right and duty of the Zimbabwean people to make a constitution by themselves and for themselves." On the contrary, the process was beset by "deadlocks" and disputes. It was dominated by political parties and they produced a compromised negotiated document, thus the so-called people-driven process became questionable (Raftopoulos, 2013).

Again, ONHRI was set up under Article 7.1 (c) of the GPA (2008: 7) which stated that,

> The parties hereby agree that the new Government: . . . shall give consideration to the setting up of a mechanism to properly advise on what measures might be necessary and practicable to achieve national healing, cohesion and unity in respect of victims of pre and post-independence political conflicts.

ONHRI was a very significant institution towards wider reconciliation in Zimbabwe. It provided for a peace architecture through partnerships with churches whereby peacebuilding trainings were to be carried out in communities. Overall, ONHRI, a product of the Global Political Agreement, attempted to come up with procedures to be followed to bring to book political parties whose supporters would be responsible for political violence. In support of peace, the late Vice President John Landa Nkomo (co-chairperson of the Organ on National Healing, Reconciliation, and Integration representing ZANUPF) said: 'Peace Begins with Me, Peace Begins with You, Peace Begins with all of Us' (Chitando and Mukenge, 2015).

In this light, the GNU (made up of the three principals, cabinet, co-ministers, and legislators) helped considerably in providing a stage for inter-party dialogue amongst the political parties. Essentially, negotiations at the behest of SADC facilitated by then President Thabo Mbeki of South Africa eased the Zimbabwean political turmoil. However, sticky issues remained regarding the sharing of ministerial positions, constitutional and electoral reforms, the demilitarisation of the Zimbabwean politics, and media reforms.

Through its Victims Commemoration Day, the MDC party donated food hampers, wheel barrows, shovels, and roofing sheets to victims of political violence in 2012 (Chitagu, 2012: 2). A day before the July 2013 harmonised elections, ZANU PF had an advert in the *Daily News* newspaper with the message: "What a Peaceful campaign! Thank you Zimbabwe for heeding our call for tolerance and brotherliness. Vote Cde Robert Gabriel Mugabe For President, Vote ZANU PF, Bhora Mugedhi, Ibhola Egedini" (Daily News, 2013: 14). The 2013 elections were peaceful compared to the previous election held in June 2008. ZANU PF surprised everyone by preaching peace and tolerance, the very components that had eluded the country for more than a decade. Peacebuilding is achievable if political parties commit themselves to it.

To end violence Zimbabwe's leaders must take cognisance of the late Prime Minister Morgan Tsvangirai's observation that efforts towards peace were defeated by supporters of President Robert Mugabe who "did not want to let go of the culture of violence." He concluded that, "it is difficult to convince the world that you have turned the corner when others are perpetuating the same culture of violence in the countryside; the same culture and behaviour that brought us where we are" (Hove, 2012a: 82). In this regard, we urge all the political parties in Zimbabwe to remain mindful of the fact that political parties are crucial in peacebuilding. They can play an imperative role in brokering an end to conflict, through mediating or negotiating.

The international community

Increasingly, the international community has taken keen interest in conflict resolution through engaging parties involved in conflict via the use of regional and continental organs. The implementation of the protection of civilians remains a priority and a challenge for many multilateral organisations, including the North Atlantic Treaty Organisation (NATO), the United Nations (UN), and the African Union (AU) (Keenan and Beadle, 2015: 1). On 2 June 2000, Sierra Leone's President Ahmad Tejan Kabbah wrote a letter to United Nations Secretary General Kofi Annan. The president asked the United Nations for assistance in bringing to justice those responsible for the crimes perpetrated during the conflict between 1991 and 2002. Consequently, on 16 January 2002, the UN and Government of Sierra Leone signed the agreement which led to the creation of the Special Court for Sierra Leone (SCSL) (Trial International, 2016). The United Nations established a Peacebuilding Fund as one of several multilateral funds to pre-position resources for rapid and early disbursement (United Nations, 2010: 15). The Fund provides quick monetary assistance for critical institution building, political dialogue, and rule of law initiatives. The challenge, however, is the absence of longer-term and larger-scale support (United Nations, 2014: 2). In the eastern Democratic Republic of the Congo, coordinated efforts by the World Food Programme and UNICEF helped in the reintegration of child soldiers through schooling, feeding, and protection programmes (United Nations, 2014: 9). The office of the UN secretary general thus strongly endorses national capacity development as the cornerstone of all peacebuilding efforts (United Nations, 2014: 7). The international community can equally play significant roles in a drive to promote healing in Zimbabwe through encouraging tolerance. The politics of intolerance was fundamental in the occurrence of violence since 1980. In addition, the international community can be crucial in restituting the victims of politically-motivated violence.

Academia

The field of peacebuilding is vast and academia joined in the conversation with a rapidly growing body of literature whose works are consumed by research analysts spanning the practitioner-scholar divide. Accordingly, the academic fraternity is an important player in national healing through provoking thought. Knowledge production borne out of research gives policymakers a reservoir from which informed decisions can be made. However, those who use research in peacebuilding must be able to distinguish which research may undermine or support the cultivation of peaceful relations in divided societies. It means that the skill to select and use research contextually and appropriately is a vital requisite.

The term "peacebuilding" was devised by Johan Galtung in 1975 with the publication of three strategies to peace: "Peacekeeping, peacemaking, and peacebuilding." Galtung created several of the essential concepts that remain critical and of use in peacebuilding work today. Galtung reflected on negative peace, positive peace, structural violence, root causes of conflict, and sustainable peace. Linked to this, so many works have been written outlining the causes, course, and effects of Zimbabwe's major conflict watersheds and how peacebuilding can be achieved in Zimbabwe. These include the works by Masipula Sithole (1999), Josephine Nhongo-Simbanegavi (2002), Terence Ranger (1985), Lloyd Sachikonye (2011, 2012), Norma Kriger (2003), Mediel Hove and Tawanda Mukurunge (2014), Mediel Hove (2012a, 2012b), Mediel Hove and Enock Ndawana (2016), and Cyprian Muchemwa et al. (2013), among others. Undeniably, the humanities and social sciences play a prominent role in peacebuilding. Perhaps in an effort to accomplish the objective of building peace in Zimbabwe, different state and private universities (University of Zimbabwe, Bindura University of Science Education, the National University of Science Technology, Chinhoyi University of Technology, Great Zimbabwe University, Midlands State University, Africa University, and Solusi University) are running peacebuilding and related courses in a drive to resolve the ongoing Zimbabwean conflict (Hove, 2019: 157–158). The need for continued support for these different initiatives (research and education) need not be overstated in light of the polarisation that prevails in Zimbabwe.

Conclusion

The chapter asserts that conflict resolution is a multi-stakeholder process, not a preserve of an individual or a single institution. Likewise, the government of Zimbabwe should be encouraged to take the strategy of inclusivity seriously in its endeavour to heal, reconcile, and integrate Zimbabweans. This means the church and the civil society among other stakeholders have significant roles to play in an attempt to realise sustainable peace in the country. Above all, everything that is done concerning peacebuilding should be guided by what the citizens (and specifically what the victims) suggest. Stakeholders should be there to regulate (and unconditionally assist materially) the demands of both the perpetrators and the victims. The stakeholders can also relate different experiences to the contending parties with the view of sharing the experiences of others who resolved their conflicts before. Accordingly, stakeholders are forbidden from dictating in any of the processes that are initiated to find pragmatic and sustainable solutions to the conflicting parties. The approach of listening to the victims is important because there is no single way of achieving national healing and reconciliation in any given polity and Zimbabwe is no exception. People's experiences and violent watersheds are different. That is why national healing and reconciliation processes should be context-specific thus being people-centred.

References

Bloomfield, D. 2003. "Reconciliation: An Introduction," in David Bloomfield, Teresa Barnes, and Luc Huyse (eds.), *Reconciliation After Violent Conflict*. Stockholm: International Institute for Democracy and Electoral Assistance.

Catholic Commission for Justice and Peace in Zimbabwe and Legal Resources Foundation. 1997. *Breaking the Silence Building True Peace: A Report on the Disturbances in Matabeleland and the Midlands 1980–1988*. Harare: CCJP.

Chari, T. 2010. "Salience and Silence: Representation of the Zimbabwean Crisis in the Local Press," *African Identities* 8(2), 131–150.

Chibaya, M. 2013. "PM Echoes Mugabe's Peace Calls," *The Standard*, 21–27 April.

Chinowaita, M. 2012. "Macheso Charms Mugabe," *Daily News*, 15 August.

Chitagu, T. 2012. "Tsvangirai Mulls GNU Pullout," *The Standard*, 7–13 October.

Chitando, E. and C. Mukenge. 2015. "'Peace Begins with Me, Peace Begins with You: Peace Begins with All of Us': Assessing the Potential of the Slogan to Promote National Healing and Integration in Zimbabwe," *Southern Peace Review Journal* 4(1), 11–26.

Chitando, E. and L. Togarasei. 2010. "June 2008, Verse 27': The Church and the 2008 Zimbabwean Political Crisis," *African Identities* 8(2), 151–162.

Colvin, C. J. 2007. "Civil Society and Reconciliation in Southern Africa," *Development in Practice* 17(3), 322–337.

Daily News. 2013, 30 July.

De Waal, V. 1990. *The Politics of Reconciliation: Zimbabwe's First Decade*. London: Hurst and Company; Cape Town: David Philip.

Eyre, B. 2015. *Lion Songs: Thomas Mapfumo and the Music That Made Zimbabwe*. Durham: Duke University Press.

Fischer, M. 2011. "Transitional Justice and Reconciliation: Theory and Practice," in B. Austin, M. Fischer, H. J. Giessmann (eds.), *Advancing Conflict Transformation*. Opladen, Farmington Hills: Barbara Budrich Publishers (The Berghof Handbook II).

Gumbo, B. 2013. "Peace Concert Tonight," *Daily News*, 30 July.

Global Political Agreement (GPA). (2008).

Hayner, P. B. 2011. *Unspeakable Truths: Transitional Justice and the Challenge of Truth Commissions*. Oxon: Routledge.

Hove, M. 2012a. "The Debates and Impact of Sanctions: The Zimbabwean Experience," *International Journal of Business and Social Science* 3(5), 72–84.

Hove, M. 2012b. "War Legacy: A Reflection on the Effects of the Rhodesian Security Forces (RSF) in South Eastern Zimbabwe During Zimbabwe's War of Liberation 1976–1980," *Journal of African Studies and Development* 4(8), 193–206.

Hove, M. 2016. "Review of Banning Eyre. 2015. *Lion Songs: Thomas Mapfumo and the Music that Made Zimbabwe*. Durham: Duke University Press," *African Studies Quarterly* 16(3–4), December, 190–191.

Hove, M. 2019. "The Necessity of Peace Education in Zimbabwe," in Hove, Mediel and Harris, Geoff (eds.), *Infrastructures for Peace in Sub-Saharan Africa* (pp. 147–163). Zurich: Springer Publishers.

Hove, M. and E. Ndawana. 2016. "Regional Mediation Strategy: The Case of Zimbabwe," *African Security Review* 25(1), 63–84.

Hove, M. and V. Chenzi. 2017. "'Prophets of Doom': The Zimbabwean Christian Community and Contemporary Politics," *Insight on Africa* 9(2), 173–195.

Hove, M. and G. Harris. 2015. "Free and Fair Elections: Mugabe and the Challenges Facing Elections in Zimbabwe," *International Journal of Human Rights and Constitutional Studies* 3(2), 157–170.

Hove, M. and T. Mukurunge. 2014. "Revolutionary Songs as a Strategy of Transforming Listeners' Mindset: The Zimbabwean Practice After 1999," *Alternatives: Turkish Journal of International Relations* 13(3), Fall, 12–30.

Hudzerema, F. 2015. "All Souls Church Donates to the Needy," *Avondale and Mt Pleasant Suburban*, 13–19 November.

Hutchison, E. and R. Bleiker. 2013. "Reconciliation," in R. M. Ginty (ed.), *The Limits of Peacebuilding Theory (Routledge Handbook of Peacebuilding)*. Abingdon, Oxon: Routledge.

Kandimire, J. 2015. "Victims of Political Violence to Meet in Masvingo on World Peace Day," *Voice of America*, Zimbabwe, 18 September. www.voazimbabwe.com/content/political-violence-victims-to-meet-in-masvingo-monday/2969689.html (accessed on November 2015).

Keenan, M. and A. W. Beadle. 2015. "Operationalizing Protection of Civilians in NATO Operations," *Stability: International Journal of Security & Development* 4(1), 44, 1–13. http://dx.doi.org/10.5334/sta.gr.

Kriger, N. J. 1992. *Zimbabwe's Guerrilla War: Peasant Voices*. Cambridge: Cambridge University Press.

The Legal Monitor. 2012a. "Buhera Villages Fight Violence," 7 May, 142.

The Legal Monitor. 2012b. "On World Press Freedom Day Zimbabweans Deserve a Free Media and Diverse Information," 7 May, Edition 142.

The Legal Monitor. 2012c. "Zimbabwe's Retrogressive Decades," 7 May, Edition 142.

The Legal Monitor. 2013a. "Dreadful 2008 Imminent," 1 April, 186.

The Legal Monitor. 2013b. "On World Press Freedom Day, ZLHR Urges Government to Advance Media Freedom Package," 6 May, Edition 191.

Mashaba, S. 2015. "Mandela Upbraids Zulu King," *Sowetan*, 17 April.

Matenga, M. 2016. "'Mugabe Must Go," *Newsday*, 7 January.

McCombs, M. E. and D. L. Shaw. 1972. "The Agenda-Setting Function of Mass Media," *Public Opinion Quarterly* 36(2), 176–187.

Muchemwa, C., E. T. Ngwerume and M. Hove. 2013. "When Will the Long Nightmare Come to an End? Challenges to National Healing and Reconciliation in Post-Colonial Zimbabwe," *African Security Review* 22(3), 145–159.

Muguwu, S. 2012. "Artists Speak on National Healing," *Daily News*, 30 September.

Murambadoro, R. 2014. "The Politics of Reconciliation in Zimbabwe: Three Times Failure – Will the Fourth Time Count?" https://kujenga-amani.ssrc.org/.../the-politics-of-reconciliation-in-zimbabwe-three-tim ... (accessed on 18 June 2018).

Ncube, C. 2014. "Civil Society and Peacebuilding During Zimbabwe's Government of National Unity, 2009–2013," *African Security Review* 23(3), 283–294. doi:10.1080/1024 6029.2014.930056.

Ndlovu, N. 2017. "ACCZ Ready to Lead Gukurahundi Peace, Reconciliation Efforts," *Newsday*, 30 October.

Ndlovu, S. 2018. "Chiefs Unapologetic About Cars, Says Charumbira," *Chronicle*, 22 January.

Raftopoulos, B. (Ed.) 2013. *The Hard Road to Reform: The Politics of Zimbabwe's Global Political Agreement*. Harare: Weaver Press.

Sachikonye, L. 2011. *When a State Turns on Its Citizens: Institutionalized Violence and Political Culture*. Johannesburg: Jacana Media.

SADC Gender Protocol Barometer. 2014.

The Standard. 2012. 26 August–1 September.

The Standard. 2013. "Police Hold Keys to Peaceful Polls," 21–27 April.

The Sunday Mail. 2012. "Kunonga Hails Empowerment," 26 February–3 March.

The Sunday Mail. 2013a. "Church Pledges Allegiance to President Mugabe," 5–11 May.

The Sunday Mail. 2013b. 3–9 March.

Trial International. 2016. Foday Sankoh. https://trialinternational.org/latest-post/foday-sankoh/.

Tromp, B., N. Olifant and M. Savides. 2015. "Kill Thy Neighbor: Alex Attack Brings Home SA's Shame," *Sunday Times*, 19 April.

United Nations. 2010. "Women's Participation in Peacebuilding: Report of the Secretary-General," A/65/354 – S/2010/466, 10–50820.

United Nations. 2014. "Peacebuilding in the Immediate Aftermath of Conflict, Report of the Secretary-General," A/69/399 – S/2014/694, 14–61476. www.un.org/en/peace building/pbso/pdf/SG%20report%20OCT%202014%20EN69_399.pdf.

Van Binsbergen, Wim. 1999. *Reconciliation: A Major African Social Technology of Shared and Recognized Humanity*. Ubuntu. www.shikanda.net/african_religion/reconcil.htm (accessed on 18 June 2018).

Zimbabwe Press Statement 204/80/JEM.

Zimbabwe Press Statement 463/80/SFS.

4 The government of national unity and national healing in Zimbabwe

Tobias Marevesa

Introduction

The Government of National Unity (GNU) (2009–2013) was the product of the Global Political Agreement which was signed between the major political parties in Zimbabwe, namely, ZANU PF of Robert Mugabe, MDC-T of Morgan Tsvangirai, and MDC-M of Arthur Mutambara with the mandate of forming a transitional government in preparation for a free and fair election. The GNU was necessitated by the politically-motivated violence which rocked the country between 2000 and 2008. The purpose of this chapter is to interrogate the conflict which led to unprecedented violence which was caused by a number of factors such as food riots, inflation, war veterans' compensation fund, post-independence wars, the economic structural adjustment programme and sanctions, among others. The chapter argues that the GNU could have done better in bringing about reconciliation if the Organ on National Healing, Reconciliation, and Integration could have incorporated people with expertise in dealing with conflict transformation rather than depending on politicians. The chapter concludes that the inclusion of civil society organisations, traditional leaders, church leaders, academics, local communities, and other relevant stakeholders could have brought the much needed reconciliation and peace in Zimbabwe.

The background to the GNU

This section discusses the factors and situations that gave birth to the Government of National Unity (GNU) in Zimbabwe. The purpose of this section is to put the GNU in its proper political context. ZANU was formed in 1963 after it parted ways with the Zimbabwe African People's Union (ZAPU) which was led by Joshua Nkomo. Reverend Ndabaningi Sithole was the first president of ZANU, and was replaced by Robert Mugabe in 1975 (Chung, 2006: 115).

The two MDC formations are the offshoot of the MDC, which Meredith (2002: 70) states, was formed in September 1999 as a brainchild of the Zimbabwe Congress of Trade Unions (hereafter ZCTU) and civic movements, with the aim of dislodging ZANU PF's monopoly in ruling Zimbabwe. The MDC split because they could not agree on whether to participate or not in

Senatorial elections of 2005. However, some critics and analysts such as Kriger (2012: 11); Raftopoulos (2010: 705), claim that the issue of the senatorial election was a symptom of a deeper problem, as there was a power struggle among the party leaders.

The problems of Zimbabwe, which resulted in the "Zimbabwean Crisis," dates back to 1980. Zimbabwe's post-colonial period was characterized by an economic boom and reconciliation in the early 1980s (Raftopoulos, 2007: 79). However, the political problem of Gukurahundi resulted in the political instability in the Matabeleland and Midlands regions from 1982 to 1987. The economic boom of the immediate post-independence period did not last long. Zimbabwe's economy experienced mixed fortunes throughout the 1980s, as it went through the negative effects of drought, weakening terms of trade, and high interest rates and oil prices (Bond, 2003: 163). All this impacted negatively on the government's capacity to finance its programmes. Muzondidya (2009: 40) argues that the International Monetary Fund and World Bank mounted pressure on the government to abandon some of its social policies between 1983 and 1984 which had free social services.

The land reform programme

The land resettlement programme occurred in two phases. The first was from 1981 to 1987 (Chung, 2006: 296). About two million hectares were acquired by the government on the "willing seller-willing buyer" system which was funded by the British government during Margaret Thatcher's tenure. This was done according to the Lancaster House agreement of 1979, according to which the British Government was supposed to fund the redistribution of the land in Zimbabwe (Sachikonye, 2013: 9; Chung, 2006: 298). During the first phase of land redistribution, the process was well organized and the intended beneficiaries, the poor peasant farmers, benefited. After the 1987 land redistribution, the British government had a new leadership after the fall of Margaret Thatcher. Her successors stopped funding land resettlement, and gave the excuse that there was corruption and patronage in the land redistribution programme.

In reaction to Tony Blair's government, the government of Zimbabwe enacted a constitutional reform which gave the government powers to repossess land for redistribution from white farmers to poor peasants (Gono, 2008: 95). The British reportedly also retaliated by funding local people, media, civic societies, and political parties to try to dislodge the ZANU PF regime. According to Kanyenze (2004: 131), when financial support was not forthcoming to finance land redistribution this resulted in *jambanja* or the fast-track programme. It can be pointed out that there was a deep-rooted conflict between Zimbabwe and the United Kingdom. The conflict led to Zimbabwe being sanctioned by the West (Britain, USA, and the EU), and accused being of not observing the rule of law when repossessing the land. The *jambanja* or fast-track resettlement programme was also named the Third Chimurenga. It was an episode where people were fighting for their birthright, thus the land.

The economic structural adjustment programme

Another contributing factor towards the meltdown of the economy of Zimbabwe was the adoption of the ESAP in the early 1990s, (Chung, 2006: 304; Sadomba, 2011: 40; Mlambo, 1997: 97). By 1991, the ruling ZANU (PF) Party had drifted from its former socialist ideology when it adopted ESAP. This programme was initiated by the government under the pressure and assistance from the World Bank (WB) and International Monetary Fund (IMF). The adoption and implementation of ESAP as a free-market system implies an abandonment of the government's socialistic policies of 1980 (Verstraelen, 1998: 25). From 1980–1990, the government had a socialist policy for the benefit of the black majority: Expansion of educational facilities in rural areas, free health services, the subsidy of basic consumer goods, and a minimum-wage system (Mlambo, 1997: 97). It can be pointed out that the ESAP was the major contributor to the Zimbabwe crisis. According to Sadomba (2011: 206), Muzondidya (2009: 188), and Chung (2006: 2990), a number of workers lost their jobs as industries closed down, and public spending was cut, in line with structural adjustment policies.

The revolt of the war veterans

The other notable factor that led Zimbabwe into a crisis was the demands by the war veterans in 1997, where they were given Z$50,000,00 each as pension gratuities for their involvement in the liberation war. Chung (2006: 243) posits that the collapse of the Zimbabwean dollar was primarily caused by the plunder of the War Veterans' Compensation Fund in 1996–1997. About Z$41 billion was given to the ruling ZANU PF elite. This resulted in the revolt by war veterans and the subsequent handouts of about Z$44 billion to silence them (Mhanda, 2011: 225). It can be argued that the money which was given to the war veterans was unbudgeted for and therefore it eroded the economy. The government gave in to the temptation of printing money, leading to the collapse of the Zimbabwean dollar. In fact, President Mugabe was trying to gain political advantage, because the war veterans were the backbone of his party but they were complaining of not being recognized.

Food riots

In 1998, the ZCTU organized food riots which paralysed the economy. These riots were mainly caused by the hiking of fuel prices and increased inflation. This resulted in the formation of the "broad based movement for change" (Kanyenze, 2004: 136). This movement was later called the MDC and was launched in September 1999. After the launch, the ruling party resorted to terror tactics on realizing the massive support which the MDC had, after the experience of the referendum of 2000. Raftopoulos (2009: 222) posits that another major effect of the economic meltdown was the dizzying speed of hyperinflation, which resulted in the "dollarization" of economic transactions.

Wars after independence

There were three wars which Zimbabwe went through after 1980. The first one was an internal conflict between ZANU and ZAPU which lasted from 1982 to 1987. The problems between ZANU and ZAPU went back to 1963, when ZANU split from ZAPU during the liberation struggle (Eppel, 2013: 44; Chung, 2006: 3, 14). The conflict between the two, went on until Zimbabwe got its independence in 1980. From 1982, there was an insurgence of the dissidents in the Matabeleland and Midlands provinces. This insurgence was swiftly and brutally stopped by the 5th Brigade (Eppel, 2013: 45). The former President of Zimbabwe, Canaan Banana, played a pivotal role in brokering the peace, by persuading the two parties ZANU and ZAPU to lay down their arms for the sake of Zimbabwe (Chung, 2006: 315). It can be argued that this war aroused bitterness against ZANU PF. This was seen in the 2000 and 2002 elections when the whole of Matabeleland voted against ZANU PF.

The second Zimbabwe war was Zimbabwe's involvement in the Mozambique war, supporting the FRELIMO government against the Renamo insurgence. This happened from 1980 and continued until 1994. This was actually a solidarity war, because Mozambique had supported the liberation struggle of Zimbabwe and so Zimbabwe had an obligation to help militarily.

The third was Zimbabwe's participation in the Democratic Republic of the Congo (DRC) war, from 1998 until 2003, supporting initially the government of Laurent Kabila, and later Joseph Kabila. The war benefited several business people, and some individuals became billionaires (Chung, 2006: 244). According to Eppel (2013: 44), as had taken place in Mozambique, Zimbabwe as a country did not benefit much from the post–war recovery period in the DRC. Instead, the South Africans benefited because they had a strong industrial and commercial sector, while Zimbabwe had superior armed forces but weak industrial and commercial sectors.

The Church's role in promoting conflict

The church was divided during this period of the "Zimbabwe an Crisis." Some churches supported Mugabe's exhausted nationalism, while others aligned themselves with the critical civic movements (Sachikonye, 2011: 75). For instance, some church leaders in the Anglican Church, such as Bishop Nolbert Kunonga, expressed support for President Mugabe and his ZANU (PF) party. There was then a split in the Anglican Church, probably because of Bishop Kunonga's endorsement of the regime. Following Bishop Kunonga's excommunication from the Anglican Church of Province of Central Africa (CPCA), he then refused to return the assets of the Church (Sachikonye, 2011: 78). This resistance brewed into a conflict within the Church led by Bishop Kunonga and Bishop Gandiya. State authorities and the police supported Kunonga for political reasons. Generally, the African independent churches were accused of being partisan. According to Hofisi, Manyeruke, and Mhandara (2013: 110), the two denominations, led respectively by Johanne Masowe and Johanne Marange, caused conflict because they publicly supported ZANU PF. Most of the ZANU PF leadership were seen fellowshipping with them, probably because they wanted to lure them into ZANU PF. Even the opposition leader Morgan Tsvangirai was also seen being part of the Johanne Marange church, fellowshipping with them (Hofisi et al., 2013: 110). However, other African indigenous churches such as Paul Mwazha condemned sanctions just like other church leaders such as Kunonga and a Pentecostal leader, Emmanuel Makandiwa. Meanwhile, the Pentecostal churches taught their congregants to "make the best of rapid social change" (Maxwell, 2006: 351). Really, the church did not play its prophetic role in the crisis because she feared being victimized. In March 2007, the police brutally disrupted a prayer meeting of the Christian Alliance Church in Highfield, Harare (Raftopoulos, 2009: 227). The publicity of this event globally resulted in international condemnation and pressure on President Mugabe's regime, putting more pressure on the Southern African Development Community (SADC) to deal with the Zimbabwe crisis.

Politically motivated violence 2000–2008

Politically motivated violence can be understood as an illegitimate use of force or violence against people or property with the aim of pressing or intimidating an individual, in order to advance a political or social mandate (www.thefreed ictionary.com/Politically+motivated+violence-Accessed on 10–02–2016). Political violence can be traced back to the pre-colonial era, where violence was mainly caused by the struggle for land and chieftainship. While in the colonial period, violence was centred on the fight for land and ethnic recognition and supremacy, in the post-colonial dispensation, violence was prevalent in the struggle for political dominion and hegemony (Sachikonye, 2011: 13). These forms of political violence were witnessed before, during, and after elections. A case in point is the Matabeleland massacre of 1982 to 1987, which was referred to as Gukurahundi, where civilians were killed; some were buried alive, and some burnt in their homes, while others were knifed (www.sokwanele. com). This did not end with Gukurahundi, and the situation only worsened when the MDC was formed in 1999. The MDC became a threat to ZANU PF in the 2000 Parliamentary elections and the subsequent elections which were held in 2002, 2005, and 2008 (Research and Advocacy Unit, 2011: 2).

The 2008 general election began in a very peaceful way. All the observers spoke with one voice that elections were free, fair, and peaceful (Maruta, 2013: 7). The main contenders were, ZANU PF, led by Robert Mugabe, MDC-T led by Morgan Tsvangirai, and the other MDC-M led by Arthur Mutambara. These elections were referred to as harmonised elections because they combined local government, parliamentary, and presidential elections (Hofisi et al., 2013: 103). The results of the local and parliamentary elections were published immediately after vote counting. For the first time in the history of Zimbabwe, ZANU PF was defeated by an opposition party in national elections. However, the presidential election results were delayed and there were many allegations that it could be that the election results were tampered with, Tsvangirai having gained 47.9%, while Mugabe had 43.2% (Raftopoulos, 2009: 229; Tatira and Marevesa, 2011: 188). According to Ndlovu-Gatsheni (2013: 158), after the announcement of the results that the MDC-T candidate had won, but did not exceed the 50% plus one threshold which was a prerequisite by new electoral law for one to be an outright winner, a run-off was mandatory (Masunungure, 2009: 79). ZANU PF was only narrowly defeated. A likely analysis of this scenario is that these results could have been a reflection of what had happened in 2000, where ZANU PF was defeated in the constitutional referendum. These two episodes shocked ZANU PF. The national rejection technically pointed to the results of March 2008.

Maruta (2013: 7) and Raftopoulos (2009: 230), posit that during the period towards the run-off, the campaign was characterised by organised politically-motivated violence against the opposition. The violence inflicted by the ruling party can be seen as a punishment for the electorate for voting for the opposition, and it was also a warning that the electorate should not vote for the opposition again. Maruta (2013: 7) claims that the situation in the country was uncertain, "[a]lmost everybody felt unsafe, unsure where the sword will fall next." The magnitude of the violence, intimidation, displacement and elimination was so intense to an extent that the other contender Morgan Tsvangirai of the MDC-T had to quit the race, leaving Robert Mugabe of ZANU PF to "run a one-horse race" (Hofisi et al., 2013: 105). However, the media were divided in their coverage, with the state media generally supporting Mugabe, while the private media tended to side with the opposition. This disparity intensified conflict among the political parties.

Sanctions

Sanctions are mechanisms which are employed by countries and international organizations to persuade a particular government or group of governments to change their policy by restricting trade, investment or other commercial activities (Gono, 2008: 91). In the case of Zimbabwe, sanctions were widened to include other elements such as diplomatic isolation, culture, and sport. Gono (2008: 91) claims that the sanctions which were imposed on Zimbabwe were illegal because they were not sanctioned by the UN Security Council, but by Britain and her allies, while Mashakada (2013: 2), an MP for MDC-T, alleges that these sanctions could be referred to as "restrictive measures." The opposition did not see sanctions as a reality, but as targeting individuals in government who did not uphold the rule of law and human rights. According to MDC-T, the UN could not impose sanctions on Zimbabwe because they were blocked by China and Russia. The sanctions which were imposed on Zimbabwe affected financial relations, trade, and financial flows.

The United States and other Western countries imposed sanctions on Zimbabwe's government in 2002 because of the reports of election rigging and gross human rights abuses (Duzor and Zulu, 2015: 1). In addition, the land redistribution programme angered the West who imposed sanctions in the name of human rights abuse in Zimbabwe (Maruta, 2013: 6). What can be confirmed by a number of scholars such as Ndlovu-Gatsheni (2013: 144), Raftopoulos (2013: 16), and Nyakudya (2013: 174) is that from 2000 to 2008 there was a lot of politically motivated violence which may have forced the US and the West to impose sanctions on Zimbabwe. There is an element of truth in this claim because it is from 2000 that there was a sharp decline in net capital flows, grant flows, external loan flows, and foreign direct investment inflows in Zimbabwe (Gono, 2008: 111).

The government of national unity in Zimbabwe

The conflict-resolution in Zimbabwe should be understood in terms of the signing of the GPA among the main political parties. The GPA is a political agreement which was signed among three major political parties in September 2008, the Movement for Democratic Change – Tsvangirai (hereafter MDC-T) led by Morgan Tsvangirai, the Movement for Democratic Change – Mutambara (hereafter MDC-M) led by Arthur Mutambara, and the Zimbabwe African National Union Patriotic Front (hereafter ZANU PF) led by Robert Mugabe. The GPA gave birth to the GNU which started its operations in February 2009 (Chipaike, 2013). This brought a lot of hope and relief to Zimbabweans after years of economic and political difficulties. The GNU was put in place as a conflict transformation with the mandate of crafting a new constitution and preparing a credible fresh election but, the dictates of the GPA were not fully implemented because of the political bickering over the control of the government.

Chiwara et al. (2013) argue that the GNU which is also known as the Inclusive Government has received different interpretations For example, those who support the GNU argue that it reduced inflation which had brought economic meltdown for almost a decade. It is true that the introduction of the multicurrencies brought significant progress in addressing the economic challenges which be devilled the country for almost a decade. In addition, the dollarization helped to bring stability in the economy in that business ventures stabilised and recovered. Many Zimbabweans were seen with smiles on their faces because basic commodities and food were now available in shops and the provisions of some social services had also improved. According to Zimbabwe Institute (2011), there was a notable number of workers who were back at work because the economy had improved.

Politically, the formation of the GPA government helped in reducing polarization and tension in Zimbabwe. Critics of the GNU argue that it prohibited a situation where the Zimbabwean political landscape would start on a new page. They posit that, "the inclusive government has failed, among other failures, to address issues relating to transitional justice, healing and reconciliation" (Chiwara et al., 2013: 36). The Zimbabwe Institute (2011) argues that during the GNU, there was a notable decrease in politically motivated arrests, violence, abductions, and murders as it can be compared to the period before the GNU. However, there were isolated pockets of violence, intimidation, and political tension nationally which were dealt with by the police.

The GNU brought a number of key constitutional commissions which were established in consultation with all the GPA political parties. These commissions include Media Commission, Anti-Corruption Commission, and Human Rights Commission. In addition, there were some reforms in some sectors of the government such as the economy, media, and politics which brought a new page of democracy, progress, and development. The constitutional reform process has been very slow because of political bickering among the political parties, but under the GPA, it succeeded to complete its major mandate of doing public outreach programme that led to the drafting of the constitution. Manyeruke and Hamauswa (2013) posit that the constitution from the Constitutional Parliamentary Select Committee (COPAC) came as a people-driven document, which means that it was a product of prolonged negotiations among the major political parties in Zimbabwe.

The inclusive government was a fragile political agreement which did not yield very good fruits because it did not solve all the challenges which the country was facing. There was extreme contestation for the control of the government and state power within the GNU. This resulted in the slowdown of the political and economic growth and development of the country (Maisiri, 2013). Tatira and Marevesa (2011) proposed that the GNU was also adversely affected by the outstanding issues which went unresolved throughout the whole period of the inclusive government. The issues were the appointment of the reserve bank governor, attorney general, and provincial governors, among others, this resulted in the tensions within the inclusive government.

The Organ on National Healing, Reconciliation, and Integration and the Joint Monitoring and Implementation Committee

In the GPA document, article VII there are provisions which promotes the ideas of equality, national healing, and unity. This is specifically enshrined in section 7.1 where the GNU was directed among other things to:

1 give consideration to the setting up of a mechanism to properly advise on what measures might be necessary and practicable to achieve national healing, cohesion, and unity in respect of victims of pre- and post-independence political conflict;
2 strive to create an environment of tolerance and respect among Zimbabweans and that all citizens are treated with dignity and decency irrespective of age, gender, race, and ethnicity, place of origin or political affiliation.

It is on the basis of section 7 (c) of the GPA document, that a National Healing Committee was put in place to lead national healing programmes. The GNU could have done better in the quest for transitional justice, healing, and reconciliation if the Organ on National Healing, Reconciliation, and Integration could have incorporated people with expertise in dealing with conflict-resolution rather than depending on politicians. Section 7 (c) of the GPA shows that it (GPA) has approached the transitional justice, national healing, and reconciliation in a casual way. The clause appears to be a mere promise to "give consideration" to what would look like *an advisory mechanism* in the context of the past violence (Eppel, 2013). It can be argued that this casual approach by the GPA may have resulted in the poor performance of the ONHRI during this period of the GNU. The chapter highlights the potential contribution of the inclusion of civil society organisations, traditional leaders, church leaders, academics, local communities, and other relevant stakeholders to bring the much needed transitional justice, national healing, reconciliation, and peace in Zimbabwe.

As an organ of the GPA government, the ONHRI had the mandate of advising the government on measures to be taken to promote national healing, cohesion, and unity. The organ has demonstrated minimum expertise in being able to advise the GPA government and the communities in creating conditions that promoted peace (Chipaike, 2013). It can be observed that the major problem in the failure of the ONHRI to achieve its mandate was the lack of conflict transformation expertise. The political parties made a mistake that they presumed that politicians would be able to lead a programme of national healing and reconciliation. Therefore, it can be argued that conflict transformation in Zimbabwe could have been more effective if both the elite and those in the grassroots level with the blessing of the state could have been implementing national healing and reconciliation processes.

Civil society organisations could have played a pivotal role in bringing about conflict transformation programmes in Zimbabwe if they were roped in with their expertise. These civil society organisations include Zimbabwe Community Conflict Resolution Agenda, Zimbabwe Human Rights, and Women's Coalition of Zimbabwe, among others. The inclusion of these civil society organisations could have made a tremendous difference in bringing peace, healing, and reconciliation. This could have also build a firm foundation for elections without violence in the future. According to Chipaike (2013), these civil society organisations could not be roped in because ZANU PF was suspicious to include these organisations because they (ZANU PF) thought that they were the agents of the West who had a regime change agenda. However, if these civil society organisations were included in national healing and conflict transformation, it was going to be instrumental in ushering in a new dispensation of peace, healing, and reconciliation.

The church could also have played a pivotal role in conflict transformation in the GNU. After high levels of violence and political polarisation which was experienced in Zimbabwe, the church could have been very useful in bringing

national healing and peace. The church could have been an instrumental platform to bring about national healing and conflict transformation had it been
included to participate in bringing about peace in the GNU. There are church
organisations like Evangelical Fellowship of Zimbabwe (EFZ), the Zimbabwe
Catholic Bishops' Conference (ZCBC), and Catholic Commission of Justice
and Peace (CCJP). These church organisations were the voice of the voiceless
to the people of Zimbabwe before, during, and after the GPA.

According to Chiwara et al. (2013), the ZCBC acted as the voice of the
voiceless in 1983 when they wrote a communique entitled *Reconciliation is Still
Possible* showing that they (ZCBC) vehemently denounced and condemned the
atrocities of the Gukurahundi and encouraging the government to respect and
maintain law and order in Matabeleland and Midlands provinces. In addition,
the CCJP members played a crucial role in the negotiations between ZANU
PF and ZAPU in order to bring unity in Zimbabwe. Furthermore, the heads of
Christian denominations approached the then President Canaan Banana, who
was a minister of religion, to intervene and mediate on the political conflict
which was there between ZANU PF and ZAPU. This resulted in the signing of
an agreement between ZANU PF and ZAPU on 22 December 1987 bringing
peace in Matabeleland and Midlands provinces (Chiwara et al., 2013).

Chitando argued that the churches remained marginalised by the ONHRI,
partly because of its internal squabbles (Chitando, 2011: 267). Chiwara et al.
(2013) correctly note that "national healing and reconciliation are embedded
in moral obligations, the church-based individual organisations can claim moral
authority and legitimacy to lead the National Healing and Reconciliation Process, as politicians are viewed as not having the moral integrity to remain neutral
and/or separate national issues from party politics agendas." It can be observed
that politicians are not experts of conflict transformation and healing. Chitando
(2011) further contends that the churches did not position themselves to be visible and to show that they were potential players in the inclusive government in
resolving conflict. Therefore, if the church had been given space in the inclusive
government, it could have played a major role in bringing national healing and
conflict transformation in Zimbabwe.

Another key element that could have been very important in bringing about
conflict transformation, national healing, and peace was the involvement of the
traditional leadership as represented by the chiefs (*ishe/mambo*). In the Shona
religion and customs, the chief is an embodiment of tradition and culture (Chiwara et al., 2013: 41). He is the leader of all the people in his community and is
the custodian of the land where people get life. According to Nkomo (1998: 14),
chiefs are a combination of executive, ritual, and judicial power and always enjoy
the support of his subordinates and the people under his jurisdiction. The role
of the chiefs therefore would stabilize societies for development. The major role
of chiefs is to resolve conflicts and disputes through his traditional court (*dare*).
Chiwara et al. (2013: 42) note that the chief is the last court of appeal for the
village headmen refer cases to him which are difficulty for them to settle. As the
chief presides over his traditional court he is helped by his advisors (*machinda*)

who advise the chief and make it a point that there is peace, harmony, and unity within his kingdom. Bourdillon (1976) argues that the chief's court deals with a variety of cases which include divorce, quarrels, compensation, breaking taboos, and theft of cattle, among others. The chief is both a "religious and political ruler" (Bourdillon, 1976: 137). Among other roles of the chief is to mediate between his subjects and the spirit guardians in his area of jurisdiction (Shoko, 2007: 10). Given the importance of the traditional leaders to indigenous societies, the GNU could have utilised the involvement of traditional leadership in national healing, conflict transformation, and reconciliation. What usually happens is that, chiefs are only used by some politicians to make sure that they remain in power.

The Shona religion and customs are rich in principles of conflict transformation and reconciliation – among them are the role and respect of the spirits, cultural values, and customs. For the purposes of this chapter, the role and respect of the spirits will be discussed, particularly focusing on the avenging spirits (*ngozi*) (see also the chapter by Jeater in this volume). According to Sibanda (2016) and Chiwara et al. (2013), the avenging spirits are the spirits of the dead people who died in anger, such as victims of murder, who may want to seek revenge. The family of the person who murdered the person would consult the n'anga who would help to settle the problem between the angry spirit and the family. Sibanda (2016: 353) argues that the Shona say: "*Mushonga wengozi kuiripa.*" (The solution to ngozi is restitution or compensation.) When not appeased the ngozi can cause mayhem in a family, even to the extent of wiping out the whole family. The avenging spirits/ngozi can only be compensated with the payment of blood money, a herd of cattle, or a girl child (Sibanda, 2016). The element of the avenging spirits could have been handy if it had been utilised by the GNU. The traditional chiefs could have been used to spearhead national healing and reconciliation in Zimbabwe. This is so because the spirits of the victims of politically-motivated violence may rest in peace provided the persons who killed them are brought to book; traditionally, this would be done by paying compensation. Chiwara et al. (2013) rightly pointed out that the inclusive government could have initiated the traditional ceremonies that were meant to silence the spirits of the victims of politically-motivated violence. If the cleansing ceremonies were undertaken during the GNU spearheaded by the ONHRI, there could have been reconciliation and conflict transformation between the families who were involved in political violence from 2000 to 2008.

The academics could have been versatile in conflict transformation, national healing, and reconciliation during the GNU in Zimbabwe. These academics could have been experts in conflict resolution. Chipaike (2013) rightly notes that at times governments and organisations have a propensity of addressing the symptoms of a conflict without looking at the root causes of the conflict. The ONHRI and JOMIC could have embraced the academics during the GNU to ensure that there was a successful conflict transformation drive that could have resulted in peace and national healing. The fact that the academics were not embraced, means that politically-motivated violence is continually witnessed up to the present day.

Conclusion

The GNU brought joy and happiness to the people of Zimbabwe after years of economic and political suffering. The period between 2000 and 2008 can be referred as the "darkest period" in the history of Zimbabwe. The crisis eventually gave birth to the GNU. The GNU was brokered by the SADC with the mandate of forming a transitional government in order to prepare for fresh election. There were positive developments which were witnessed by the coming in of the GNU. These included the decrease of political violence, bringing warring parties together, bringing food on the table among other things. However, the ONHRI which was tasked by the Global Political Agreement to promote national healing and reconciliation did not perform well to what was expected by the people of Zimbabwe. The chapter argues that the GNU could have done better in bringing about reconciliation if the Organ on National Healing, Reconciliation, and Integration could have incorporated people with expertise in dealing with conflict-resolution rather than depending on politicians. The chapter concludes that the inclusion of civil society organisations, traditional leaders, church leaders, academics, local communities, and other relevant stakeholders could have brought the much-needed reconciliation and peace in Zimbabwe.

Bibliography

Bond, P. and Masimba Manyanya. 2002. *Zimbabwe's Plunge: Exhausted Nationalism, Neoliberalism and the Search for Social Justice*, 2nd ed. Pietermaritzburg and London: University of Natal Press and The Merlin Press.

Bourdillon, M. F. C. 1976. *The Shona People: Ethnography of the Contemporary Shona with Special Reference to their Religion*. Gweru: Mambo Press.

Chipaike, R. 2013. "The Zimbabwe Government of National Unity as a Conflict Transformation Mechanism: A Critical Review," *Southern Peace Review Journal* 2(1), 17–34. (Special issue with OSSREA Zimbabwe Chapter).

Chitando, E. 2011. "Prayers, Politics and Peace: The Church's Role in Zimbabwe's Crisis," *Open Space* (1), 43–48.

Chiwara, A., T. Shoko and E. Chitando. 2013. "African Traditional Religion and the Church: Catalysts for National Healing in Zimbabwe in the Context of the Global Political Agreement," *Southern Peace Review Journal* 2(1), 35–54. (Special issue with OSSREA Zimbabwe Chapter).

Duzor, M. and B. Zulu. 2015. US Sanctions Against Zimbabwe to Stay in Place. voanews. com/Africa/US-sanctions-against-zimbabwe-stay-place.

Chung, F. 2006. *Re-living the Second Chimurenga: Memories from the Liberation Struggle in Zimbabwe*. Harare: Weaver Press.

Eppel, S. 2013. "Repairing a Fractured Nation: Challenges and Opportunities in the Post-GPA Zimbabwe," in Brain Raftopoulos (ed.), *The Hard Road to Reform: The Politics of Zimbabwe's Global Political Agreement*. Harare: Weaver Press.

Gono, G. 2008. *Zimbabwe's Casino Economy: Extraordinary Measures for Extraordinary Challenges*. Harare: ZPH Publishers.

The Government of Zimbabwe. 2008. *Global Political Agreement*. Harare: The Ministry of Constitutional and Parliamentary Affairs.

Gunduza, M. L. and C.W. Namusi. 2004. *Negotiation in Conflict Management Module LIR 303.* Harare: Zimbabwe Open University.

Hamauswa, S. and P. Chinyere. 2015. *Unpacking the Complexities of Mediation in Africa: Some Lessons from SADC's Mediation Role in Zimbabwe Between 2008 and 2013,* University of Pretoria. http://www.ac.za/media/shared/237/PDFs.

Hofisi, S., C. Manyeruke and L. Mhandara. 2013. "The Church and Political Transition in Zimbabwe:The Inclusive Government Context," *Journal of Political Administration and Governance* 3(1), 103–114.

Kanyenze, G. 2004. "The Zimbabwe Economy 1980–2003: A ZCTU Perspective," in D. Harold-Barry (ed.), *Zimbabwe: The Past and the Future.* Harare: Weaver Press.

Kriger, N. 2012. "ZANU PF Politics Under Zimbabwe's 'Power–Sharing' Government, " *Journal of Contemporary African Studies* 30(1), 11–26, doi:10.1080/02589001.2012.644947.

Maisiri, T. 2013. "Zim's Elusive Reconstruction Agenda: The Zimbabwe Independent," www.theindependent.co.zw/2016/04/26/zims-elusive-reconstruction-agenda (accessed on 26 April 2016).

Manyeruke, C. and S. Hamauswa, 2013. "Rethinking the Concept of a 'People-Driven' Constitution in Zimbabwe: The Case of COPAC's Constitution Making Process," *Southern Peace Review Journal* 2(1), 197–215. (Special issue with OSSREA Zimbabwe Chapter).

Mashakada, T. J. 2013. "Macroeconomic Consequences of Fiscal Deficits in Developing Countries: A Comparative Study of Zimbabwe and Selected African Countries (1980–2008)," Stellenbosch, Sunscholar Research Repository.

Masunungure,V. D. 2009. "Voting for Change:The 29 March Harmonised Elections," in E.V. Masunungure (ed.), *Defying the Winds of Change.* Harare: Weaver Press.

Maruta, S. 2013. "The Global Political Agreement as Game Changer: For Better or for Worse?" *Southern Peace Review Journal* 2(1), 5–17. (Special issue with OSSREA Zimbabwe Chapter).

Maxwell, D. 2006. *African Gifts of the Spirit: Pentecostalism and the Rise of Zimbabwean Transnational Religious Movement.* Harare: Weaver Press.

Media, Monitoring Project Zimbabwe. 2009. *A Report on Media Coverage of Political Violence and Human Rights Abuses in Zimbabwe's 2008 Election Campaigns,* Harare.

Meredith, M. 2002. *Our Votes, Our Guns: Robert Mugabe and the Tragedy of Zimbabwe.* New York: Public Affairs.

Mhanda, W. 2011. *Dzino: Memories of a Freedom Fighter.* Harare: Weaver Press.

Mlambo, A. S. 1997. *The Economic Structural Adjustment Programme: The Case for Zimbabwe, 1990–1995.* Harare: University of Zimbabwe Publications.

Muzondidya, J. 2009. "From Buoyancy to Crisis, 1980–1997," in B. Raftopoulos and A. Mlambo (eds.), *Becoming Zimbabwe: A History from the Pre-Colonial Period to 2008.* Harare: Weaver Press.

Ndlovu-Gatsheni, S. J. 2013. *Empire, Global Coloniality and African Subjectivity.* Oxford: Berghahn.

Nkomo, J. 1998. "Compiling Specialised Dictionaries in African Languages: Isichazamazwi SezoMculo as a Special Reference," in E. M. Chiwome and Z. Gambahaya (eds.), *Culture and Development: Perspectives from the South.* Harare: Mond Books Publishers.

Nyakudya, M. 2013. "Sanctioning the Government of National Unity: A Review of Zimbabwe's Relations with the West in the Framework of the GPA," in Brain Raftopoulos (ed.), *The Hard Road to Reform: The Politics of Zimbabwe's Global Political Agreement.* Harare: Weaver Press.

Raftopoulos, B. (ed.). 2013. *The Hard Road to Reform: The Politics of Zimbabwe's Global Political Agreement.* Harare: Weaver Press.

Raftopoulos, B. 2010. "The Global Political Agreement as a 'Passive Revolution.' Notes on Contemporary politics in Zimbabwe", *The Round Table*, 99:411, 705–718.

Raftopoulos, B. 2009. "The Crisis in Zimbabwe 1998–2009," in B. Raftopoulos and A. Mlambo (eds.), *Becoming Zimbabwe: A History from the Pre-Colonial Period to 2008*. Harare: Weaver Press.

Raftopoulos, B. 2007. *Nature, race and history in Zimbabwean Politics*. Cape Town: Institute of Reconciliation and Justice, pp. 160–175.

RAU. 2011. "Politically Motivated Violence Against Women in Zimbabwe 2000–2010: A Review of the Public Domain Literature," http://archive.kubatana.net/docs/women/ran-politically-motivated-violence-lit- (accessed on 11 May 2016).

Sadomba, Z. W. 2011. *War Veterans in Zimbabwe's Revolution: Challenging Neo-Colonialism Settler and International Capital*. Harare: Weaver Press.

Sachikonye, L. 2011. *When a State Turns on Its Citizens: Institutionalized Violence and Political Culture*. Auckland Park: Jacana Media.

Shoko, T. 2007. *Karanga Indigenous Religion in Zimbabwe: Health and Well-Being*. Aldershot: Ashgate Publishers.

Sibanda, F. 2016. "Avenging Spirits and the Vitality of African Traditional Law, Customs and Religion in Contemporary Zimbabwe," in P. Coertzen, M. C. Green and L. Hansen (eds.), *Religious Freedom and Religious Pluralism in Africa: Prospects and Limitations*. Stellenbosch: SUN Media.

Tatira, L. and T. Marevesa. 2011. "The Global Political Agreement (GPA) and the Persistent Political Conflict Arising There From: Is This Another Manifestation of the Council of Jerusalem?" *Journal of African Studies and Development* 3(10), pp. 181–191, Academic Journals.

Vestraelen, F. J. 1998. *Zimbabwean Realities and Christian Responses*. Gweru: Mambo Press.

ZESN. 2008. "Report on the Zimbabwe 29 March Harmonised Elections and 27 June Presidential Run-off," Harare.

Zimbabwe Institute: Innovative Thinking for a Sustainable Future, 2011. Two Years of Political Inclusivity in Zimbabwe? A Review of the Global Political Agreement Government, ZI Policy Brief No. 2, Harare.

5 Tinkering with the commission

Zimbabwe's use of commissions of inquiry as a transitional justice mechanism[1]

Everisto Benyera

Introduction

The need for transitional justice in communities that experience cyclic human rights abuses such as Zimbabwe's cannot be overstated. Tools used to establish historical accountability include truth commissions and commissions of inquiry. Both these commissions have been generally regarded as indispensable tools in the establishment of the truth and the seeking of accountability for human rights abuses. The commissions' efficacy as fact-finding tools is often taken for granted and accompanied by an assumption of impartiality that is thought to be commensurate with the appointment of legalistic truth-finding mechanisms such as commissions of inquiry and truth commissions. The challenges associated with the deployment of commissions as institutions that impede rather than enhance historical accountability have not been fully addressed in scholarship. These commissions are often religiously embraced without questioning their efficacy. The end results, as was the case in Zimbabwe between 1980 and 2014, are that commissions were used by the state to officially hinder truth finding and consequently blame apportionment. In this discussion, truth commission and Truth and Reconciliation Commission will be used interchangeably but will essentially denote the same thing.

This chapter will begin by defining the commission as an institution used not only in transitional justice but also in other cases and circumstances deemed to be warranting a nuanced scrutiny by those deemed to be impartial and in possession of the prerequisite craft competence and craft literacy to address the objectives as laid down in the terms of references for such commissions. In the second part, the chapter discusses the general uses of commissions of inquiry followed by a third part which addresses the three generic stages in the work of commissions as postulated by Ashforth (1990). These stages are the investigative, persuasive, and archival phases. The fourth part discusses the four commissions used in Zimbabwe between 1980 and 2014. These are the Dumbutshena Commission of Inquiry, the Chihambakwe Commission of Inquiry, the Zimbabwe Human Rights Commission, the Organ on National Healing and Reconciliation, and finally the embryonic National Peace and

Reconciliation Commission (NPRC). It must be acknowledged from the onset that there are current debates on whether the NPRC is indeed a truth commission. This chapter makes no distinction between commissions of inquiry and truth commissions, based on the fact that they both serve the same purpose, which is establishing historical accountability.

Defining a commission of inquiry

By definition, a commission of inquiry is a formal group of experts brought together either on a regular or *ad hoc* basis to investigate matters within their expertise and with regulatory or quasi-judiciary powers such as the powers to search, seize, and subpoena. One of the major defining traits of a commission is its composition and the legalistic manner in which its members are appointed. Burton and Carlen (quoted in Ashforth) aptly characterised the composition of commissions of inquiry as, "representing a system of intellectual collusion whereby selected, frequently judicial, intelligentsia transmits forms of knowledge into political practices" (1990: 2). Thus, in this regard, the commission is used as a source of knowledge about political practice useful in future related cases. While unstated in most commissions' mandates, the shaping of legal jurisprudence by commissions is probably their second most influential function after the apportionment of blame for human rights abuses. Theoretically, the work of the commission is governed by norms and rules of independence, impartiality, decorum, impermanence, and speed (Ashforth, 1990: 9).

Common traits of commissions are: Their ability to seize, search, and subpoena; their formality, that is, that they are formally constituted body, their source (appointed in most cases by the head of state, although some commissions were appointed by the church); their mandate is time bound; they produce reports, usually with recommendations at the end of their investigations; they tend to be quasi-judicial; commissioners are usually experts at the matter under investigation. Based on this broad characterisation, it can be argued that past commissions instituted in Zimbabwe which from the crux of this chapter are, indeed, commissions. These include the 1982 Commission of Inquiry into Events Surrounding Entumbane (also known as the Dumbutshena Commission of Inquiry); the Zimbabwe Commission of Inquiry into the Matabeleland Disturbances, also known as the Chihambakwe Commission of Inquiry; the Human Rights Commission appointed in 2009; the Organ on National Healing, Reconciliation, and Integration (ONHRI) 2008–2013; and finally the nascent NPRC.

Uses of the commission of inquiry

A discussion on the uses of a commission of inquiry is complicated by the fact that who uses the commission matters, given the fact it has many stakeholders. The commission is used by different stakeholders for various, usually self-serving, reasons. This chapter will, therefore, first enumerate the various key stakeholders who constitute the political landscape in Zimbabwe. These are the state, victims, perpetrators, and private capital. In discussing the usefulness of the commission, Bulmer (1981: 353) was spot on in noting that the political context in which the commission operates predetermines its success as evaluated by the various stakeholders. Bulmer also noted the central role played by three factors in the work of the commission. These are the procedural and technical issues such as the commission's preferred modes of taking evidence, the way in which commissions are staffed and the internal dynamics of their workings (Bulmer, 1981: 353).

Viewed from the position of the victims of human rights abuses, it can be noted that, "Commissions produce a rational and scientific administrative discourse out of the raw materials of political struggle and debate" (Ashforth, 1990: 3). The links between the commissioners and the state which appointed them is taken as an innocent and apolitical event with little or no impact on the work of the commission. Peta Sherriff notes that the most important role of the commission is harmonizing society and not policy formulation (Peta, 1983: 672). In this case the form, and not the content of the commission, is its most important aspect. Reduced to its most basic terms, every problem that faces society must have three components. It must have a name, a cause, and a solution (Ashforth, 1990: 7). The commission, therefore, exists to name the problem, identify the causality, and come up with solutions to the problem.

Another important function of the commission, according to Ashforth, is its ability to mediate when powerful interests clash. In this case the interests of the labour unions, the state, and private capital came to a head such that the state concluded that only a commission could be deployed to mediate a common ground through the gathering of facts from these stakeholders. Ashforth notes that there are four reasons why the state appoints the commission. These are: Its ability to transcend politics, limitations of resources within the statecraft, lack of trust between stakeholders, and conflicts from within the statecraft.

Besides the legitimate uses of truth commissions, unpopular regimes and dictatorships have also used these bodies for their own benefit, such as creating a narrative consistent with their own views which at times would have caused the human rights abuses under investigation. This instrumentalisation and politicisation of the truth commission was unavoidable and needs to be managed in order to protect the integrity of the commission.

For the objectives of truth commissions to be achieved, victims need to come out with their narratives, thereby providing individuals, families, and communities with their own version of historical human rights abuses. In the absence of trust between the victims and the commission, such narratives will hardly come out, thereby rendering the commissions' mandate a stillbirth. This lack of trust will block other processes such as memory, remembering, and eventually forgiveness, from ensuing. The omnipresent political bickering and mistrust in Zimbabwe which runs through the country's political edifice creates a poisonous environment for the NPRC to operate. Under such circumstances, the commission will surely fall victim to partisanship and patronage and instead of being used positively to heal communities, it will instead inhibit, short-change, and sabotage restorative justice. These are some of the moments when well-meaning instruments such as truth commissions are used to harm the very people they are meant to heal.

On Zimbabwe's proclivity towards the commission

Zimbabwe's proclivity towards the commission deserves to be qualified. This will be undertaken via a discussion of the advantages which such fact-finding and blame-apportionment instruments accords to the state. This will be followed by a section which demonstrates the concomitant challenges in the use of the commission. It is imperative to note that perceptions on the efficacy of commissions is a subjective one, influenced by one's position. For example, a government official's position and that of a victim or perpetrator are likely to be divergent, given the nature of their expectations of the commission. This section is, therefore, framed from the logic and perspectives of the perpetrators and victims and not that of the state.

The major advantage of commissions is their ability to be a useful tool in shaping public opinion and policy. Once such public opinion would have been influenced, the outcome is usually an enhanced fact-finding process which enhances healing, reconciliation, and most importantly post-conflict or post-dictatorship nation building. Secondly, commissions of inquiry are famed for their particularity. The commission enjoys the distinct advantage that it can delve into a particular problem and analyse its causality in relation to its peculiar environment. Its ability to isolate a problem and concentrate time, expertise, witnesses, and resources in unearthing hitherto unknown facts has resulted in achieving historical accountability. Thirdly, the commission is very useful in striking political accommodations between contending powerful interests. This is the case where the source of the problem can be traced and located in differing group values and ideologies. The commission has the distinct advantage in that it has the institutional capacity to operate as a vehicle to foster cohesion between various opposing interests such as the warring labour unions, the state and the unions, and the unions and private capital.

The major argument against the use of the commissions is that putting an issue before a commission effectively closes other avenues of establishing the truth. Commissions can also be criticised for their over judicialisation and intellectualisation at the cost of other stakeholders such as traditional leadership structures. Regarding the application of law in practise and study of transitional justice, Sriram et al. (2012: 52), posited that the "judicialisation" of fact-finding endeavours tended to render such efforts procedural and almost superfluous. The main criticism of this "judicialisation" of fact-finding is that it tends to create fairly individualised accounts of human rights abuses which deprives the victims and their families of a chance to know the complete picture about what actually transpired, which in most cases will be part of larger well-coordinated and orchestrated patterns of human rights abuses.

Continuing the same argument against the use of commissions as fact-finding tools, Burton and Carlen (1979) characterised this system as "representing a system of intellectual collusion whereby selected, frequently judicial, intelligentsia transmit forms of knowledge into political practices." The crux of the argument here is that, "Commissions produce a rational and scientific administrative discourse out of the raw materials of political struggle and debate." Viewed from this point, the commission becomes a tool for legitimising state actions. Legitimisation of state actions refers to actions of the commission when it provides explanations of state actions in a manner that justifies possible and desirable ends for state power.

Dumbutshena commission of inquiry

The 1982 Commission of Inquiry into Events Surrounding Entumbane (also known as the Dumbutshena Commission of Inquiry) was the first Commission to be appointed in Zimbabwe to look into human rights violations. It was chaired by Justice Enoch Dumbutshena and was mandated to look into the clashes between former Zimbabwe African National Liberation Army (ZANLA) and Zimbabwe People's Revolutionary Army (ZIPRA) forces at Entumbane and the related killings in Matabeleland in 1983 (Catholic Commission for Peace and Justice and Legal Resources Foundation, 1997: 53). According to the lawsuit which pitted the Zimbabwe Lawyers for Human Rights and the LRF against the president of the Republic of Zimbabwe and the attorney general (Civil Application No. 311/99), the terms of reference for the Dumbutshena commission were to:

> inquire into the mutinous disturbances which took place during February 1981 at Glenville Military Camp, Ntabazinduna Military Camp, and Entumbane ZANLA and ZIPRA Camps for the purposes of determining the causes underlying, or which led to, the mutinous behaviour and of identifying, if possible, the persons and organisations responsible for planning or promoting the disturbances; and to make recommendations for the resolution of the problems identified.

The circumstances which gave rise to the Dumbutshena Commission were disturbances which emanated from efforts made to integrate the three armies, namely, ZIPRA, ZANLA, and the Rhodesian Armed Forces. There were open confrontations, especially between ZANLA and ZIPRA forces at Chitungwiza, Connemara, Ntabazinduna, and Entumbane Assembly Points, which resulted in open warfare (Nyarota, 2006: 132). Like the Chihambakwe Commission of Inquiry Report, the Dumbutshena Commission of Inquiry Report was never published (Catholic Commission for Justice and Peace and Legal Resources Foundation, 1997: 53; Compagnon, 2011: 283), and its concealment meant that the nation was deprived of an opportunity to learn the truth and to find healing and closure. This applies particularly to the families of the combatants who died in the confrontations at these Assembly Points. It is imperative to note that under the *Commissions of Inquiry Act [Chapter 10: 07]*, the prime minister (subsequently the president) was not obliged to publish the report of a commission. This law has since changed with the coming into effect of the new Constitution which under Chapter 1, Section 62(1) says:

> Every Zimbabwean citizens or permanent resident, including juristic persons and the Zimbabwe media, has the right to access to any information held by the State or by any institution or agency of government at every level, in so far as the information is required in the interest of public accountability.

Chihambakwe commission of inquiry

The Zimbabwe Commission of Inquiry into the Matabeleland Disturbances, commonly known as the Chihambakwe Commission of Inquiry, was set up by the government in November 1983. It was chaired by Simplicius Julius Rugede Chihambakwe. The Commission's mandate was basically to investigate atrocities in Matabeleland following disturbances at Glenville, Ntabazinduna, and Entumbane military camps (Eppel and Raftopoulos, 2008: 16; Kriger, 2003: 79; Catholic Commission for Justice and Peace and Legal Resources Foundation, 1997: 53). Public interest in the work of the Commission was very high as citizens came forward with their testimonies. The Commission commenced collecting evidence of army atrocities in Bulawayo in January 1984 (Auret, 1992: 156; Catholic Commission for Justice and Peace and Legal Resources Foundation, 2008: 97) and found hundreds of people waiting to give evidence, with the result that it had to return in March to hear more testimonies (Catholic Commission for Justice and Peace and Legal Resources Foundation, 1997: 15). Enough and credible evidence was collected as "the Commission was given plenty of evidence of atrocities involving hut burning, mass beatings and executions by the 5 Brigade" (Catholic Commission for Justice and Peace and Legal Resources Foundation, 1997: 97). However, against the expectations of the nation, in November 1984 the government announced that the Chihambakwe Commission's report would not be made public (Auret, 1992: 156; Catholic Commission for Justice and Peace and Legal Resources Foundation, 1997: 98; Nyarota, 2006: 142). In November 1985, the then Minister for State Security Emmerson Mnangagwa made a further announcement that the report would not be released (Compagnon, 2011: 58; Nyarota, 2006: 142). The CCPJ and the LRF took the government to court, demanding the right of the nation to see the Chihambakwe Report.

The court ruled in favour of CCPJ and the LRF, but the government then announced that there was only one copy of the report and that it had been lost, so they were unable to comply (Eppel and Raftopoulos, 2008: 18). To date, the contents of the Chihambakwe Commission of Inquiry Report are unknown to the public. This represents a gross miscarriage of justice, both for the victims and for those who gave testimonies to the Commission. The state squandered a propitious moment to make the truth known and officially recognised as a part of the families', communities', and the country's history.

The Zimbabwe human rights commission

The Human Rights Commission was appointed in 2009 when the Zimbabwe *Human Rights Commission Act of 2009* came into effect. It was one of many commissions resulting from the formation of the Government of National Unity (GNU). The Human Rights Commission was established to, "counter the large scale orchestration of alleged violations and the falsification, exaggeration, orchestration, and stage-managing of human rights violations by detractors" (du Plessis and Ford, 2009: 7). While it had noble goals, the biggest flaw in the Human Rights Commission was that its enabling Act, the *Human Rights Commission Act of 2009*, only allowed it to investigate cases of human rights abuses committed after 13 February 2009. Part III Clause 9 (4) (a) which addresses the jurisdiction of the Human Rights Commission reads:

> The Commission shall not investigate a complaint unless the complaint is made within three years from the date on which the action of omission occurred; provided that such investigation shall not relate to an action or omission that occurred earlier than 13th February 2009.

This rendered all cases of human rights abuses committed between 1980 and 12 February 2009 inaccessible to the Human Rights Commission. The Bill should have been given a mandate that enabled it to investigate the 2008 violations, which according to many were the most violently contested elections in Zimbabwe. The Commission had the potential to strengthen human rights protection in Zimbabwe and in order to fulfil this potential, the Commission should be in harmony with international human rights law and international standards and best practices (Zimbabwe Human Rights Non-Governmental Organisation Forum, 2011: 7). It preposterous birth notwithstanding, the Commission failed to get off the ground in what civil society argued was not a genuine failure, but a deliberate and engineered one. It is disappointing to note that the Human Rights Commission was eventually disbanded without having done anything tangible to achieve justice and reconciliation in a country desperately in need of such an institutional safeguard. Nothing concrete occurred to the Commission between its announcement by the Zimbabwe African National Union Patriotic Front (ZANU PF) politburo in 2006 and the Constitution Amendment Act No. 19 of February 2009, which made provisions for the Commission.

The Commission lay dormant, only to resurface in September 2009 when the Parliamentary Committee on Standing Rules and Orders merely shortlisted candidates to serve as Human Rights Commissioners. In October 2009, a final list of 16 prospective commissioners was submitted to the president in line with the constitutional provisions. The president only made the appointments five months later in March 2010. This lack of urgency on the part of the government is indicative of the peripheral status that justice and reconciliation issues enjoy in its priorities.

The Zimbabwe Human Rights Commission needs to operate cognisant of the international standards which regulate the setting up and mandates of such commissions. The international norm is that human rights commissions are set out according to the five United Nation's Paris Principles. According to the United Nations Handbook of 1995 (Paragraph 14: 7), international standards in the setting up of human rights commissions were defined and agreed upon at the first International Workshop on National Institutions for the Promotion and Protection of Human Rights held in Paris between 7 and 9 October 1991. These Principles were adopted by the United Nations Human Rights Commission as Resolution 1992/54 of 1992 and Resolution 48/134 of 1993 and related to the status and functioning of national institutions for the protection and promotion of human rights including issues of broad post-conflict justice and reconciliation. They contained recommendations on the role, composition, status, and functions of national human rights instruments. The principles are:

1   the institution shall monitor any situation of violation of human rights which it decides to take up
2   the institution shall be able to advise the Government, the Parliament and any other competent body on specific violations, on issues related to legislation and general compliance and implementation with international human rights instruments
3   the institution shall relate to regional and international organisations
4   the institution shall have a mandate to educate and inform in the field of human rights
5   that some institutions may be given quasi-judicial competence.

These shortcomings notwithstanding, there is still hope that Zimbabwe's Human Right Commission will be more effective in the near future. The new constitution made provision for the establishment of the Zimbabwe Human Right Commission under Chapter 12, Part 3, Sections 242, 243, and 244. Of particular importance to those seeking historical accountability is Section 243 (f) and (g) which mandates the Commission to investigate human rights violations and to secure redress for victims and prosecution of offenders. This also presents a strategic opportunity for the Commission to align itself with international human rights standards and principles such as the previously mentioned Paris Principles. Otherwise, the Commission risks creating further injustices in the process of attempting to remedy them.

The organ on national healing, reconciliation, and integration

The fourth attempt by the state at justice and reconciliation after the three commissions and the policy of reconciliation and collective amnesia was the establishment of the ONHRI. The mandate of the ONHRI was contained in Paper 7, Section 1, Subsection (c) of the Global Political Agreement (GPA) which provides that:

> The Parties hereby agree that the new Government shall give considera-
> tion to the setting up of a mechanism to properly advise on what measures
> might be necessary and practicable to achieve national healing, cohesion
> and unity in respect of victims of pre and post-independence political
> conflicts.

Masunungure (2009: 1) partly noted that the origins of the term "Global Political Agreement (GPA) is unknown as it appears nowhere in the official document that constitute the now GPA." He further noted the term used in the
legal instrument (The Constitutional Amendment Number 19) was Interparty
Political Agreement. This chapter will refer to this Agreement as the GPA.
Formed in 2009, the Organ comprised three ministers, one each from the three
parties to the GPA. As an approach, this representation of the three main political parties was intended to give the Organ a universal appeal, thereby enhancing
its effectiveness. The blurred mandate which set up the Organ notwithstanding,
a number of inevitable pitfalls awaited this peacebuilding institution (Masunungure, 2009). The Organ's work was complicated by the fact that it was set in the
context of a temporary GNU and most problematic, in the midst of animosity
at the highest political level. The functions of the Organ on National Healing
were stated as:

> To study the physical, including emotional, social and mental trauma afflict-
> ing most Zimbabweans with the view to addressing it and to promote pro-
> grams to compassionately address the economic and social needs of victims
> of political violence and related maladies.
>
> (ONHRI, 2009)

Its focus areas were given as, "identifying the sources of the conflicts, identifying
a relevant national healing framework, restoration of Zimbabwe's Africanness,
unhu/ubuntu" (ONHRI, 2009). It was clear that the Organ was preoccupied
with identifying the causes of violence and describing what had happened.
Whilst it is important in justice and reconciliation to establish causality, it
should not be allowed to overshadow the prime issue of redressing past wrongs.
No mention was made of the need to document past atrocities; rather, the
Organ spoke of *identifying* sources of conflict, *examining* national healing frameworks, *focusing* on gender and youths, *involving* the diaspora, and *restoring* African
traditional values. While these factors need not be ignored, they need not be
pursued at the detrimental expense of the provision of justice and truth-telling.

The Organ listed its strategies for conflict resolution as anchored in Zimbabweans admitting their violent past and exhibiting a willingness to forgive and
to be forgiven. Of interest is the strategy of "engaging victims and perpetrators of violence to achieve pledges of forgiveness and reconciliation." For the

Organ, simply pledging to forgive someone who harmed one was an adequate strategy to resolve past conflicts. The provision of engaging victims and perpetrators appears to be so trivial that it is listed as item number 17 out of 19.

In a case akin to the proverbial putting the cart before the horse, the state appeared obsessed with memorialisation before it had established the truth. The norm in justice and reconciliation is that, reparation (where applicable) and reconciliation precedes memorialisation. The state initiated a series of new memorialisations, particularly after the formation of the GNU. Chief among these was a presidential proclamation published in the *Government Gazette Extraordinary* of 15 July 2009, General Notice 92 of 2009, in which the president proclaimed that:

> In the spirit of the Interparty Political Agreement, I do hereby declare, set out and dedicate the 24th, 25th, and 26th July 2009, as a period during which the nation may dedicate the Inclusive Government, our new found peace, our freedom, our new spirit of nation building, National Healing, Reconciliation and Integration to inspire the nation going forward.
>
> (Government Gazette Extraordinary, 15 July 2009, General Notice 92 of 2009)

The state's lack of commitment is also evident in the use of phrases such as, "the government *will ensure*" (GPA Paper 7.1 (a) and (b), 2008). Key words such as justice and reconciliation were missing in the wording of the paper, with the word reconciliation appearing only in the name of the Organ. There is general lack of clarity as conflicts from different governments and episodes of gross violation of human rights are lumped together and not individually acknowledged or addressed. Paper 7 of the GPA was littered with examples of unwillingness and lack of government commitment, which bordered on casting a blind eye on impunity. For example, Section 7.1(c) stated that "the government *shall ... in consideration*." If something is in consideration, it implies that the resultant action or lack of action is acceptable and failure or lack of action will be equally acceptable. Section 7.1 9(d) stated that, "the government *will strive*." Again, striving to end intolerance and politically motivated human rights violations implies that the government was prepared to fail in its endeavours to end violence and intolerance.

Explaining the use of commissions of inquiry by Zimbabwe

The popularity of the commission of inquiry as a fact-finding tool is down to its malleability and manipulability. Commissions offer an opportunity which no other fact-finding tool such as prosecutions do not which is the ability to be politically manipulated. This occurs at various level throughout the lifespan of the commission from the drawing of the terms of reference to the appointment of commissioners.

The second reason why commissions are popular, especially in Zimbabwe, is because of their protracted nature. Commissions take time to be appointed, hear testimonies, write their reports, etc. This affords regimes an opportunity to literally buy time. With Zimbabwe's NPRC having a lifespan of ten years, this time would have been sufficient for those in power to have weakened the NPRC and watered down the impact of the NPRC. If it manages somehow to serve the genuine transitional justice needs of the survivors, its likely challenge will be how to publicise its findings, bearing in mind the fate of other commission reports that were never made public by the state. Another reason that explains Zimbabwe's proclivity to commissions is that such bodies are so technical that at times they are tantamount to sentencing the matters before it to death by burial under too many facts. However, there are cases where, after years of conducting hearings and carrying out other due processes, commissions' reports do meet the expectations of the survivors.

Lessons for Zimbabwe from elsewhere

It must be stressed from the outset that there is no perfect model of a commission and that each commission is adopted for a specific domestic situation. Owing to the vast extent of the truth commission as a subject of study, this section will only cover lessons that pertain to three areas, namely, the time frame, the mandate, funding and key operational issues. The general lesson pertains to the nature of truth commissions as historical accountability instruments. Simpson (2010) noted that the major lessons from the SA TRC are that TRCs are at least double-edged swords. While TRCs avoid blanket amnesia, their overreliance on negotiations compromises the future of the post-conflict state in that it sets precedence that any matter of political substance must be negotiated between the former belligerents. The lesson for Zimbabwe from South Africa would be therefore to capacitate a single body so that it awards both reparations and amnesty in order to ensure that justice is also seen to be done. In that regard, an amnesties and reparations body would be an ideal suggestion for consideration by the NPRC.

Time frame

The lifespan of any truth commission must not be perpetual, so must be the time frame for investigating historical human rights abuses. Zimbabwe's NPRC has a life span of ten years, the most that any truth commission has ever been awarded. This risks rendering the processes of the commission protracted and seemingly *ad infinitum*, more so given the importance accorded to the final report of such commissions. Therefore, prolonging the life span of a truth commission beyond three years is tantamount to sentencing the commission to death by slowly chocking from the unreformed political environment in which it will operate, which was described by Simpson (2010) as a "tip toe" vehicle of reconciliation, within an increasingly robust and combative political environment.

Zimbabwe's NPRC functions include:

> developing and implementing programmes to promote national healing and unity, developing procedures to facilitate inter-party dialogue, and developing mechanisms for detecting areas of future conflict.

While the previous statement is a noble mandate of the commission, one is forced to ask the following question. If the NPRC manages to develop such programmes, procedures, and mechanisms, how will they be implemented or maintained after the Commission has ceased to exist? Logically, there is need for someone to be appointed to run and maintain these programmes, procedures, and mechanisms after the Commission has ceased to exist. Therefore, there is need for mechanisms to be put in place, right from the onset, so that the recommendations of the Commission are implemented after the Commission's ten-year life has run its course. In the absence of such a continuation contingency, the recommendations of the NPRC will most likely not be implemented. There are critical lessons from the South African TRC whose well-thought-out recommendations remain only on paper today, decades after they were drawn.

Operational challenges

A major challenge is that the NPRC is viewed as a politicised institution created by the elite to formally exonerate the executive for its impunity and historical human rights abuses. What more when the NPRC will be reporting to the executive which in Zimbabwe is the prime accused for benefiting from human rights abuses. Also, top officials might refuse to appear, leaving the truth commission to deal with "small cases" committed by runners and foot soldiers at the expense of getting the full story and accountability from the kingpins, that is, those who ordered the shots.

The mandate

Regarding the mandate of Zimbabwe's NPRC, the major lesson from the SA TRC is that the mandate must not be broad and vague. Unfortunately, these markers are already there if the mandate as laid out in the constitution is anything to go by. Investigating nearly all forms of human rights abuses is virtually impossible, more so given the extent of human rights abuses in Zimbabwe which occurred since the pre-colonial period. The NPRC will certainly be overwhelmed by volumes of testimonies if communities respond positively to calls to bring their stories forward. A key Achilles for the NPRC is the absence of enabling legislation granting amnesties in exchange of the truth as was the case with the SA TRC. Without such a provision in the new Constitution which states expressly that the NPRC can grant amnesties to people who tell the truth about historical human rights abuses, it is highly unlikely that perpetrators will find the motivation to make submission before the Commission. This is complicated by the fact that no such power to summon, seize, and *subpoena* can be legally implied. Such powers were supposed to be constitutionally provided and in their absence the NPRC has no power even to force witnesses to appear before it. Additionally, the Commission will be unable to demand information from state institutions such as the army, police, and the state security agencies in the absence of such powers. The enactment of the National

Peace and Reconciliation Commission (NPRC) Act in January 2018 provides some hope, provided that the NPRC is allowed to act independently, and to pursue its mandate in full.

Conclusion

The commission of inquiry has emerged over the years to be a very favourable tool for establishing historical accountability. It has been used variously in Latin America and Africa, with the South African model of a truth commission emerging as a role model in this regard. The chapter argues that the commission has found ample use in Zimbabwe since 1980 as a mechanism deployed by the state to investigate human rights abuses. What rendered the appointment of the Chihambakwe, Dumbutshena, and the Human Rights Commissions problematic is that the state, which is the prime accused and benefactor of these abuses, took the lead role in appointing these commissions. This compromised the commissions' effectiveness, with their reports, in one way or the other, remaining inaccessible to the public. This has greatly affected the NPRC even as it commences its mandate as the general population, especially the victims, feel short-changed by past commissions, more so when they see no essential differences between the NPRC and previous commissions.

The commission, therefore, remains a popular transitional justice mechanism among unpopular regimes primarily due to its political manipulability. In this regard, the truth commission becomes a resource available in the toolkit of unpopular and repressive regimes used to further perpetrate human rights abuses. Depending on its political willingness, going forward, the state in Zimbabwe needs to devise inclusive mechanisms in which major stakeholders such as victims' bodies, opposition political parties, non-governmental organisations, and other institutions such as academic think tanks can make a meaningful contribution into the formulation and running of such bodies. The depoliticisation and non-instrumentalisation of truth commissions is, therefore, highly recommended.

Note

1 This chapter was part of the author's PhD study: Benyera, E. 2014. *Exploring Zimbabwe's Debating the efficacy of transitional justice mechanisms: The case of national healing in Zimbabwe, 1980–2011*. Pretoria: University of South Africa.

References

Ashforth, A. 1990. "Reckoning Schemes of Legitimation: On Commissions of Inquiry as Power/Knowledge Forms," *Journal of Historical Sociology* 3(1), 1–22.

Auret, D. 1992. *Reaching for Justice: The Catholic Commission for Justice and Peace Looks Back at the Past Twenty Years 1972–1992*. Gweru: Mambo Press.

Bulmer, M. 1981. "Applied Social Research? The Use and Nonuse of Empirical Social Inquiry by British and American Governmental Commissions," *Journal of Public Policy* 1, 353–380.

Burton, F. and P. Carlen. 1979. *Official Discourse: On Discourse Analysis, Government Publications, Ideology and the State*. London: Routledge & Kegan Paul.

Catholic Commission for Justice and Peace and Legal Resources Foundation. 1997. *Breaking the Silence, Building True Peace: Report on the Disturbances in Matabeleland and the Midlands, 1980–1989*. Harare Catholic Commission for Justice and Peace and Legal Resources Foundation.

Catholic Commission for Justice and Peace and the Legal Resources Foundation in Harare. 2008. *Gukurahundi in Zimbabwe: A Report on the Disturbances in Matebeleland and the Midlands, 1980–1988*. Columbia: Columbia University Press.

Compagnon, D. 2011. *Predictable Tragedy: Robert Mugabe and the Collapse of Zimbabwe*. Philadelphia: University of Pennsylvania Press.

Compagnon, D. 2011. *Zimbabwe: Twelve Years of Democratic Struggle for Nothing?* Alternatives South.

du Plessis, M. and J. Ford. 2009. "Transitional Justice: A Future Truth Commission for Zimbabwe?" *International and Comparative Law Quarterly* 58(1), 73–117.

Eppel, S. and B. Raftopoulos. 2008. *Political Crisis, Mediation and the Prospects for Transitional Justice in Zimbabwe*. Solidarity Peace Trust. www.idasa.org.za/gbOutputFiles.asp?WriteContent=Y&RID=2541 (accessed on 13 November 2015).

Government of Zimbabwe. 2009. *Government of Zimbabwe Gazette Extraordinary, General Notice 92 of 2009*, issued on 15 July. Harare: Government Printers.

Human Rights & National Institutions Report, December 2011 – July 2012. Harare and London: Zimbabwe Human Rights NGO Forum.

Kriger, N. 2003. *Guerrilla Veterans in Post Zimbabwe: Symbolic and Violent Politics: 1980–1987*. Cambridge: Cambridge University Press.

Masunungure, E. 2009. "Zimbabwe's Power Sharing Agreement," Paper Prepared for a Workshop on "The Consequences of Political Inclusion in Africa" 24–25 April, American University, Washington, DC. www.american.edu/sis/africacouncil/upload/Paper-3-Political-Inclusion_Zimbabwe.pdf (accessed on 21 May 2015).

Nyarota, G. 2006. *Against the Grain: Memoirs of a Zimbabwean Newsman*. Cape Town: Zebra Press.

ONHRI. 2009. Organ on National Healing Reconciliation and Integration Concept Paper. *Organ on National Healing Reconciliation and Integration Concept Paper*. Harare: Organ on National Healing Reconciliation and Integration.

Peta, E. S. 1983. "State Theory, Social Science and Governmental Commissions," *American Behavioural Scientist* 26(5), 669–680.

Simpson, G. 2010. "A Brief Evaluation of South Africa's Truth and Reconciliation Commission: Some Lessons for Societies in Transition," Paper Presented at the Witwatersrand University History Workshop: The TRC – Commissioning the Past, 11–14 June 1999. http://wiredspace.wits.ac.za/bitstream/handle/10539/8084/HWS-383.pdf?sequence=1&isAllowed=y (accessed on 12 April 2012).

Sriram, C., J. García-Godos, J. Herman and O. Martin-Ortega. 2012. Eds., *Transitional Justice and Peace Building on the Ground: Victims and Ex-combatants*. New York: Routledge.

Zimbabwe Human Rights Non-Governmental Organisation Forum, 2011. Zimbabwe Human Rights NGO Forum.

6 Theorising reconciliation and national healing in Zimbabwe

Joram Tarusarira

Introduction

Having gone through conflictual and violent experiences in their various forms, including colonialism and liberation war struggle before independence the Matabeleland massacre (1982–1987), electoral violence, violent fast-track land reform programme (2000–2003), Murambatsvina (2005), Chiadzwa diamond fields violence since mid-2000s, and political violence after independence, Zimbabwe (and its people) has been wounded severely. As such, it is in dire need of healing to arrest the socio-economic and political quagmire that it is mired in and place it more strategically to work towards economic recovery and growth. National healing after conflict and violence is a key objective of the reconciliation processes. Thus, national healing cannot be discussed outside the realm of reconciliation. Tensions, contestations, and endless debates exist around how to best conceive of national healing and reconciliation.

This chapter argues that people act on the basis of how they conceive of a situation. That is to say, on the basis of ideas. For a comprehensive, sustainable, and successful healing and reconciliation process to be implemented, there must be a clear understanding of what the concepts themselves mean in a particular context and time. Thus, it is the task of this chapter to theorise national healing and reconciliation in the context of Zimbabwe. For the most part, scholars tend to discuss reconciliation and healing, and democratization processes as independent categories. In this chapter, I argue that alongside reconciliation and healing must be a democratization process because the two safeguard the existence of the other. The simultaneous pursuit of these two has, however, been a cause of contention in Zimbabwe, thus has stifled the reconciliation process. Political actors, especially those who have been part of the violence, hence fear incrimination, prefer reconciliation talk, sidestepping democratization. This already hints on their conception of reconciliation, which is basically equating reconciliation with forgiveness. Thus, advancing reconciliation is to ensure that they go scot-free. This is a parochial reading of reconciliation and national healing because to search for democracy is to search for reconciliation and healing and vice versa, and one without the other is minimalist, if not vacuous, shallow, and hollow. This chapter begins by articulating the basic tenets of democracy, how it is legitimate to apply this "Western" concept to Zimbabwe and proceeds to link the concept of democracy to reconciliation, before delving deep into the dynamics of reconciliation and national healing.

Democracy and reconciliation

Democracy is a contested concept in Africa because for some it is an extension of the Western global imperial designs meant to advance global coloniality (Ndlovu-Gatsheni, 2013). Deploying this concept, however, in Zimbabwe, remains legitimate because Zimbabwe has adopted the configurations of the modern-state which is based on liberal democracy. This makes it susceptible to evaluation against these principles. Zimbabwe is configured as a modern nation-state committed to liberal democracy. Dahl (1989: 221–222) lists ten elements as constituent of liberal democracy which by extension should safeguard or ensure reconciliation and national healing: rule of law, individual liberty, independent judiciary, rights to information, freedom of association, minority rights, strong opposition, uncertainty of a party or individual to win an election, accountability of state officials, and competitive and free elections. Haynes (2001: 10) describes three forms of democracy, namely, façade, electoral, and full democracy. Façade democracy involves rulers having few real pretensions to democracy. There are regular but controlled elections and rulers work closely with the armed forces. Electoral democracy involves some plausible claims to democracy insofar as there are formal criteria of democracy but a number of societal freedoms are limited. Political stability in electoral democracy is based not on respect for democratic rules but personalised power of the principal leader. A full democracy is one that goes beyond formal mechanisms of electoral democracy. It includes real and sustained, as opposed to rhetorical and intermittent, stress on individual freedoms. Representation of interests is via elected public officials and group participation. There is a high degree of equity, justice, civil liberties, and human rights. The armed forces are subservient to civilian rule. There is not only genuine participation, but consistent effective channels of accountability between ordinary people and public officials.

Linking democracy and reconciliation

After conflict it is imperative to address past human rights abuses, atrocities, or other forms of social trauma to facilitate a smooth transition into a sustainable democratic and peaceful future (Tarusarira, 2016). While it is difficult to refer to Zimbabwe as a country in transition, as was assumed during the period of the power-sharing government (2009–2013), its instability can be seen as a transitional phase, from the military action against then President Robert Mugabe in 2017 to the post-Mugabe era. Although there were elections in 2018, these were highly contested and sustained the transition. Thus, the logic of transitional periods can be deployed. "Transitions are both defining and formative events that have lasting consequences on the quality and duration of democracy (Stradiotto and Guo, 2010). This is born out of society's desire to heal, that is, to rebuild social trust, repair a fractured justice system, and build a democratic system of governance. Transitions entail structural (institutional design) and behavioural change (political culture) (Makulilo, 2010: 20). With human rights becoming the accepted core of governance, democracy becomes more clearly the most effective way of implementing requisite principles such as equality, representation, participation, and accountability (Bloomfield, 2003: 10). Democracy is a way of managing conflicts without recourse to violence. It does not remove differences or exclude other groups who differ. It rather functions as a process through which differences are brought out, acknowledged, and dealt with in a way that permits them to exist without threatening the whole system. It is a way of managing debate, argument, disagreement, compromise, and cooperation within a system that permits opposing views to exist together without recourse to violence. In Zimbabwe, this has been extremely difficult to achieve, as violence appears to be the default response to contestation.

A functioning democracy is built on a dual foundation of a set of fair procedures for peaceful handling of the issues that divide society (political and societal), and secondly a set of working relationships between the groups involved (Bloomfield, 2003: 12). Under post-conflict situations former enemies face the challenge of implementing new negotiated structures. However, because of the violence of the past, their relations are based on antagonism, distrust, and disrespect. This was so evident in how the power-sharing government in Zimbabwe worked. It was marred by political parties trying to outdo the other in government and claim credit at the expense of the other. This makes the need to address the negative relationships imperative, to engender the minimum requirements of trust necessary for cooperation. This need is not only for politicians, but also for the entire population. Political democracy without the support of the population lacks foundation. Reconciliation therefore underpins democracy and vice versa. Against a background of conflict, violence, and dictatorial rule, the two are intertwined and interdependent. Reconciliation is not a luxury or add-on to democratic transition (Bloomfield, 2003: 12).

The democratisation process is one of the key aspects of reconciliation. Reconciliation transcends institutional or procedural recovery after conflict. It deals with attitudes which are broken during conflict (see Tarusarira, 2016). Reconciliation oils the wheels of democratisation, and democracy safeguards reconciliation, because the provisions of reconciliation will be enshrined in the constitution. The two are interdependent, but the concept of reconciliation is often left out of discussions on democratisation, allegedly because of its religious overtones. Transition theory has neglected the importance of coping with the past as a prerequisite for the implementation of democratic institutions and the development of civic virtues within civil society (Arenhovel, 2008: 571).

Zimbabwe falls short of full democracy. The militarisation of elections and government institutions underlines this. Public Order and Security Act (POSA) and the Access to Information and Protection of Privacy Act (AIPPA) have stifled and restricted people's freedoms. The ever-contested election results indicate how electoral democracy has been merely formal. Let alone the Political violence permeates political activities in Zimbabwe and has destroyed the tapestry of social and political relationships, thereby engendering the need to deal with the legacies of a violent past.

The definition of reconciliation gained international salience since the 1990s, but a fixed definition for it remains elusive. No wonder Du Toit asserted that: To define it too closely would be to destroy the vitalising energy of differing voices converging. Excluding divergent opinions on reconciliation forfeits it. To leave it undefined may again prevent focused and effective interventions. Continuously postponing the definition of reconciliation may in itself be escapist (Du Toit, 2003: 295). Its Latin derivation, "concilium," describes how antagonists would meet in council to settle their disputes (Villa-Vicencio, 2004: 5). Reconciliation means restoring and transforming relationships that have been harmed by conflict so that they reflect a shared humanity and seek a shared future based on truth, justice, mercy, and peace (Lederach 1997: 30). Restoration of broken relationships is generally believed to be at the centre of reconciliation. Therefore reconciliation has to do with various forms of brokenness and woundedness.

What runs across these definitions is restoration, that is, establishing things to their original state. In certain situations, however, there is no desirable previous order to go back to. (cf. Moellendorf, 2007: 210). The case of South Africa, illustrates this scenario as Krog (1999: 165) observes: "But in this country there is nothing to go back to, no previous state or relationship one would wish to restore." She argues that under such circumstances, the term reconciliation does not even seem the right word, but rather "conciliation." Philpott (2006: 14) notes that instead of being understood retrospectively, reconciliation can be understood as a state towards which to move. In the case of Zimbabwe there was a time when the country was fairly peaceful, but a future-oriented process may be productive as well.

Definitions of reconciliation are based on various disciplines which include politics, law, theology, psychology, and sociology. Loizdes et al. (2010: 5), identify four generic categorisations of four but not exclusive clusters of reconciliation, which are shown in Table 6.1:

Reconciliation is contextual, rather than a "one size fits all." Each context determines what slant the process should take. Healing as an objective of reconciliation emanates from the fact that conflict and violence create a state of "woundedness," of which Philpott (2006: 16–18) names six dimensions:

1   brute harm i.e. the physical, psychic, economic, or emotional harm to the victim's personhood
2   suffering due to ignorance, willingly sustained by the perpetrators of violence, with questions such as "Who was behind the gun? How was my daughter or son abducted?" Not knowing the truth of one's past is itself a form of torment
3   violation of a person as a subject of justice, as a member of the political order from which the person is entitled to human rights, interpreted as social death or political death

Table 6.1 Approaches to reconciliation

Approaches	Focus/Unit of analysis	Instruments	Objectives
Legal	Individual (perpetrator)	Retributive justice (tribunals, policies of lustration)	Reconciliation (deterrence and rule of law)
Political	Society	Amnesties	Reconciliation (democratic consolidation)
Theological	Individual (victim and perpetrator) and society	Restorative Justice (forgiveness, grassroots activities – Ubuntu, Gacaca, Truth and Reconciliation Commissions)	Reconciliation (restoration of broken social relations)
Political psychology	Collective/National identities	Truth recovery (truth commissions, revised history textbooks)	Reconciliation (reconstruction of collective identities)

Source: Loizdes et al., 2010: 5

4 withheld regard, that is failure to recognise the victim as a legitimate member of the order but as a victim suffering in the name of the order
5 lack of accountability by the perpetrator of the wound inflicted
6 failure to confess, apologise, atone for, and make amends for the perpetration of political violence

It can be distilled from this aforementioned list that reconciliation and healing are attitudinal and institutional processes and goals. Lundy and McGovern (2008: 267) capture these dimension in their understanding of transitional justice, which is part of reconciliation. They observe that transitional justice includes "inter related principles and processes centered around the imagined role of law and law making in constituting transition toward a range of goals and ends. These goals and ends include, amongst others: the restoration of the rule of law; judicial retribution designed to counter a culture of impunity; recompense and restoration of dignity to victims; reform of institutions; social and political reconciliation; nation building and re-constitution of the past on the basis of a shared narrative." Murphy (2010: 28ff) conceptualizes reconciliation in terms of three elements, namely rule of law, development of political trust, and enhancement of capabilities. The general condensed definitions of reconciliation conceal numerous dynamics which are perceived as facilitating healing. These include justice and reparations, truth-telling and truth commissions, and repentance, apology, and forgiveness.

Justice and reparations

Arguments raised against reconciliation in post-conflict situations assume that it suppresses or stifles justice, particularly retributive justice. For some victims and survivors of violence, healing, also understood as coming to terms with their tragic past, can only be when perpetrators of violence receive retributive punishment. While justice is closely associated with the rule of law, it is one aspect that has the potential to stall the reconciliation and healing process. The debate segues into the distinction between retributive justice and restorative or reparative justice. Retributive justice, the "criminal, procedural, or legalistic justice which focuses on crime as the violation of law" (Brounéus, 2007: 8) is particularly delicate to implement during reconciliation processes. In transitional power-sharing governments, as was the case in Zimbabwe from 2009 to 2013, the former power holder remains in government, as did the ZANU PF government. This can be seen as a serious compromise, as it leads to avoidance of full criminalization of human rights abuses committed during the conflict. One reason why implementing retributive justice or locking up perpetrators of violence has been difficult is that during political crises and violence, many people get involved in human rights abuses and prosecution may be seen as vengeance. If prosecution is to proceed it is challenging to balance this type of punishment and the need for reconciliation. Mass punishment can lead to a new cycle of resentment. Trying to establish justice when huge numbers of people are involved is expensive and time consuming and can be counterproductive in terms of reconciliation when too many wounds are exposed.

However, war crimes and serious human rights abuses are thought to require some form of punishment for justice to be seen to be done and for peace to hold and for healing to begin. An alternative way to understand retributive justice is not to understand it only within the logic of retribution, since punishment can also be restorative. It can be a way to communicate to the offender the evil they have committed in the hope that they will come to positive remorse. Punishment acknowledges the dignity of the victim and makes reconciliation not cheap. Retributive justice or accountability can also take various forms, not necessarily imprisonment; it can be condemnation spoken by a public authority, shame imposed by the public, reparations, or lustrations (Philpott, 2006: 21).

Linked to justice is amnesty. Amnesty can be a useful way to recognize the moral justice of acts which are illegal but if not handled well can threaten peace and scatter prospects of healing. It can be interpreted as impunity which can trigger further conflict thus scuttle healing prospects. Victims may feel their suffering is belittled should they see people who perpetrated violence against them walking scot-free. To avoid this amnesty should not be seen to come cheap. In the South Africa Truth and Reconciliation Commission (TRC), the perpetrator of the violence had to appear before the public, recount his evil deeds, face the cries of the victims, and endure the censure of the commissioners (Philpott, 2006: 23). But the decision as to which acts to punish and which people to prosecute are political choices to be left to the citizens of a particular country. When the citizens are involved in determining the benchmarks of amnesty they will spell out those parameters with which they will allow amnesty without compromising their healing. The fear of retributive justice in Zimbabwe stalls the reconciliation and healing process. It stalled the work of the Organ for National Healing, Reconciliation, and Integration. Truth-telling, another dynamic of reconciliation, has not been preferred, for it has been thought to prepare the ground for prosecution. Hence human rights organizations and activists that have attempted to document such ills have been subjected to legal sanctions by the state.

Restorative justice focuses on "crime as conflict between individuals as well as on injuries crime inflicts on all parties: the victim, the perpetrator, and society" (Brounéus, 2007: 8; Zehr, 2001: 4). This is the form of justice that is easy to identify with reconciliation and healing. It focuses on reconciling and healing conflictive relationships in order to end the vicious circle of crime, revenge, and recurring crime. Truth commissions have been known to move in this direction. Recent conceptions of restorative justice have called for extra-judicial mechanisms to deploy restorative justice. These have included local systems rooted in local culture and politics. Gacaca courts in Rwanda and community courts in East Timor are cases in point. This has been amplified by the increased questioning of the extent to which justice as advanced by the international community is politically neutral. There are increased calls for justice mechanisms which do not exclude the locals so as to ensure legitimacy, local ownership, and participation (Lundy and McGovern, 2008: 266, Salter and . . . . With reference to Africa, Sarkin and Daly (2004: 671) state that "The notion of reconciliation has been part of the African systems of dispute resolution. In these traditions, the restoration of balance, rather than punishment of the guilty, is the main focus of law enforcement." However, Pankhurst (1999: 243) warns that some local systems of justice tend to reflect the local power structures with no inherent virtue or necessary commitment to egalitarian principles. The case of politicized traditional leaders in Zimbabwe who now support overtly the ruling regime proves the point. Moral qualities are not inherently embedded in simply being traditional leaders. Such qualities are not a priori but a posteriori. That they are traditional and part of people's culture is no guarantee that they embody moral qualities. In Zimbabwe they can only work if the institution of the traditional leaders is depoliticized.

The pursuit of justice can contribute to democratization and reconciliation by cultivating forms of interaction premised on the rule of law, reasonable default for trust and trust-responsiveness, and the capacity to be respected and recognized as a member of one's political community, which includes the capability to participate in the economic, political, and social life of a community (Murphy, 2010: 32). This means "equal respect for individuals and their agency, a commitment to reciprocal sharing of benefits and burdens of social cooperation and an institutional structure that is based on the rule of law and on political economic and social institutions in which all individuals have a genuine opportunity to participate" (Murphy, 2010: 34). Reconciliation is a response to injustice, hence it must provide what justice institutionally requires. It provides a guide to establish the institutional requirements of justice for a political community of equals. This involves reinforcing practices consistent with the rule of law or crafting a system of declared rules if there have been none in place, changing the way citizens and officials view and respond to each other in respect of political trust. Such a community requires an institutional order that ensures formal equality of rights, liberties, and protections under the law. A just political community treats everyone equally, is self-governing since it is held by the people rather than by egocentric elites, and it honours principles of equal citizenship and inclusion (Moellendorf, 2007: 208). The victim is healed from violation as a subject of justice and ongoing failure of the political community to acknowledge them as legitimate subject. Through this act they are "resurrected" from political or social death (Philpott, 2006: 17). Democratization is about creating an environment in which individuals are able to exercise their agency without fear or favour.

To enhance harmed capabilities there is a need to increase personal and external resources, and to change social and material structures to be inclusive to allow all citizens to equally participate in all dimensions of life. Examples of doing this include healing technologies such as psychological medical intervention to address trauma, stress, and anxiety that inhibit agency; education and training to develop capacities of citizens, avail resources through reparations and compensation, and strengthen social networks and familial support. Laws that prohibit discrimination can support social and material support (Murphy, 2010: 138). As I have observed elsewhere (Tarusarira, 2016), reparations may heal the victim from brute harm, which is physical, psychic, economic, or emotional. They can be paid by a public authority or by the offender. When the offender pays, that act fulfills accountability. In monetary terms reparations can alleviate victims' brute suffering by enabling medical care and economic relief. The reparation can also be in the form of public memorial or monument and that bestows recognition of the victims' suffering and denied citizenship (Philpott, 2006: 23–24). Reparations are another form of truth-telling insofar as they acknowledge that harm was done. They are also a form of justice. Along this line Mani (2002 19; cf. Lundy and McGovern, 2008: 274) talks of legal, rectificatory, and distributive justice. Legal justice is concerned with restoration of the rule of law, rectificatory with human rights abuses suffered by individuals, while distributive justice addresses structural and systematic injustices caused by political and economic discrimination and inequalities of resource distribution. This aspect dovetails with Murphy's (2010: 28) concept of capabilities restoration.

Truth-telling and truth commissions

Truth-telling is one of the worldwide acclaimed aspects of reconciliation processes. It is argued that there should be acknowledgement of the past conflict as opposed to denial. Denial can take place at the level of officials and citizenry, during and after the conflict. It may be general or specific, reflecting either a wholesale repudiation of the idea that political relationships need rebuilding or more specifically, that is, refusing to acknowledge a particular form of damage. There are three types of denial, namely literal, interpretive, and implicatory. Literal denial refers to disputing the truth or recovery of factual claims, for instance officials refusing claims of torture during conflict. Interpretive denial refers to a scenario where actions or events are re-described so as to appear less profound. This is done using technical jargon such as 'regrettable excesses' instead of torture, 'transfers of populations' instead of forced expulsions. The state-controlled media have been instrumental in doing this in Zimbabwe. Implicatory denial refers to a failure to recognize and acknowledge the significance of what one witnesses, knows, or does (Murphy, 2010: 128). Acknowledgement is needed to counter denial during transitions and it allows for agency since the problem is outlined outright.

Truth-telling has been conceived to be cathartic, thus directly connected to victims' healing. But as Brounéus (2007: 12) notes, psychological research also suggests that instead of facilitating reconciliation, truth-telling can retraumatise victims. A public expression of the traumatic wounds which often have feelings of humiliation, shame, and guilt is difficult and may lead to stigmatisation. Public revelation and airing of political crimes may open old wounds and create new ones for victims. Those who may have been prepared to forget the past may find themselves reminded. Hence care should be taken in the talking and in the listening and the victim may have to know that truth-telling does not instantly lead to healing. Truth-telling becomes a self-defeating exercise if it is carried out just for the sake of it, and if is dissociated from "decommissioning the past." This means being a basis for either change or administration (purging/lustrations), prosecution of perpetrators, reparations/restitution or revelation/remembering (Campton, 2008: 7). On the other hand truth-telling provides the basis of the process. Numerous secrets, such as unrevealed disappearances, remain unknown. Relatives want to know what happened to their beloved ones. Citizens want to know the extent of the economic disruption so as to redress the economy. They need to know how the army, police, and secret agencies operated. This ensures lasting reconciliation by guarding against such activities in the future. That also provides a basis to mete out justice. Truth-telling addresses the wounds of ignorance (Philpott, 2006: 17) by revealing the truth about their circumstances. It provides public recognition that the victim's rights were violated.

Official acknowledgement validates past experiences and may help restore the dignity and self-esteem of the victims. Public recognition is not only restorative in itself, but also restores the victim's citizenship. Knowledge about the truth is the first step towards forgiveness. The ability to forgive or let go is the most concrete demonstration of having healed. Hence truth-telling can contribute more to transformation towards stable democracies than sowing seeds of division and opening wounds. Truth commissions have in recent times been increasingly created to deal with violent pasts. They are not the same in all contexts. They are charged with terms of reference by the authorities that establish them, be they parliaments, presidents, or whatever. Common reasons for setting up these commissions include: "to discover, clarify, and formally acknowledge past abuses; to respond to specific needs of victims, to contribute to justice and accountability; to outline institutional responsibility and recommend reforms;

and to promote reconciliation and reduce conflict over the past" (Hayner, 2002: 24). In Zimbabwe, there are disappearances that have not been accounted for and tortures whose extent still remains only known to the victims. *Gukurahundi* and unknown mass graves are a case in point. In 1985 a Zimbabwe commission of inquiry known as the Chihambakwe Commission was set up to investigate governmental repression of "dissidents" in Matabeleland and Midlands Provinces. However, after promising to release the report, the government did not make it public and no explanation was given. Later it was said that releasing the report could spark violence (Hayner, 2002: 55).

Repentance and forgiveness

Repentance can come in the form of an apology, where the offender expresses contrition and sorrow and assumes responsibility for their violence. Silence can be counterproductive by separating the offender and the victim. Repentance is an inward act to which an offender can be encouraged. However, it is more than an apology, remorse, or regret. It includes all of these, as well as a deliberate turning from patterns of behaviour that led to those past wrongs, and often involves attempts to make appropriate reparation or restitution for the past. In this way it is linked to reparations. Repentance has always been linked to forgiveness, as some have wanted to stress,[1] though it carries religious connotations. Desmond Tutu employed Christian metaphors to facilitate forgiveness during the South African TRC (Campton, 2008: 12). Meetings and hearings were opened with church hymns and prayers, candles were lit and crucifixes used in an act of consecrating space. If the offender is the state, a public authority can apologise, as President Clinton did to Rwanda for not intervening during the genocide (Philpott, 2006: 24) and David Cameron in Londonderry, Northern Ireland, on behalf of British troops who fired at civil marchers (Stratton, 2010; Loizdes et al., 2010: 1). Such gestures are also known as corporate apologies and repentance. While apologies by non-participants have been questioned, they can have symbolic power of their own. However, these apologies need to be accompanied by an interactive process of engagement between the relevant organizations and communities (Campton, 2008: 28). The closest that the Zimbabwean state has gone in expressing an apology has been with regard to Gukurahundi to which former President Mugabe said, that was a moment of madness. However, this has not been accompanied by engagement with the communities. Instead any efforts to engage communities affected by Gukurahundi has been met with incrimination and tribal attacks by the ruling regime.

Together with forgiveness, repentance is blamed for making reconciliation sound religious because the two words (forgiveness and repentance) use religious metaphors, considering that Zimbabwe, in this case, while predominantly Christian, is not a religious but religiously pluralistic or multi-religious country. The Bible is awash with verses that link repentance and forgiveness. Examples include Luke 17 verse 3, "If your brother or sister sins against you, rebuke them;

and if they repent, forgive them" and Acts 2 verse 38, "Repent and be baptized, every one of you, in the name of Jesus Christ for the forgiveness of your sins. And you will receive the gift of the Holy Spirit." It is for this reason that many societies have expected religious people and churches to play a significant if not leading role in the reconciliation process. While this need not be, if the affected society feels religion is important for it and can facilitate the process, so be it. What is out of order is to impose a particular religious tradition on the process without the assent of all parties involved. Further, it will be as well out of order to reduce reconciliation to forgiveness, a key theme in Christianity.

Some people have conceived reconciliation strictly speaking as forgiveness, defined as overcoming negative emotions such as anger, hatred, and resentment, which are natural responses to wrongdoing (Murphy, 2010: 9). But others argue that forgiveness only makes sense in a situation where wrongdoing is an exception and not where wrongdoing is both systematic and ongoing, as is the case during politically motivated violence. In these cases it can actually be naïve complicity in the maintenance of oppression and injustice. Not to have feelings of resentment can be tantamount to not respecting oneself; or it may justify what violence wanted to achieve in the first place. During the TRC in South Africa, Desmond Tutu, who was the chair of the commission, was very keen on forgiveness. As Wilson (2001: 120) observes, for Tutu forgiveness did not have to depend on the wrongdoer expressing remorse. While forgiveness which is not contingent on the wrongdoer's remorse can be liberating, if it is not voluntary from the victim or survivor, it can be pressurizing and unfair for victims if they are expected to forgive, and failing to do so is viewed as moral deficiency on their part (Campton, 2008: 14ff). To put pressure on a victim to forgive or overcome resentment (internal changes) may overlook the external changes that are needed in the aftermath of war or conflict. The primary concern should be ending injustice or oppression and addressing conditions that facilitate and support injustice or oppression (Murphy, 2010: 9). Chief among them is violence. In Zimbabwe the dominant view of reconciliation has been based on forgiveness and until this conception is reformed or reconstituted, reconciliation and healing will remain shallow and elusive.

While forgiveness is an internal process undertaken by an individual, it has to be expressed to the offender for it to be part of the reconciliation process, which is a mutual process. The act restores the perpetrator as a person in good standing. What is important is that it has to be fashioned in a restorative manner. If it means unconditional general amnesty, it can make reconciliation cheap. For it not to be cheap, it has to be linked to accountability and truth-telling. Forgiveness can also coexist with harsher forms of punishment like imprisonment. It is possible for a victim to forgive someone while the perpetrator of violence remains in prison. Instead of being the basis of reconciliation, the stage at which forgiveness enters the reconciliation process should be determined by the context. For some contexts apologies and forgiveness should come first, for others in the middle or at the end (Tarusarira, 2016).

The liberal objections

Liberals argue that the concept of reconciliation runs against one of the oldest tenets of liberalism, that crimes must be punished. This is a perspective that seems to drive human rights organizations in Zimbabwe. Against the backdrop of truth-telling, they argue that it is natural that when one knows who committed a crime, they want retributive justice. Dynamics of reconciliation such as forgiveness and repentance cannot be dealt with by the state and do not resonate with retributive justice. Instead they are an affront to it. They require one's confrontation with their soul and inner transformation. Liberals argue the private and the public have to be separated. As a result they only support dimensions of reconciliation that advance the citizenship of victims and foster a stable, healthy, and just democracy (Philpott, 2006: 25ff). From a liberal perspective, forgiveness implies "some sense of release from a debt, or penalty, or threat of retribution, leading to the perception that it is unfair, or a substitute for justice, or at least weakens the deterrent aspect of the judicial process" (Campton, 2008: 14–15). Philpott's contention can as well be applied to human rights activists in Zimbabwe. He contends that what the liberals are advocating is not reconciliation. It can simply be called non-lethal existence, democratic reciprocity, deliberative democracy, or human rights culture. This approach focuses on the political aspect of dealing with the past but does not adequately take into account the social and interpersonal aspects, which distinguishes reconciliation from other political and technical mechanisms of dealing with the past. Retribution alone does not heal or restore relationships. In fact, it risks perpetuating the culture of violence. But forgiveness might help to break cycles of revenge and recrimination within and between communities. It empowers the victims, allowing them to act according to their free will and not just react to what is being done to them. This helps them claim true agency and identities as individuals rather than being defined by past wrongs. Forgiveness is not about forgetting, but about remembering differently, transforming memories; not forgetting the past but redeeming it (ibid.: 20–21).

By now it has become clear that the meaning of reconciliation and the possibilities it raises vary considerably. The meanings proffered by John Paul Lederach (1997: 30) and David Stevens (2004: 22–23) sound comprehensive by capturing both attitudinal and institutional dimensions of reconciliation. Lederach speaks of reconciliation as both 'a perspective' and 'a place' (a focus and a locus) that bring together truth, justice, mercy, and peace. The dynamics of truth-telling are honesty, transparency, clarity, accountability; those of justice-seeking are responsibility, rectification, restitution, reparation, and retribution; those of mercy-offering are compassion, dignity, forgiveness, acceptance; and those of peace-building are harmony, unity, well-being, sustainability. Conceiving reconciliation as a perspective (focus) implies seeing it as a process in which former conflicting parties are engaged towards a shared future; place-locus implies viewing reconciliation as a goal or a state that can be reached that is a state of a desired future, which when reached is the present. Building upon Lederach's conception, Stevens (2004) discusses the meaning of reconciliation using six different approaches, namely reconciliation:

1 as living together in difference
2 in terms of the inter-related dynamics of forgiveness, repentance, truth and justice
3 as a place where different conflicting parties meet and face together the claims and tension between truth and mercy, and justice and peace
4 in the context of new forms of respect instead of revenge for heroic sacrifices of past generations
5 in the context of a set of attitudes and practices that are necessary for dealing with plurality, for fair interactions between members of different groups, for healing divisions and finding common purpose and
6 as creating and sustaining conversation.

Conclusion

In conclusion, it is difficult to reduce reconciliation and healing to a fixed and neat definition. It centres on the restoration and transformation of relationships, takes place at various levels, is voluntary, is a goal and a process and a focus and a locus. It can be distinguished from already established conflict-handling mechanisms such as mediation, arbitration, and negotiation by its focus on the social and interpersonal aspects and is not simply non-lethal existence, democratic reciprocity, deliberative democracy, or human rights culture. It is a comprehensive process that facilitates national healing by its interlinking dynamics of truth, justice, forgiveness, peace, and mercy which in themselves are contested. It is a place of encounter where the conflicting parties meet to face the claims of justice, peace, truth, and mercy. It takes place at different levels, ranging from the individual to relations between states. Tied to reconciliation are moral perspectives which influence ideological biases. Hence reconciliation depends highly on the context of the conflict (nature of political transition, historical, political, social, economic, geographical, ethnic, religious, and cultural outlook). It is a complex concept that can be reflected upon from different paradigms and dimensions to the extent of even saying one thing theoretically and noting another in practice.

In Zimbabwe reconciliation should be seen as a process aimed at restoring social and political trust through attitudinal and institutional reform. The social dimension addresses broken relationships between individuals and communities. This might involve truth-telling, justice, apology, forgiveness, and reparations, as many people had their livelihoods destroyed during the conflict. The political dimension restores trust in political institutions for them to be at the service of all without fear or favour. In this way democratization and reconciliation are intertwined.

Note

1 Rev. Ian Paisley, former leader of the Democratic Unionist Party in Northern Ireland, is renowned for his strong statement "there is absolutely no forgiveness without repentance." But as is demonstrated later, waiting for repentance so as to forgive makes one not an agent of one's life. If repentance does not come, then one will remain stuck in anger indefinitely (cf. Campton, 2008: 26).

References

Arenhovel, Mark. 2008. "Democratization and Transitional Justice," *Democratization* 15(3), 570–587.

Bloomfield, David. 2003. "Reconciliation: An Introduction," in David Bloomfield, Teresa Barnes and Luc Huyse (eds.), *Reconciliation After Violent Conflict*. Stockholm: IDEA, 10–18.

Brounéus, Karen. 2007. *Reconciliation and Development. Dialogue on Globalization Occasional Paper*. Berlin: Friedrich Ebert Stiftung, available at http://library.fes.de/pdf-files/iez/04999.pdf (accessed on 17 March 2011).

Campton, David. 2008. "Divine and Human: Nurturing a Spirituality and a Culture of Forgiveness," in David Campton and Nigel Biggar (eds.), *Divided Past: Shared Future: Essays on Churches Addressing the Legacy of the Troubles*. Belfast: Centre for Contemporary Christianity in Ireland.

Dahl, Robert A. 1989. *Democracy and Its Critics*. New Haven: Yale University Press.

Du Toit, Fannie. 2003. *Learning to Live Together: Practices of Social Reconciliation*. Cape Town: Institute for Justice and Reconciliation.

Haynes, Jeffrey. 2001. "Introduction: The 'Third World' and the Third Wave of Democracy," in Jeffrey Haynes (ed.), *Democracy and Political Change in the 'Third World'*. London: Routledge, 1–21.

Hayner, Priscilla. 2002. *Unspeakable Truths: Facing the Challenges of Truth Commissions*. New York: Routledge

Krog, Antjie. 1999. *Country of My Skull*. London: Vintage.

Lederach, John Paul. 1997. *Building Peace: Sustainable Reconciliation in Divided Societies*. Washington, DC: United States Institute of Peace Press.

Loizdes, Neophytos, Losif Kovras and Kathleen Ireton. 2010. "Introduction: Federalism, Reconciliation and Power-Sharing in Post-Conflict Societies," *Federal Governance* 8(2), 1–14.

Lundy, Patricia and Mark McGovern. 2008. "Whose Justice? Rethinking Transitional Justice from Bottom Up," *Journal of Law and Society* 35(2), 265–292.

Makulilo, Boniface Alexander. 2010. "State-Party and Democracy: Tanzania and Zambia in Comparative Perspective," Unpublished Dissertation, University of Leipzig.

Mani, Rama. 2002. *Beyond Retribution: Seeking Justice in the Shadows of War*. Cambridge: Polity Press.

Moellendorf, Darrel. 2007. "Reconciliation as a Political Value," *Journal of Social Philosophy* 38(2), 205–221.

Murphy, Colleen. 2010. *A Moral Theory of Political Reconciliation*. Cambridge: Cambridge University Press.

Ndlovu-Gatsheni, Sabelo. J. 2013. "The Entrapment of Africa within the Global Colonial Matrices of Power: Eurocentrism, Coloniality, and Deimperialization in the Twenty-first Century," *Journal of Developing Societies* 29(4), 331–353.

Pankhurst, Donna. 1999. "Issues of Justice and Reconciliation in Complex Political Emergencies: Conceptualising Reconciliation Justice and Peace," *Third World Quarterly* 20(1), 239–256.

Philpott, Daniel. 2006. "Beyond Politics as Usual: Is Reconciliation Compatible with Liberalism?" In Daniel Philpott (ed.), *The Politics of Past Evil*. Notre Dame, IN: University of Notre Dame Press, 11–44.

Sarkin, Jeremy and Erin Daly. 2004. "Too Many Questions, Too Few Answers: Reconciliation in Transitional Societies," *Columbia Human Rights Law Review* 35, 661–728.

Stevens, David. 2004. *The Land of Unlikeness: Explorations into Reconciliation*. Blackrock, CO and Dublin: Columba Press.

Stradiotto, Gary A. and Guo Sujian. 2010. "Transitional Modes of Democratisation and Democratic Outcomes," *International Journal on World Peace* 27(4), 5–36.

Stratton, Allegra. 2010. "David Cameron Condemns Blood Sunday Killings and Makes an Apology," Guardian, 15 June, available at www.guardian.co.uk/commentisfree/June 15, 2010/david-cameron-bloody-sunday-apology (accessed on 15 March 2012).

Tarusarira, Joram. 2016. *Reconciliation and Religio-Political Non-Conformism in Zimbabwe*. London: Routledge.

Villa-Vicencio, Charles. 2004. "Reconciliation," in Charles Villa-Vicencio, Erik Doxtader and Richard Goldstone (eds.), *Pieces of the Puzzle*. Cape Town: Institute for Justice and Reconciliation, 3–7.

Wilson, Richard A. 2001. *The Politics of Truth and Reconciliation in South Africa: Legitimizing the Post-Apartheid State*. Cambridge: Cambridge University Press.

Zehr, Howard. 2001. "Doing Justice: Healing Trauma – The Role of Restorative Justice in Peace Building," *Peace Prints: South Asian Journal of Peacebuilding* 1(1), 1–16.

7   Violence as a peace repellent

The politics of Zimbabwe and hate language during the "Old Dispensation"

Francis Matambirofa

Brief background

In historical terms, for close to two decades, Zimbabwe, in an exorable advance in the wrong direction, grew increasingly infamous for reasons that robbed most Zimbabweans of basic peace. The restive and troubled state of the nation could not be envied by anyone seeking after the truth, irrespective of their political affiliation. The situation then, even as it is still now (at the time of writing), was characterised by a moribund economy which relied upon other countries' currencies to transact business – an economic (in)convenience sticking out like a thorn in the flesh of national pride; unbridgeable political polarisation and vilification of political opponents using virulent invective in easily accessible spaces such as political rallies, the public media, in addition to visiting intermittent installments of violence upon political opponents for which no apologies were made. In this analysis, we shall, however, place emphasis only on the historical culture of violence, and to a comparatively limited extent, on the reckless use of language that was calibrated to inflict emotional injury on political opponents.

In the current exegesis, we are of the entrenched view that national success dictates that the leadership at various levels of governance, indeed, starting from the very bottom, right up to the topmost, must be of the highest calibre in regard to individual integrity and honesty, because, perching on the pinnacle of power, its example provides to all and sundry the very brick and mortar of a successful nation-building project. We posit that even in the New Dispensation, the promise of peace will largely remain a pipedream as long as the baggage of both the pre-colonial, colonial, and post-colonial psyche which still haunts the nation is not boldly confronted and jettisoned overboard. It is a very welcoming development that President Mnangagwa Emmerson has so far (early 2018) shown a positive ability to change with the times by abandoning reference to the opposition as merely barking dogs – in his trademark mantra *pasi nemhand-uuuu* "down with rebels/traitors" and *kuvukura*, "to bark."[1]

Zimbabwe as a modern African state has for far too long attracted both regional and world attention, the magnitude of which is proportional neither to its "small" size nor relative global significance. This discussion shall for the most part, unless only for illustrative purposes, *not* concern itself with the current political personages *per se*. Given the tenuous politics of Zimbabwe, the chances of being misconstrued to be advancing some hidden political agenda are high, when in fact nothing could be further from the truth. The intriguing scenario that engenders anxiety is paradoxically worthy of exploration and explanation given the country's relative global "insignificance." The Old Dispensation (or the First Republic) left in its wake not a few pages of writing and analysis by global citizens from various walks of life and disciplines who have tried to make sense of its melodrama. Hammar and Raftopoulos (2003: 1) have highlighted the need for serious academic engagement on Zimbabwe's crisis.

Language as the fuel of violence

In this section, we argue that language is a tool that can effectively be used to inflict violence in a psychological way (Matambirofa, 2016). Demeaning and hate speech are some of the apparatus that dominated the political speech style of the First Republic as it was used to discredit and pour scorn as well as scoff at the opposition. Making reference to the potency of language as a tool for violence, Matambirofa (2016: 126–127) avers that, "language is . . . not only a vehicle, but it is also the fuel that powers the consuming fire of violence." However, before examining language and violence in relation to how it was deployed during the Old Dispensation, we will gently remind the reader of its dehumanising and demonising deployment in racist Rhodesia.

There is an extricable link between language and violence which characterised white settler racism in Zimbabwe. The lingo used by the Rhodesian settlers certainly did not originate with them *per se*. They used epithets that had been "invented" in Europe itself as an excuse for the invasion and colonisation of Africa. Martin and Johnson (1980: 36) remind us that explorers and missionaries had negative views of Africa.

It hardly comes as a surprise that apart from firearms, the white settlers had in their stock the following denigrating terms and clauses which they freely hurled at Africans such as: *savages, tribes, kaffirs, barbarians, cowards, heathens,* in addition to "warlike,"[2] "uncivilized," and "heathen hordes" living on the "Dark Continent" from the previous quotation. Given the wanton invasion of African territories and attempted exterminations, of say the Herero in Namibia and the Congolese in King Leopold's Belgium Congo, as well as the dynamiting of rock enclaves in which the Shona people sought refuge during the First *Chimurengas*, just to mention a few regarding the genocide that was perpetrated by "civilised," "Christian" colonisers on "savage" blacks, one is left wondering who was indeed uncivilised and heathen between the settler murderers and their African victims. The irony and hypocrisy that accompanies it is nothing short of monumental. However, with hindsight, like Achebe (2000: 33) talking in direct relation to his native Nigeria, we now know that the "holy desire" to "civilise Africa" was after all only a smokescreen made "in order to make our colonization possible and excusable."

From the hate language used during the First Republic in relation to its perceived enemies, both real and imagined, one may pessimistically be led to the conclusion that human nature is irredeemably egoistic and evil, irrespective of race, creed, or whatever else. Power and privilege seek to protect its gains either by hook or crook and ironically, therein lies its very own self-destruction. This is partly what led to the ignominious ouster of Robert Mugabe and the concomitant demise of the First Republic. In regard to language, it must be noted that some of the denigrating language used during the First Republic was crafted way back, during the struggle for liberation itself where some "recalcitrant insults" instinctively sneaked into the lingo of the New Dispensation. This includes concepts such as *mutengesi/kapurikoni*[3] "sell-out," *bhunu* "white person," *zvigananda* "counter revolutionaries," *mu/vapanduki* "rebel(s)," and *isikhotamathe* "puppet," among others. White (2003: 17) points out that regarding the formation of FROLIZI[4] "Chitepo used to call it 'influenza.'" The demeaning and derogatory terms come in great profusion, especially from an onomastic point of view as regard the *nom de guerre* which the comrades gave themselves after crossing into Mozambique for training. Some names go like PasiNemasellout, "Down with sell-outs," and Musatanyoko, "Mother-fucker" (Nhongo-Simbanegavi, 2000: 60), among many others.

Following bitter disgruntlement with how ZANU PF was badly conducting government business when the fortunes of the First Republic begun to flounder, a plethora of small political parties were cobbled together. One such party was called Zimbabwe Unity Movement (ZUM). It was formed by a onetime close ally of Mugabe, Edgar Tekere. Tekere and many others were, during the politics of this time, going to make free use of the term *mafia* several times. Meredith (2002: 86) writes thus "[Tekere] accused cabinet ministers . . . and security chiefs of stashing away money in Swiss bank accounts 'just like the *mafia*.'" Tenders were awarded fraudulently and there was a nepotistic group connected to the Mugabe ruling oligarchy which was sometimes "referred to as the Zezuru *mafia*" (Meredith, 2002: 99). Regarding the MDC, it was often vilified as a *puppet* and a *front* for white interests.

When the idea of holding talks to form the 2009 Government of National Unity (GNU) was floated, ZANU PF was initially adamant that it wanted to negotiate directly with the British who it alleged were the handlers of the MDC. To underline the contempt with which MDC was held, Mugabe often derogatorily called its late leader, Morgan Tsvangirai, *Tsvangson* so that it sounded English, instead of his actual Shona name, Tsvangirai. The innuendo is that Tsvangirai was perceived as a traitor on the payroll of the British who was bent on reversing the gains of independence. The same leader was also lampooned as *Chamatama* (Big Cheeks). Slogans referring to *mhandu* "rebels" and *kuvukura* "to bark" were also used by President Emmerson Mnangagwa as recently as the entry into the Second Republic in November 2017. But, the MDC in turn was not going to be outdone in throwing insults at the ruling ZANU PF party and its leadership as it made references to *mazi ZANU*, "huge, ugly ZANU people" and *Mhondoro* Mugabe, "Guardian Lion Spirit." Mugabe was in late 2017 also mockingly called *Asante Asana*, "Thank you," following an address to the nation in November 2017 during which the vast majority of people thought that he would announce his resignation. It was such an anti-climax for the nation when he simply ended his address with a nonchalant routine "thank you very much," in addition to the uncharacteristic use of the KiSwahili equivalent, "Asante Asana."

Diagnosing other sources of violence in the First Republic

The First Republic was not only unprepared, but it was also entirely unaccustomed to unconditional peace. A number of factors can be invoked to account for such an unfortunate state of affairs. The factors, which are numerous and variegated, are in the first instance broadly locatable within the country's chequered history – in both its pre-independence and post-independence epochs. Some of the major signposts point towards as far back as Zimbabwe's pre-colonial political, social, and economic formations which inferably must have celebrated violent upheavals as they specifically relate to the establishment of now famous empires and polities such as Great Zimbabwe, the Mutapa State, the Torwa State, and the Changamire State which was eclipsed by the last and most powerful of all the indigenous polities, that is, the Ndebele State. It would be downright dishonest to ever imagine that these "great states" on what Beach (1980) has called the Zimbabwean plateau were crafted on the basis of peaceful coexistence and the respect of fundamental human rights, though the concept is a recent construct. It is certainly far from the actual truth. It is probable that they were based on violence, bloodshed, and ferocious conquests.

Another devastating landmark scar in the history of Zimbabwe relates to the informal "school of violence" that blacks were inducted into by the racist denigration and humiliation by British settlers. The occupation was masterminded by Cecil John Rhodes's British South Africa Company (BSAC), which was an imperialist arm of British rapacious expansion and hegemony. The BSA Company was granted the Royal Charter by the Queen of England which illegally gave it the mandate to rule and engage in extractive business chiefly concerned with the exploitation of mineral and other natural resources. Settler invasion and the naked provocation of blacks subsequently led to the first *Chimurenga/Umvukela* of 1896–1897 war of resistance by indigenous people. This is the epoch about which Ndlovu-Gatsheni (2009: 39) writes about as follows:

> The 1890s also saw both Ndebele and Shona reacting violently to the provocative interventions of early colonial rule in what became known as the Ndebele-Shona Rising of 1896–97: the *First Chimurenga* or *Umvukela Wokuqala*.

Whilst erecting a stage and setting a time bomb for further and more consuming violence, the white settlers were at the very core of their hearts evidently bereft of any regard for the humanity of conquered blacks. In their language, they gave free course to denigrating descriptions of indigenous people as *savages*, *tribes*, *kaffirs*, *barbarians*, *uncivilised*, *boy*, and *cowards*, among a litany of other derogatory epithets from whose insulting tenor a deranged fringe from amongst them inferably must have drawn sadistic pleasure. Giving explication to the Anglo–Ndebele war of 1893, one white supremacist called Gale, remarked, as quoted by Martin and Johnson (1980: 47), "It was [not] natural for a nation of *savages* . . . to discard the cloak of racial independence for the sackcloth of servitude without a struggle." The same author is quoted once again by Martin and Johnson (1980: 48–49) describing the Shona in perhaps even worse and non-redeeming terms as follows:

> Cowardice was their besetting sin. A *sjambok* in the hand of a determined man was sufficient to send them scurrying in all directions. As a race they lacked courage and spirit, and from the white man's point of view, possessed few redeeming qualities. Any suggestion that so spineless a people could have perpetrated the outrages they committed during the Rebellion would have been laughed to scorn.

The previous quote reinforces the principal point of this chapter, namely, that white colonial rule inadvertently schooled blacks in the excesses of how to deal with a defeated people through the coarse manner in which Africans were treated. This included, among other injustices: Massive land expropriations, taxation, incarcerations, detentions, house arrests, long working hours and poor working conditions, forced labour and serfdom, and being driven into concentration camps by the Rhodesian army which was coupled with all manner of slights and racial slurs. Whilst it would be dishonest to describe pre-colonial Zimbabwe as pervaded by perpetual paradisiacal peace, however, settler violence and brutality exacerbated the situation by availing more powerful and brutal methods of inflicting pain and injury such as automatic weapons and *sjamboks* – tools manufactured industrially for the killing and dehumanisation of humans.

Thus coming full circle, two decades subsequent to independence, not only would the same blacks ill-treat white commercial farmers through farm seizures and other injustices, but would also use more or less the same methods of inflicting physical and psychological violence on those opposed to their whims, whether black or white. Regarding white commercial farm seizures, Matambirofa (2015: 339) observes as follows, "Land was simply taken as spoils of the Second *Chimurenga* – along the same fashion that white settlers had done subsequent to the 1893 Anglo–Ndebele war and First *Chimurenga* of 1896–97."

Colonial racism and oppression which was brought to bear upon Africans became, in time, the very seed of its own self destruction as it stung the oppressed to turn to militant retaliatory measures that radically were aimed at the revolutionary overthrow of the violent system.[5] This became a historical reality during the bloody and protracted armed guerrilla war of liberation – the second *Chimurenga/Umvukela* which was spearheaded by the nationalists fighting against an intransigent white supremacist Rhodesian regime led by Ian Douglas Smith. He is the one who, in 1965, made the Unilateral Declaration of Independence (UDI) from Britain, arrogantly declaring that his white supremacist party, the Rhodesia Front (RF), would not concede black rule – "*not in a thousand* years," thereby infuriating the nationalists by his firmly closing the door to a political settlement. Ironically, the country attained majority rule in 1980, as it were, hardly before the echo of his deluded pronouncement had faded away.

Tracing the history of violence in Zimbabwe, which has ceaselessly acted as a barrier against peace, a lack of which has thus necessitated the current clarion call for national healing, it would be recalled that even when waging war against a common enemy, the nationalists' guns were intermittently trained at the jugular of other liberation formations evident in the fights between ZANLA and ZIPRA,[6] both in Tanzania and Zambia, as well as in overlapping operational areas in Zimbabwe itself. The Nhari Rebellion and the purges subsequent to the death of Herbert Chitepo in 1975 when a cadre of rebels was crushed by military action at Chifombo by Josiah Tongogara – the ZANLA commander, and the subsequent escape of Simpson Mutambanengwe to Malawi, speaks of black-on-black violence in the heat of the liberation struggle itself. This infighting is what inspired Sithole's (1999) *Zimbabwe: Struggles Within the Struggle*. We make brief mention of these historical issues because they have continued to dog us since. In uncensored reality, human beings rarely make a clean break with their past habits – much of course in theory it is thought to be achievable through a revolution. But we here argue that revolutions are nothing more than accelerated and/or unregulated evolutions. The lack of peace that was experienced during the First Republic (or Old Dispensation) had its roots deep in the trajectory of our history of violence which dissipated the prospects of enjoying peace.

A diagnosis of a lack of peace in the Old Dispensation is also traceable to the ushering in of a ZANU PF-led nationalist government in 1980 – coming as it were straight from war camps into government. The violence and fighting associated with the founding stages of Zimbabwe give ample testimony to the fact that both ZANU and ZAPU[7] failed to wholly transit from being liberation movements to national democratic parties. Monumental violence directly linked to a trigger-happy war-psyche witnessed the emergence of the dissident phenomenon and the subsequent venomous unleashing of the North Korean-trained 5th Brigade in Matabeleland and Midlands under the notorious Operation *Gukurahundi*, "First-rains-that-wash-away-chaff," in which an estimated 20,000 citizens are reported to have been brutally liquidated (Muzondidya, 2009).

The Old Dispensation resorted more and more to violence, as it gradually drifted even further away from the prospect of peace as its poor management of the country's economic fortunes commenced to unremittingly pile pressure on the citizenry. The failed Economic Structural Adjustment Programme (ESAP) of the early 1990s that was underwritten by the IMF and the World Bank, resulted in the first post-independence massive labour layoffs, inflation ominously started to steadily climb conversely resulting in political anxiety, agitation, and activism that came to a head with the formation in 1999 of the first potent opposition party, the Movement for Democratic Change (MDC), which was led by the late Morgan Richard Tsvangirai and whose strongest support base was the labour movement and/or the Zimbabwe Congress of Trade Unions (ZCTU) in particular, for which he was the former leader; disgruntled urban dwellers whose ranks had been swelled by both the retrenchees and the unemployed; in addition to the increasingly agitated and/or militant student movement.

As can be seen, the spectre of peace grew more and more dim in covariance with the inflationary pressures that were mounting rapidly and which saw a rapid increase in the prices of basic commodities. In order to stem the political agenda and menacing political advance of the MDC, the Old Dispensation, true to the spirit of its intransigent leader, Mugabe, who once boasted of having "degrees in violence," unleashed unmitigated reverse-racism on the white citizenry[8] by embarking on a chaotic white commercial farms seizure escapade which was christened the Fast Track Land Reform Programme (FTLRP). It seems that the whole plan was to dramatically pull the rug from below the MDC's feet, thereby depriving it of both its alleged financial base and political support from white farmers who, it was alleged, by virtue of supporting the MDC had necessarily therefore spurned the overtures for reconciliation and were unrepentant and thus unwilling to politically come to terms with the reality of a black majority government. The bitter allegation was that white commercial farmers' political project was to bankroll and inaugurate a weak puppet MDC government and foist it on the seat of political power in order to frustrate ZANU PF's national black empowerment and other entrepreneurial projects.

The punitive and retributive state-orchestrated violent seizures of white-owned commercial farms by the so-called[9] war veterans and villagers, purportedly in order to restore land, thereby fulfilling one of the cardinal aims of the war of liberation, surprisingly, twenty years after the attainment of independence, is deeply problematic. In the midst of all this, the first harmonised elections of March 2008 and the massive violence and intimidation of political opponents by the ruling party ZANU PF which reached a crescendo in weeks leading towards the presidential election re-run in June of the same year ushered in Zimbabwe a low-intensity war situation that witnessed South Africa sending a contingent of retired army generals to assess the situation on a fact-finding mission that was spearheaded by the grouping of Southern African countries called SADC. The intensity of politically-motivated violence that pitted the veteran Mugabe of ZANU PF against Tsvangirai of the MDC was such that in order the save the skins of his supporters, the latter, Tsvangirai, decided on withdrawing altogether from the deadly contest.

Violence and its fruitlessness during the old dispensation

Much as it is perhaps tantalising to explore and examine more factors in which the seeds of violence were broadcast whilst awaiting germination, this discussion will not purport to be exhaustive of all possible manifestations of violence during the Old Dispensation (or the First Republic). The historical signposts and events chronicled previously are individually well-documented elsewhere in a manner that we are unable to improve upon. The canvass upon which this entire discussion proceeds from is the assumption that the sum total, as well as the extremely adverse consequences of all these challenges are so well-known and are undisputed by anyone who is familiar with any rudiments of current Zimbabwean history, even as it captured by the general media. However, before we get any further, we are in total agreement with Raftopoulos (2009, 202) who broadly diagnoses and sums up the upheavals of the worst years of the First Republic as follows:

> the key aspect of the crisis was the rapid decline of the economy, characterised by among other things: steep decline in industrial and agricultural productivity; historic levels of hyperinflation; the informalisation of labour; the dollarization of economic transactions, displacements and critical erosion of livelihoods.

The bottom line is that there is no nation that can be visited by a litany of self-inflicted troubles as Zimbabwe was, and which still can, sphinx like, defiantly continue to enjoy peace and prosperity. In view of that, our humble submission is that there is scholarly merit in dissecting the causes of this grim picture as a means through which we may perhaps foresee and prevent the recurrence of these too frequent and costly installments of avoidable disharmony, violence, and butchery. A sincere interrogation of how it all began and finding where the rain started pummeling us will help in healing the nation, as well as predict events and processes that brew trouble. Armed with that kind of knowledge, it is potentially possible to be proactive and help maintain equanimity and peace in the Second Republic and others reposing in posterity.

When puzzling over and interrogating the *trouble with Nigeria*, the renowned Nigerian writer, critic, and intellectual, Chinua Achebe (1983: 1) was forthright when he saw it as "simply and squarely a failure of leadership." We have, however, thus far dissected the *"trouble with Zimbabwe"* from a broader, perhaps multidimensional perspective, in our conviction that rarely can one factor single-handedly determine the destiny and fortunes of an entire nation. However, in respect of leadership, unlike Achebe, we would like to lay blame not solely on it alone but, maybe with comparatively less culpability, also on the general citizenry. Our hypothesis in relation to this dimension of leadership is predicated on the thinking that both the leaders and the led are products of a milieu and a philosophy of governance that is deeply embedded in the collective psyche of a people.

We argue that the conceptual incompatibility and philosophical gulf dividing these two systems of governance, that is, traditional and democratic governance as stated in the earlier paragraph and the concomitant inability to successfully syncretise them, constitutes one of the major ingredients of the overall failure of African politics in general and Zimbabwe's First Republic in particular. It is these two powerful cultures of political governance that are representative of the cleavages and fissures between continuities and discontinuities of statecraft in Zimbabwe. In this chapter, we are insistent that to therefore dissect and explore how these precepts interact and/or counteract is not only a prerequisite, but also a practical pathway eventually leading to the achievement of lasting peace in the country. Here, we take a leaf from the advice that is extended to us by experts versed in the treatment of psychological and emotional trauma (Smith and Segal, 2011[10]) who instruct thus:

> In order to heal from psychological and emotional trauma, you must face and resolve the unbearable feelings and memories you have long avoided. Otherwise they will return again and again, unbidden and uncontrollable.

Zimbabwe is a nation that has for successive generations, experienced psychological and political trauma and is, therefore, in dire need of healing in order to enjoy lasting peace. The country does not seem to have had a genuine and serious appetite to reflect with due discipline upon the people's easy resort to political violence and how to put a gag on it. Following the inauguration of the Government of National Unity in 2009, some feeble attempts were made by the formation of what was called the Organ on National Healing, Reconciliation, and Integration (ONHRI) which was superintended by the late Vice President John Nkomo. Although it achieved some level of visibility, it suffered from a top-down approach.

The lamentations and/or prayer for Zimbabwe by some clergyman pleading for psychological and spiritual healing of the nation in the aftermath of the 2008 election violence and callous butchery would summarise the trauma that the Old Dispensation made people go through. Cried the clergyman, (The Bible Society of Zimbabwe, 2009: ii)

> Whatever happened to Zimbabwe towards the June 27th 2008 Presidential Re-run Elections is unexplainable . . . The state of the Nation during the last few weeks of June 2008 revealed intense hurt that existed for a long time in the lives of many . . . this nation needs healing . . . "Simon, Simon! (Zimbabwe, Zimbabwe!) Satan has asked for you, that he may sift you as wheat."

The antidote for this entrenched culture of politically motivated violence lies in honestly and boldly confronting its causes and manifestations with a view to uprooting it altogether from the national psyche. The corollary is that in doing so, peace can indeed be sought and found. Although the avoidance of violence in itself and by itself does not necessarily constitute the prevalence of peace, all the same, the proactive and active prevention of violence is a prerequisite and perhaps first principle towards the attainment of lasting peace. If the nation rests on a cushion of peace, a solid platform for national healing would have been inaugurated.

Conclusion

The foregoing exposition has preoccupied itself with the violence and politics of the Old Dispensation (or the First Republic), whose political tincture and governance style was largely a function of Mugabe and ZANU PF's political whims. It has been one of our chief concerns to retrace in historical terms the country's trajectory as it intersects and crosses paths with the chequered histories of the polity which may be demarcated into the following major epochs: Pre-colonial, colonial, the liberation struggle and, more importantly, the post-independence period. The historical dimension was necessitated by the desire to locate where things went wrong in order to avoid the same pitfalls in the future. We argued that national healing and peace are largely achievable by boldly looking ourselves in the mirror as a people and being uneconomic with the truth in relation to the causes of violence and where exactly we went wrong.

From our dissection and study of the past, it became apparent that violence, anguish, and anxiety which account for the lack of peace are tendencies that have stalked Zimbabwe for far too long. In inference, this might have started prior to the establishment of strong and centralised states such as Great Zimbabwe, Mutapa, Torwa, Changamire, and the Ndebele state. The founding of such powerful and enduring states could never have been a stroll in the park. They were built on blood and sweat – the fuel of which must have been the enactment of ruthless violence. In elaboration, we argued that this violence must have, with time, became ingrained in the collective psyche of our forebears and that as a culture, it transited through successive generations of which our own is not exempted.

We also rested our analytical microscope on the issue of language use and arrived at the conclusion that language is indeed a potent resource which is exploited and harnessed to emotionally sting political opponents and paralyse them. It can be mischievously deployed, like was the case during the colonial times, to call into question the full membership of black people in the family of homo sapiens who, apartheid-style, were ring-fenced outside the settlers' enclave of opportunity and privilege. In interpretation, to dehumanise is to strategically lock out the conscience of the perpetrator of violence as a prerequisite to allow for the optimum infliction of injury on the "object" of abuse. During the colonial period, white settler racists reinforced their dehumanisation of blacks by taking recourse to all manner of linguistic paraphernalia that availed scaffolding to their perception of blacks as: *warlike, savages, heathen hordes, dirty, cowardly*, and many other racist epithets that they hurled at Africans in order to anesthetise their conscience and justify their brutal and uninhibited relieving of wrath upon blacks.

Ironically, the First Republic was not going to be outdone by their erstwhile colonial masters in the denigration of their political foes in the opposition and whoever else was opposed to their ruinous policies. These are some of the political behaviours that deprived the denizens of Zimbabwe of enjoying permanent peace. In view of these facts, we are of the positive view that national healing is achievable if we, *inter alia*, break with the culture of violence as well as sanitise our language vis-à-vis those with whom we are in political polarity.

Notes

1 *Kuvukura*, "to bark," is invocative of the proverb attributed to the Arabs which goes like "The dogs may bark but the caravan goes on." The insinuation is that the opposition will make no political dent on the ruling ZANU PF party – an attitude that is arrogant and disrespectful of the former, which might be taken by some as a sign of confidence in the party's political stamina. However, it also carries intonations of abuse and of being inconsequential.

2 When one considers European classical times' protracted Peloponnesian wars of attrition, and in the twentieth century, the European WW1 and WW11 which witnessed the slaughter of millions of people in addition to the genocide committed of six million Jews in Auschwitz, Dachau, and other concentration camps' incineration ovens in which the killing of humans was done at an unprecedented industrial scale by "civilized whites," then bigotry and racism is straightaway exposed for its total irrationality.

3 Capricorn is a failed multiracial social experiment that was tried during the years of the Federation from 1953–1963 to bridge understanding between liberal whites and educated blacks. For some reason, it would seem that, by a semantic shift, Africans who fraternized with whites were, later, regarded as traitors during the liberation struggle.

4 FROLIZI stands for Front for the Liberation of Zimbabwe which was formed to integrate all the liberation forces fighting against the Rhodesian regime. It was a flop since ZIPRA and ZANLA were unable to work together.

5 This is succinctly demonstrative of the adage that *Violence begets violence* or the biblical equivalent of it that *He who fights with a sword, dies by the sword* (Matthew 26:52).

6 ZANLA stands for Zimbabwe African National Liberation Army while ZIPRA stands for Zimbabwe People's Revolutionary Army.

7 ZANU stands for Zimbabwe African National Union and ZAPU stands for Zimbabwe African People's Union.

8 He once made the injunction to his supporters to "Strike fear in the heart of the white man" in a manner that clearly departed from elementary dignity befitting the office of a head of state and government.

9 It was politically correct and sound to claim that war veterans who had fought for land during the liberation war had had their patience exhausted by the *willing-buyer willing-seller* clause for legally acquiring land because Britain, in abrogation of the Lancaster House agreement, had abruptly stopped financing land acquisition from willing white sellers and therefore war veterans morally had the right to take what rightfully belonged to the people. In reality, however, while there may have been a significant sprinkling of genuine war veterans, there were in addition, rented hordes of peasants, party supporters, nondescript ruffians, scoundrels, and other rabble-rousers, among whom some eked a living singing for their supper at the hands of their state handlers.

10 www.helpguide.org/mental/emotional_pyschological _trauma.htm and it is titled: *Healing Emotional and Psychological Trauma: Symptoms, Treatment and Recovery*. Accessed 25 February 2018.

References

Achebe, C. 1983. *The Trouble with Nigeria*. Portsmouth: Heinemann.

Achebe, C. 2000. *Home and Exile*. Edinburgh: Canongate.

Beach, D. N. 1980. *The Shona and Zimbabwe*. Gweru: Mambo Press.

The Bible Society of Zimbabwe. 2009. *Healing to the Nation*. Harare: The Bible Society of Zimbabwe.

Hammar, A. and B. Raftopoulos, et al (ed.). 2003. *Zimbabwe's Unfinished Business: Rethinking Land, State and Nation in the Context of Crisis*. Harare: Weaver Press.

Martin, D. and P. Johnson. 1980. *The Struggle for Zimbabwe: The Chimurenga War*. Harare: Zimbabwe Publishing House.

Matambirofa, F. 2015. "Sowing Political Capital and Harvesting Economic Regression: White Commercial Farm Seizures in Zimbabwe," in E. Osabuohien (ed.), *In-country Determinants and Implications of Foreign Land Acquisition*. Hershey, PA: Business Science Reference, 338–352.

Matambirofa, F. 2016. "Language Use and the Depiction of Violence in Pre-Colonial Shona Folk Narratives," *Journal for Studies in Humanities and Social Science* 5(2), 126–138.

Meredith, M. 2002. *Robert Mugabe: Power, Plunder and Tyranny in Zimbabwe*. Johannesburg: Jonathan Ball Publishers.

Muzondidya, J. 2009. "From Buoyancy to Crisis, 1980–1997," in B. Raftopoulos and A. Mlambo (eds.), *Becoming Zimbabwean: A History from the Pre-Colonial Period to 2008*. Harare: Weaver Press, 167–200.

Ndlovu-Gatsheni, S. J. 2009. "Mapping Cultural and Colonial Encounters, 1880s–1930s," in B. Raftopoulos and A. Mlambo (eds.), *Becoming Zimbabwean: A History from the Pre-Colonial Period to 2008*. Harare: Weaver Press, 115–166.

Nhongo-Simbanegavi, J. 2000. *For Better or Worse? Women and ZANLA in Zimbabwe's Liberation Struggle*. Harare: Weaver Press.

Raftopoulos, B. 2009. "The Crisis in Zimbabwe, 1998–2008," in B. Raftopoulos and A. Mlambo (eds.), *Becoming Zimbabwean: A History from the Pre-Colonial Period to 2008*. Harare: Weaver Press, 201–250.

Sithole, M. 1999. *Zimbabwe: Struggles Within the Struggle, 1957–1980*. Harare: Rujeko Publishers.

Smith, M. and J. Segal. 2011. "Healing Emotional and Psychological Trauma: Symptoms, Treatment and Recovery," www.helpguide.org/mental/emotional_pyschological_trauma. htm (accessed on 25 February 2018).

White, L. 2003. *The Assassination of Herbert Chitepo: Texts and Politics in Zimbabwe*. Bloomington and Indianapolis: Indiana University Press.

8 The Shona proverbs as a resource for reconciliation

Liveson Tatira

> *Henceforth you and I must strive to adapt ourselves, intellectually and spiritually, to the reality of our political change and relate to each other as brothers bound one to the other by a bond of comradeship. If yesterday I fought you as an enemy, today you have become my friend and ally with the same national interests, loyalty, rights and duties as myself. If yesterday you hated me, today you cannot avoid the love that binds you to me and me to you. Is it not folly, therefore, that in these circumstances anybody should seek to revive the wounds and grievances of the past? The wrongs of the past must stand forgiven and forgotten*
> — Independence reconciliation message by the then Prime Minister of Zimbabwe, Robert, Gabriel Mugabe in Kaulemu (2011: 9)

Introduction

This chapter basically touches on two issues, namely, the Shona proverbs and reconciliation. Admittedly, the issue of reconciliation has been viewed from different perspectives covering religion, ethics, politics, sociology, or a cocktail of all the aforesaid aspects. However, this chapter dwells on interrogating how the Shona proverbs, as part of the Shona indigenous knowledge system, are able to articulate issues of reconciliation. It is important from the beginning to note that in reconciliation, no matter which form it takes, the primary tool for facilitating and achieving it is through language. Two parties who are in conflict often end their conflict through talking to each other. Obviously, there are others who think conflict can be ended through fighting, but evidence consistently shows that dialogue is the surest route to healing and reconciliation. This applies to conflicts of all types and at all levels. Fighting does not end conflict but it epitomises the boiling point of any conflict. When the other party is defeated, it does not mean that the conflict has been done away with. Generally, what it means is that the conflict has only been suppressed with greater chances of it resurfacing in the future.

Some conflicts in Southern Africa which became full blown wars ultimately ended up in negotiations. The cases in point are Zimbabwe's protracted liberation struggle which ended with the 1979 Lancaster House Constitutional Conference that ushered independence from Britain. Similarly, the Mozambican Government represented by President Chisano and RENAMO represented by its leader, Alphonso Dhlakama, ended conflict by signing a peace agreement in Rome in 1992, though after some years further conflict arose. In South Africa, Nelson Mandela negotiated with the White minority government and such negotiations led to the rainbow nation of South Africa (Ohlson, 1996).

The aforementioned are a few examples where we find that after a protracted war, people ended up talking in order to resolve their conflict. In a way, this shows the power of talks over war. It appears war drives people apart while the talks bring them closer to each other. This brings us to the importance of Shona proverbs in pursuance of reconciliation. But before we get into the details of how proverbs can be used to foster reconciliation, it is of utmost importance first to unpack our understanding of both terms, namely, reconciliation and the Shona proverbs.

Reconciliation

The term reconciliation, like democracy, is a contested one that is generally understood differently by different people. The factors or rather issues that should be put together for reconciliation to take place vary from people to people. Some advocate for retributive justice and others for restorative justice to take place before reconciliation is achieved, while others believe that people should just forgive in order to reconcile. Yet others believe that the truth should be told first before people reconcile. And yet there are those who believe reconciliation includes the search for truth, forgiveness, healing, and mercy (Bloomfield, 2006). This chapter will not be involved with the polemics of reconciliation. Having noted the contestations around the issue of reconciliation, it is still important to proffer a definition which obviously can still be subjected to contestation.

Lederach (1998: 20) notes that,

> Reconciliation can be seen as dealing with three specific paradoxes. First, in an overall sense, reconciliation promotes an encounter between the open expression of painful past, on one hand, and the search for articulation of long-term, independent future, on the other hand. Second, reconciliation provides a place for truth and mercy to meet, where concerns for letting go in favour of renewed relationship are validated and embraced. Third, reconciliation recognizes the need to give time and place to both justice and peace, where redressing the wrong is held together with the envisioning of a common connected future.

What is apparent from Lederach's (1998) definition is that a situation that begs for reconciliation will be experiencing disequilibrium, a state mostly born out of conflict. Such disequilibrium cannot be sustained as both parties need each other for their common good. There are other cocktail of different things are required for reconciliation to take place, but the issue of reconciliation as premised by the Shona philosophy of *Unhu* is underpinned by the primacy of togetherness. There is great emphasis on the idea that people need each other hence, *munhu vanhu* (a person finds full humanity through others). This philosophy predisposes the Shona people to generally seek reconciliation whenever they wrong each other.

This chapter, as earlier on alluded to, is not going into the polemics of reconciliation. It is interested in the language, Shona proverbs, used in order to achieve or foster reconciliation. Language is a key to the heart of people (Agbaje, 2002). According to Wallnork in Ademowo and Balogun (2014: 39), language has the following values,

1   for phatic communication i.e. as a social regulator
2   as an instrument of action
3   to convey order and information
4   to influence people
5   to enable self-expression, and
6   to embody and enable thought

All the previously given values make language suitable for tackling issues of reconciliation and if language is couched in proverbs, the more effective it becomes. Because of the values language possesses, Ademowo and Balogun (2014: 39) are correct to note that:

> no human society can exist to experience peace without the effective/ explorative use of and development of its metaphoric concepts/language that will encourage and teach about peace as we have in proverbs.

This leaves us to agree no less with Egenti and Okoye (2016) who note that proverbs are capable of dealing with peace and reconciliation and serve as linguistic tools for conflict management.

Proverbs

Proverbs constitutes a special genre of Shona indigenous knowledge system which occupies a very important place in Shona discourse. Proverbs are oratory linguistic tools which can be deployed in any situation, be it social, economic, political, religious, or educational, just to mention a few. They function to deride, ridicule, judge, warn, persuade, encourage, counsel, advice, and educate people. Their message is often embedded in figurative language that brings out vivid mental images that awaken the listener to the import of the discourse at hand. The images used can be animals, birds, reptiles, *flora* and *fauna*, human beings, and body parts but the ideas behind them are both penetrating and forceful. Proverbs spur listeners into action, they, in a way, breathe positive energy into people so that they act in a desirable way.

Proverbs represent abstract ideas and therefore are philosophical statements that apply to all times and in every situation when skilfully deployed. Their brevity and aptness make them appropriate in keeping the discourse focused and brief. They appeal both to the intellect and heart making them appropriate tools for handling contentious issues. Agbaje (2002: 238) notes,

> Proverbs are indispensable in conflict resolution and crisis management. As oratory and linguistic tool, when proverbs are applied to conflict situation, they can function as ice breakers in relieving tension, as therapeutic tools in facilitating trauma healing, in promoting introspection which brings about change, in promoting interpersonal communication.

For this reason, proverbs are deployed to reconcile people who might not be willing to make peace with each other. Therefore, proverbs are found to be appropriate resources in handling conflicts. The power of the proverb in facilitating peace has also been noted by Owomoyela (2012), Adeyami (2012), and Salawudeen (2012).

Conflict

Conflict, according to Ajayi and Buhari (2014) in Egenti and Okoye (2016: 56), can be described as,

> a condition in which an identifiable group of human beings whether tribal, ethnic, linguistic, religious, socio-political, economic, cultural or otherwise is in conscious opposition to one or other identifiable human group because these groups are pursuing what appears to be incompatible goals.

Reconciliation is, therefore, a process or a product of conflict resolution. In Shona society, conflict is not an issue, it only becomes an issue if it remains unresolved. The Shona are fully aware that proximity relations are bound to attract conflict, but they contend that such conflict should be resolved or kept to a low level so that the operations of society should not be affected. Generally the Shona people are not concerned about conflict but how people respond to situations of conflict. They believe that conflicts should be resolved amicably. However, they also believe that it is not every conflict that should be resolved. Minor or petty conflicts which have insignificant societal disruptions should be ignored and left to die or people should learn to live with them. It is only those that disrupt social harmony that should be attended to.

Not surprisingly, there are Shona proverbs which exhort people to ignore minor conflicts and to continue with business as usual and proverbs that try to resolve conflict by knocking sense into the disputants so that they envision the importance of reconciliation. The latter group of proverbs places emphasis on the importance of leaving the painful past and moving on with life, proverbs that celebrate unity or solidarity above everything else, and on proverbs that deal with ambivalent situations.

Proverbs that exhort people to ignore minor conflicts

The Shona people believe that wherever there are people there is bound to be conflict. Conflict is inevitable because preferences are different and humanity by its nature is imperfect. As much as people would not like to make mistakes, they do so consciously and unconsciously throughout their existence. As a result, there is no perfect society but a society which continually strives for perfection. Therefore, to human beings, conflict is a daily encounter.

The Shona people are fully aware of human imperfection. However, there is the positive side of conflict as it makes people reflect upon their weaknesses, review their actions, and correct them. If properly handled, conflict makes society mature, wiser, and better.

There are Shona proverbs that are meant to enlighten members of society who might think that life is smooth sailing and might take a minor conflict with a grudge. Such members are advised or reminded to wake up to the realities of life, to ignore minor conflicts, and continue with life as usual. Such people are encouraged by the following proverb, "*Panofamba munhu magaro anokwizirana*" (Human movement produces friction between the buttocks). The proverb informs people that proximity relations are bound to produce minor conflicts which should be ignored for the continuity of a functional society. As a person does not stop walking because of friction produced by such movements, people should not bother themselves with minor conflicts. It urges people to remain focussed and productive – walking rather than being divisive and unproductive. In this regard, paying too much attention is paralysing and prevents individuals and communities from continuing to walk and working towards more productive goals. Here, Shona wisdom is teaching that minor conflicts are part of everyday existence. People who are in proximity to each other, for example, married couples, neighbouring villages, neighbouring ethnic communities, are bound to experience minor conflicts. Proverbs in this category counsel individuals, communities, and ethnic groups to overlook minor infractions and continue to relate amicably.

The other proverb which points to the ever-presence of conflict that should be ignored in society is "*Meno nerurimi zvakagara mumuromo wani*" (The teeth and tongue reside in the mouth [though there are problems in so doing]). The proverb, like the one discussed earlier, points to the supreme importance of functionality over petty conflicts. It advocates for coexistence and ignoring minor sporadic conflicts in life. At times, in the process of chewing the teeth can bite the tongue by mistake. The biting is not a deliberate one, but is a result of an accident in the process of chewing. Therefore, in life there are conflicts which might arise through mistaken judgement. These should be ignored in the same way the tongue and the teeth continue to stay and function together in the mouth. People are reminded not to take offence and to continue to work together for the benefit of society.

In both proverbs conflict is automatically followed by reconciliation, one instantly triggers the other. However, there are instances where conflict destabilises society. Such conflicts can tear society apart if not properly handled. There are proverbs in Shona that help to reconcile people so that they reconnect and reconstruct their future as one. Oluwaseum (2009: 139–140), writing about how proverbs were used to foster peace between disputants among the Yoruba of Nigeria is correct to posit that,

> In the settlement of disputes, peaceful coexistence, harmony, and a united front were the aim of any dispute (whether civil or criminal) resolution and this was always emphasised at any trial so that fairness was exercised in the passing of judgement.

Proverbs that motivate people to leave the painful past and move on with life

As already indicated in this chapter, reconciliation is about leaving the unpleasant past experiences and moving to a shared future. Once people are in conflict, especially for a long time, they generally feel amputated, hollow, defeated, exposed, and insecure if they leave their entrenched positions. There is sometimes a feeling of self-betrayal when one considers reconciliation. Parties that are in conflict are usually bitter with each other. Though at the back of their minds they might feel that the circumstances they find themselves in are not admirable, the determination to move forward might be lacking due to the aforesaid factors. For these reasons, there are Shona proverbs which inspire people to break the circle so that they move forward with life.

There is a proverb in Shona which demands that things should be stopped forthwith. This proverb is "*Ngaisiye matambo*" (Stop forthwith). This is a terse proverb which directs the course of action that should be taken without further arguments. It is a directive, as it were, which when said in any context, means the border line has been reached. It is an oral utterance which draws a line in the sand. What it means is that in terms of conflict, disputants will be expected not to continue any further with their discordant agenda. In the context of conflict, the proverb informs the parties concerned that the stage they have reached is no longer acceptable. The parties should trace their humanity and put everything aside, deflate their ego and move forward as one. It does not matter how much one is wronged, but what matters is to arrest the direction of events. This helps people to reconsider their positions in terms of the bigger picture of their existence.

"*Ngaisiye matambo*" is an urgent injunction to people who are escalating conflict to draw back and avoid a situation where the tension gets out of hand. It is a call to the cessation of hostilities and resumption of civility and dialogue. It can be uttered by a party to the conflict, or by an outsider. When it is said, the protagonists are expected to take heed and refrain from pursuing a line that worsens the conflict. This proverb is a resource in handling conflict at the national level. It could be used to mobilise leading politicians to step back from inflammatory language and to purse the path to peace.

An almost similar proverb is found among the Yoruba of Nigeria. Mode (2015: 60) records the proverb, *A rufe tuku a ci tuwo* (Let us cover human excrement and eat food). The use of two antagonistic images in the proverb provokes people to take an urgent and inevitable action. As it is natural that no individual can partake or enjoy food in the sight of human excrement, therefore, it would be no longer tenable for people to continue in conflict but to move forward. The proverb acknowledges the wrong done and directs people affected to forget about it completely (cover human excrement) and chart a new life (eat food).

If parties dwell on the past, they are reminded that they will destroy themselves in the same way as a person who starves to death by failing to eat upon seeing human excrement.

The last proverb in this subsection that fosters reconciliation among the disputants is *Kugara kunzwana* (Harmony is necessary for good neighbourliness). The proverb speaks to the necessity of harmony between neighbours. The Shona people place great importance on harmony between individuals and between individuals and nature. Disharmony between individuals, they believe, can also cause disharmony to nature (Bourdillon, 1982; Gelfand, 1975). In situations of dispute, members are reminded to reconcile and live in harmony with each other. While the proverb was generated in the context of small communities, it can be highly useful at the national level. It can promote good neighbourliness across ethnic, racial, gender, class, and other divisions. It is a proverb that encourages citizens to know that because they occupy the same space, they have to invest in ensuring that they work across the dividing lines.

Proverbs that celebrate unity or solidarity above everything else

The Shona people believe in the strength of numbers. They do not condone individualism, hence "*Rume rimwe harikombi churu*" (One man cannot surround an anthill) and its variant, "*Gumwe rimwe haritswanyi inda*" (One thumb cannot squeeze a louse). There are many other examples of Shona proverbs which express the desirability and strength of numbers. This partly explains why traditional Shona families are large.

In the previously mentioned proverbs, the message is that a person should involve others in order for them to competently accomplish their task. It is apparent that when a hunter needs to kill an animal in an anthill, they need others so that they surround the animal in order to kill it. The same is true for killing a louse, as the thumb requires the finger to squeeze it between them.

The other proverb which extols large numbers and unity is "*Vari pachavo chikuriri*" (When people are united they are a formidable force). The proverb encourages people to remain united and it is usually deployed in circumstances where conflict threatens to tear people apart. People in conflict are reminded that unity is the mother of strength and progress. The proverb seeks to foster unity and minimise conflict or division. Similarly, at the national level it can be deployed to reinforce the saying that, "united we stand, divided we fall."

But the common trend of life is that the larger the numbers, the greater likelihood of conflict. Since large numbers are desirable but such numbers are generally a cause of strive and conflict, there should be therefore a way of dealing with conflicts.

The Shona people have proverbs which deal with such situations through their proverbs which celebrate unity or solidarity above everything else. The unity of the group takes precedence over anything else as evident in the Shona philosophical axiom, "*munhu vanhu*" (a person finds full humanity through others). Therefore, in the event of conflict, people are reminded to stop bickering and to consider the primary value of solidarity above all other considerations.

The proverb "*Ukama hahusukwi nemvura hukabva*" (Kinship cannot be washed and removed by water), speaks to the importance of unity. The proverb reminds people that no matter the misunderstanding among relatives, they should be mindful that they have a bond which they cannot easily wish away. That bond which they are reminded of should help them to reconcile as they should remain one large family. The same can be applied to a nation: The nationals should keep in mind the fact that they are bound together by their common history and nationality and hence should reconcile no matter the level of conflict between them. This can be further extended to the generality of humanity, namely, that they should not lose sight of that what should bind them together, their humanity. It is evident that the proverb functions to foster the spirit of togetherness.

The other variant, "*Ukama urimbo kudambura haubvi*" (Relationship is like a sticking stuff used to trap birds, once stuck with it you cannot remove it). The proverb points to the futility of attempting to alienate oneself from one's relatives. No matter how much one tries to do away with their kin and kith they will not succeed. This proverb is vital for forging national cohesion. It underscores the point that various ethnic and social groups belong to one larger family, namely, the nation. Consequently, they should not invest in trying to withdraw from national processes and belonging, but should be committed to having a shared national identity and vision.

Proverbs that deal with ambivalent situations

There are proverbs which deal with ambivalent situations. When the situation looks chaotic and hopeless, there is a proverb which assures people concerned that such a situation is a necessary steps that leads to sanity. One of such proverbs is, "*Mvura bvongodzeki ndiyo garani*" (The disturbed water finally clears/settles). People in a disturbed relationship are encouraged to wake up to the ambivalence of life and accept that the tension and experiences can lead to harmony after the conflict.

The other proverb which expresses ambivalence is "*Kwavira kwaedza*" (Sunset is always followed by sunrise). The proverb provokes people not to remain entrenched in the unenviable gloom and move forward. Misfortune or the state of conflict cannot be sustained as sunset always leads to sunrise. The conflict might be threatening and frightening as darkness, but through the proverb disputants are urged to see a promising future beyond the dispute.

Proverbs that deal with ambivalent situations might create the impression that there is an emphasis of glossing over the pain of conflict. There is need to recognise that these proverbs do acknowledge the pain of conflict. Their focus, however, is on the power of conflict transformation. They highlight how conflict can generate a better and more productive state that comes after the transformation of conflict.

Conclusion

It is clear that the Shona proverbs as part of Ubuntu philosophy address the issue of conflict. Language plays a very important part in human existence. It is the language which transmits the values of a particular society. When the discourse is couched in proverbs, discourses become not only animated, but oratory. When appropriately deployed, proverbs unlock deadlocks and persuade disputants to reconcile. They appeal both to the intellect and emotions, thus making them appropriate tools for settling disputes. More so, proverbs are appropriate for reconciliation as they are capable of touching every sphere of human experiences. It is critical to recover indigenous knowledge systems in the process of nation building. Zimbabwe can deepen national healing, reconciliation, and integration by appropriating proverbs such as those discussed in this essay and others.

References

Ademowo, J. A. and N. O. Balogun. 2014. "Proverbs, Values and the Development Question in Contemporary Africa: A Case Study of Yoruba Proverbs," *Antropologija* 14(2), 150–160.
Adeyami, B. A. 2012. "Utilisation of Information Communication and Technology (ICT) Facilities in the Teaching of Social Studies in Nigeria Secondary Schools," *Journal of Educational and Social Research* 2(2), 245–250.
Agbaje, J. B. 2002. "Proverbs: A Strategy of Resolving Conflict in Yoruba Society," *Journal of African Central Studies* 15(2), 37–243.
Bloomfield, D. 2006. *On Good Terms: Clarifying Reconciliation.* Berghof Report no. 14. Berlin: Berghof Research Centre for Constructive Management.
Bourdillon, M. F. C. 1982. *The Shona Peoples: An Ethnography of the Contemporary Shona, With Special Reference to Their Religion.* Gweru: Mambo Press.
Egenti, E. C. and A. N. Okoye. 2016. *On the Role of Igbo Proverbs in Conflict Resolution and Reconciliation.* Awka: Department of Linguistics, Nnamdi University.
Gelfand, M. 1975. *The Spiritual Beliefs of the Shona.* Gweru: Mambo Press.
Kaulemu, D. 2011. *Ending Violence in Zimbabwe.* Harare: The Konrad-Adenauer-Stiftung (KAS).
Lederach, J. P. 1998. *Building Peace: Sustainable Reconciliation in Divided Societies.* Washington, DC: US Institute of Peace Press.
Mode, M. A. 2015. "Proverbs as Panacea to Peaceful Coexistence in Northern Nigeria" *IOSR Journal of Humanities and Social Sciences (10SR-JHSS)* 20(V), 55–60.

Ohlson, T. 1996. "Conflict and Conflict Resolution in a Southern African Context."

Oluwaseum, F. P. 2009. "Peacemaking Proverbs in Urhobond Yoruba Marital Conflicts Part 2," *African Conflict and Peacebuilding Review*, 2(2), Special Issue on West African Research Association Peace Initiative Conference in Dakar (2009), Fall (2011), 136–152.

Owomoyela, A. 2012. *Yoruba Proverb Treasury*. http//Yoruba um.edu/Yoruba.

Salawudeen, M. O. 2012. "Role of Yoruba Proverbs in Socialisation of the Youth: Implications for Social Studies Curriculum," Paper Presented at the 3rd National Conference of School of Languages at Federal College of Education, Oyo, 5–9 March.

9 *Sahwira* and/as endogenous healing and therapy in Shona funerary rituals

Insights for national healing

Ruth Makumbirofa, Kelvin Chikonzo,
and Nehemiah Chivandikwa

Introduction

This chapter analyses the dramatic/performative act of the *sahwira* in Shona funeral rituals and how the context of such a performance and the performance itself are integral pathways for one to achieve healing. The *sahwira* in Shona funeral rituals can be defined as the funeral or ritual friend; although their functions go beyond performing at funerals. The chapter will explore the aesthetics of funerary ritual performance in Shona funerals, with particular focus on the *sahwira*, the performance of the *sahwira* and the context in which the performance takes place and the meaning that can be derived thereof.

This chapter conceptualises the *sahwira* during a funeral as a half actor performing the everydayness of life; the *sahwira* as a joker/facilitator and mediator; as well as the *sahwira* as a storyteller. The chapter demonstrates how the context set by the funeral and the role play by the *sahwira* are symbolic elements that provide room for embodiment, distancing, memory, reflection, and transformation. By context, the study analyses in this category aesthetic elements such as the transformation of the home space from private space to become public space, the use of ritualistic properties (props), the adoption of mourning attire (costuming), and the setting (scenery) created for everyday performances to take place. This chapter contends that the performative acts of the *sahwira* within the funeral context, makes provision for the bereaved; who are at this point existing in a liminal zone, to (re)negotiate meaning as they go through a painful process of loss and inevitable change. More critically, the *sahwira* institution provides a model for national healing and integration. The *sahwira* has the license to speak the truth openly and to caricature the deceased. Through drama and laughter, mourners are consoled and the memory of the deceased is cleansed. The chapter argues that the institution of *sahwira* facilitates healing, reconciliation at the family and community levels, and that it can be adopted at the national level.

Shona cosmology/worldview

Like most African cultures, the Shona people believe in an afterlife. They believe that the human being exists in two entities: the biological body, which is essentially the physical reality; and the spiritual body which is believed to be the one that separates from the physical body at one's point of death (Bojuwoye, 2013: 75). The spirit, therefore, continues to exist in an indestructible entity, a world unperceived by the human eye. In this state, the deceased can still continue as part of the family, as an ancestor, capable of interacting with the physical world, yet unseen. This worldview often has a bearing on a person and society at large as they grieve over a loved one. The belief that the deceased has transited into a different world/reality inevitably informs the manner in which rituals are carried out at a funeral, for example, the killing of a beast is partly done in the belief and intent to provide the deceased with food as they embark on a journey to the spiritual realm. Also, armed with this belief in the afterlife, the Shona can bury their dead with their favourite tools or property, for example, a great hunter could be buried with some tools of their trade. Interestingly, in the modern scenario, such tendencies are being perpetuated. At the funeral of a female sex worker observed at Granville (Mbudzi) Cemetery, the woman's body was taken underground with three carton boxes of condoms and a cot of her favourite beer. The "*sahwira*" claimed these apparatus would be useful to her friend, wherever she was going. In principle, therefore, the dead graduate into the world of ancestors, who are called the living dead and they remain in relationship with the living.

It is also customary among the Shona that when one passes on, they express sympathy. It is considered "a sacred duty" (Mwandayi, 2011) to express sympathy and pay condolences to the relatives of the deceased. Failure to do so would result in one being morally condemned or being deemed as unsociable. Furthermore, attending a funeral is considered as a sign of one's honesty and innocence regarding the death of the deceased (Muchemwa, 2007). In this regard, one finds that Shona funerals are highly communal; the funeral is not closed to close immediate family members only. Rather, the community, consisting of neighbours, extended family, friends and workmates, dutifully attend funerals, and this is considered as a social responsibility. According to Muchemwa (2007: 26), often people feel obliged to attend funerals as it is a gesture they expect to be returned in their favour one day when they pass on. The highly communal nature of these funerals also tends to determine the popularity of the deceased, as it is common to hear people use the expression, "*achemwa chaizvo*," meaning a lot of people attended the funeral of the deceased. In contrast, if the funeral is not well attended, it can be used as a measure to express that the deceased was not very popular, or was not a very good person. In the same vein, the Shona tend to believe that when one dies, they become a good person, as demonstrated in their proverb, "*wafa wanaka*." Consistent with this proverb and belief, the Shona will speak and profess mostly the good about the deceased.

Defining the *sahwira*

The *sahwira* is generally known as a family friend amongst the Shona people. Although several scholars refer the *sahwira* as "funeral friend" or ritual friend (Mwandayi, 2011; Nyota, 2008), the roles and functions of the *sahwira* traditionally went beyond performing at funerals. The *sahwira* culture was an important relationship between families and can be conceived as an integral social security network existing among the Shona to cushion families during times of hardship. The relationship of the *sahwira*s was not based on ethnicity or nationality (De Bruijn et al., 2001). Bourdillon (1987) suggests that the practice can be traced back to the Malawian peoples. This can also be evidenced by the strong visibility of the culture among the Zezuru and Korekore Shona ethnic groups, who are mostly concentrated in the Mashonaland West and Central province of Zimbabwe. It was not unusual for the *sahwira* relationships to extend to the next generation. Hence *usahwira* (the friendship) could be inherited patrilineally. This is consistent with Nyota's (2008) observation that a *sahwira* was installed. People actually went to the extent of making an agreement as in a covenant, stating the terms of their friendship and being entrusted with one's will, wishes, and secrets. In many instances, the *sahwira* was entrusted with the verbal will of the deceased, hence it was the responsibility of the *sahwira* to express the will of the deceased in the distribution of their estate.

During their lifetime, the *sahwira*s stood by each other, through all the good and the bad times. The *sahwira* could be entrusted with everything to do with the friend's life, with the exception of the friend's wife. Hence it is consequential that the *sahwira* would become the director of ceremony during one's funeral (Nyota, 2008). While other role players such as *varoora* and *vazukuru* could imitate the deceased during the funeral performance, they were limited by virtue of their positions and relationships within the family, in case they offended someone. The *sahwira* act, however, was uncensored.

The culture of the *sahwira* still continues to exist to this day, regardless of the ever-changing environment, contributing to factors such as rapid rural-to-urban migration, and country-to-country migration. Migration on the other hand, tends to disrupt and weaken the *sahwira* relationships, which were easier to maintain when people stayed closer together. Nevertheless, we can refer to at least two cases where we find the *sahwira* culture very much active, despite the variations. Wrolson recorded a modern day scenario in which the *sahwira* serves as "pallbearer, truth-teller, and jester for a family." Mukwindidza states in an interview with Wrolson, the strict selection of the *sahwira* "[she] has taken my relative to the grave. [She] is then my *sahwira*. You don't take a *sahwira* from anywhere. [She] has to go with you first in the grave and then after that [she] can do whatever [she] wants to do because [she] *achengeta amai* [looked after my mother]" (Mukwindidza in Wrolson, 2006: 28). We therefore learn how the *sahwira* relationship was not necessarily limited to a certain gender and how the *sahwira* relationship is still well-received and practiced with seriousness in modern day Zimbabwe.

Benyera (2014) also offers us insight into the various functions of the *sahwira* in facilitating transitional justice during the national healing exercise in Zimbabwe during the period 1980–2011. The *sahwira* stood as facilitator and mediator between victims (and their families) and perpetrators during the process of truth and reconciliation within communities. The institution of the *sahwira* appears to have stood the test of time through its functionality in cases of facilitating healing, mediating crises, encouraging social transformation, and alleviating pain.

Methodology

The research methodology was primarily descriptive and analytical. Using an embodied methodology, the researchers randomly selected and attended funerals. An embodied approach, otherwise known as performance ethnography, entails using participant observation, a thick description of the phenomenon as well as cultural interpretation and analysis (Denzin, 2003). Attendance at funeral sites was done randomly since the researchers had no control over variables such as when a funeral could actually occur, or which funeral to prefer over the other. We attended funerals from across different geographic areas. This was done in order to gather variations of ritual performance and determine consistency, and also for data validation. Areas where attendances were frequented are as follows: Murewa, Chinhoyi, Chitungwiza, Harare-Mabvuku, Glen Norah, Glen View, Budiriro, and Epworth.

The study also made use of archival data. Archival data analysis includes identifying evidence of corporeal experiences from past documented forms (Starbuck and Mock, 2003). In this case, extensive literature review was carried out on Shona rituals, particularly on the subject of the *sahwira*. Documented video content was used for observation. Although the videos provided invaluable insights, they were limited because the archive was "fixed" due to their historical placement; that is, the recordings were done from the vantage point of the agenda of the recorder, who happened to have their own cultural agenda. The other limitation posed by this method was the distanced perspective created as the camera directed opposed to what we could see. As researchers, we then had to think imaginatively and engage with the videos using knowledge from our past direct observatory experiences.

Theoretical framework

African thought subscribes to the ideology of a culture-based treatment for African people. Several contemporary studies have demonstrated how culture forms the rubric of holistic healing and restoration for African communities (Juma, 2011; Muchinako, 2014; Bojuwoye, 2013). In spite of geographical location, people of African descent still find their identity "centred" on a cultural reality/philosophy which then affects their sensibilities (Rosenblatt and Wallace, 2005). Present discourse in the field of psychotherapy argues for strong consideration of cultural relativism in closing the "treatment gap" in mental health cases. This suggests the need for further research in areas of health, and a reconsideration of accepted methods of healing, especially where it concerns Black African people.

Bereavement also entails a process of grieving, as pain and suffering must be experienced in order to heal and resolve the loss event. A person's grief needs to be validated in order for them to heal. African funerary ritual endeavours to validate the loss of life in the here-and-now of material existence. We submit, therefore, that grieving is a process, it is culturally contextual and not universal in its manifestations, hence the need for an Afrocentric conceptualisation of grief and bereavement care mechanisms.

The funeral context

This chapter conceptualises the funeral space as a space for performance, where the ordinary everyday acts take place. In his book, *Decolonising the Stage*, Balme (1999) problematises the tendency to create a demarcation between ritual and theatre and demonstrates how the lines between the two have been blurred by an analogue of the aesthetic values of the two. The theatrical nature of rituals is undeniably demonstrated through a study of different cultural texts and the performance of these rituals. Also using Goffman's theory on performance, we note how everyday life experiences can be related to theatrical performance. The funeral sight is a space pregnant with performative acts. Relating such performativity to Goffman's performance theory, this qualifies the funeral space as a theatrical space.

A critical look at the events and activities of a funeral shows a whole spectrum of performative acts: the arrangement of spaces, the singing and dancing that takes place all day and night, the prescribed dressing/costuming, the guided speech and movement of people, the patterned ritual of shaking people's hands as a way of showing sympathy, the viewing of "the body," and the wailing of women attending the funeral. When Goffman (1956) theorises the concept of a social front, in which people perform as expected of them, he gives an example of how a setting has influence upon a person's behaviour. Those who must use a particular setting for their performance can only begin after reaching the specific setting and have to terminate their performance upon departing from it.

The weeping act of women is an interesting example of a funeral performance. When attending a funeral, it is customary for women to wail or weep excessively in an exaggerated manner within proximity of the funeral site, as they approach. The weeping is clearly feigned and exaggerated. In actual fact, a group of women approaching a funeral will debate among each other as to who will start the wailing. When it has been agreed, the first woman will raise a high-pitched scream and starting mourning. The rest of the women will follow suit in support of the first. This is similar to Goffman's observation of how people, as social actors, will also respond in support of a feigned or pretended act. Despite knowing that the weeping is feigned, other women act as accomplices to the act. To heighten the conflict, some women will throw themselves on the floor and the others will respond by holding them up and consoling them. Such wailing performances include monologues where the weeping one will express themselves in bitter pain addressing the deceased in absentia. After a few minutes of wailing and weeping, the women will engage in a ritual of "*kubata maoko*," which is, shaking the hands of mourners gathered as a manner of showing sympathy. Thereafter, the chatter goes back to normal, with the women now engaging in everyday ordinary chattering, where non-funeral related talk is engaged in. In this regard, we submit that the funeral is a space for performance. Secondly, it is a space for the continuous expression of grief. These performative acts have the effect of triggering the emotion of mourners over and over again, during the duration of the funeral, which could take an average of three days.

Transformation of the funeral space

At the onset of someone's death, the family home space is immediately transformed from a private space to become a public space. This entails that the home is opened up for extended family members, friends, neighbours, and the community at large to come and pay their condolences to the bereaved. This new state necessitates that furniture within the home space be readjusted and redesigned so as to align to the needs of the situation/status quo. In most funeral cases observed, "empty spaces" are created; the living room which normally contains sofas, a television set, tables and chairs, etc. is emptied of these objects. Usually it is left bare, with perhaps only a carpet to cover the floor where mourners will sit and sleep. It is also within this same space where we find mourners dancing all day and night. Typically, women gather within the house, while men sit outside by the fire.

Empty spaces are typical of African performance spaces, while the emptiness is also reflective of a liminality zone. For a space to be transformed, therefore, there is need for an empty space, a truly empty space which can then be filled by needs, improvisations, and spontaneities; a performer, who tells a uniquely individual story and an audience, an audience however not passive, but engaged in a collective experience. In the empty space, "the fourth wall" in realist theatre can be broken and there can be interaction between performer and audience. In *Decolonising the Mind*, Ngugi makes a similar refers to the notion of an empty space:

> This drama (East African precolonial drama) was not performed in a special building set aside for the purpose. It could take place anywhere, wherever there was an "empty space", to borrow the phrase from Peter Brook. The "empty space" among the people was part of that tradition.
>
> (1981: 67)

Many African traditional cultures, particularly the pre-colonial forms of theatre, have shown the tendency to make use of "found spaces' or transform any empty space and subsequently define them and give them a meaning through the act of the performance that takes place within that space. For instance, the Nyau and Gule Wamkulu dances, popularly found in Malawi and Zimbabwe and performed by the Chewa ethnic groups, are secret cult dances where masked dancers move into any space and transform it into a performance space through the enactment of the ritual dances. People easily recognise that the space has been taken over, be it at a field or a marketplace, and they make way for the performance of the masked dancers. When the Nyau masquerade dancers enter a space, there is a "temporary suspension of all hierarchic distinctions and barriers among men and of certain norms and prohibitions of usual life" (Korpela, 2011: 44). In this manner, audiences begin to relate with the performer in a specific symbolic and codified manner. Similarly, the transformation of the funeral home space also makes room for the symbolic performances of the *sahwira*, *varoora*, with a fluid audience-performer relationship.

Building on Braun's concept of integrating everyday events with the scientific, in this case, the scientific being therapy, this chapter will make use of the principles propounded by Braun. The two seem to be worlds apart, with the everyday being concrete, while the therapy is quite abstract and evasive, elusive to the eye. There is therefore a need to rationalise between the two worlds, that is, the therapy and the everyday and this can be achieved through an integration of the two worlds.

The principle of integration allows us to concretise and make real the invisible and abstract phenomenon that escapes the eye, yet which people relate to in the everyday life, for example, the phenomenon of how molecules move from a particular region of concentration to the other or the process of water evaporation. Everyday performative acts can be easily integrated or made use of to embody the abstract concepts of healing and therapy. The empty space primarily offers room for an exploration/a negotiation and renegotiation of meaning as people dwell in a liminal zone. The performance which takes place within the empty space becomes an "active way of learning" or engaging with the scientific abstract principles. Performance from an empty space encourages the expression of the individual's story and begins to offer plausible and alternative way to understanding the abstract, such as death, grieving, healing. In Brook's holy theatre the "empty space" (of the stage and,

> metaphorically, for the audience) is filled by a much richer and enhanced experience, stimulating its audience by use of metaphor.
>
> (Braund, 2015: 104)

The performance that takes place in the empty space, therefore, allows mourners to access an otherwise abstract concept of healing. It becomes a space for people to face a greater reality, that of death. This is achieved though exploration of self, spontaneous reaction and expression of affective memories. This does not necessarily need a written script, nor does one make use of any particular performance skills. The empty space presents a setting for the performative acts of the *sahwira* as a dramatic performer, a joker, and the mourners as an interactive audience.

Sahwira as a story teller

The *sahwira* is first and foremost a dramatist, a performer, a character, and a sto-ryteller. The *sahwira* is a social character whose role is already established, with a pre-existing setting, costume, and properties. This chapter contends that the *sahwira* is a performer and the funeral context sets the stage for the performance of the *sahwira*. According to Mwandayi, the cultural role of the *sahwira* was "to relieve the tension at the funeral by making fun of the immediate relatives of the deceased or imitating what the deceased person used to do or wear. For a time people are as it were drawn from the intense pain of loss as they break into laughter" (2011: 97).

Fun and jest were characteristic of the *sahwira* act. The *sahwira* would often play the character of the deceased in a dramatic manner, causing people to laugh and sometimes comment on the life of the deceased. In performing the life of the deceased, the *sahwira* would imitate the everyday behaviourals of the deceased which people were familiar with, or rather, which people could easily identify and relate with as being part of the deceased's life. In this manner, the *sahwira* became a storyteller, playing back before an audience the life stories of the deceased. If, for instance, the deceased was a very talkative being, the *sahwira* would dramatically simulate that behaviour, while directly addressing the audience members, who could also respond. In a talkative and jestive manner, the *sahwira* could "act" the role of the deceased, while directly commenting on whatever was taking place at the funeral scene, in a talkative way. Hence, this role allowed the *sahwira* to comment or make social commentary on what was taking place at the funeral, in a way, also enforcing the will of the deceased. In response, the audiences would also respond and react to the act of *sahwira*, as though relating to the deceased person's life.

Also characteristic of the *sahwira* act, was non-censorship. As noted before, it was not only the *sahwira* who could perform at the funeral. The gather-ing mourners frequently engaged in singing and dancing of funerary dirges. The "*varoora*" and "*vazukuru*" could also put up dramatic performances. How-ever, it was only the *sahwira* who could perform the life of the deceased with no censorship. The *sahwira* could perform both the good and bad side of the deceased, as well as intervene directly in the activities of the funeral procession; and they had the power to do that, fully exonerated from those who could become offended. When the *sahwira* plays out the "not so lovely" side of the deceased life, this is interestingly ambivalent to the Shona saying and belief that "*afa anaka*," meaning whoever dies, becomes a good person. Guided by this belief, at a funeral, people tend to speak only the good concerning the deceased. In contracts however, the *sahwira* will show a more realistic picture of the deceased, by acting both the good and the bad. By playing out both sides of the deceased, this act served the purpose to directly intervene and encourage corrective action when things are not being done accordingly/appropriately at a funeral. Also, this served to validate the true life and existence of the deceased, providing a memory that showed the deceased's life not as forgotten but appreciated and loved in whatever good or bad.

Drawing from a systemic counselling approach, a counsellor can make use of a technique referred to as the "empty chair." We suggest that the *sahwira* serves a similar function and could have an effect relative to the empty chair technique. The empty chair is an interactive technique used to engage the client's feelings, thoughts, and behaviour. In therapy, the technique assists the clients to have a full awareness of their experience in the here and now, to work through an internalised conflict. By placing an empty chair before a client in session and allowing that person to imagine that it was their boss, husband, or parent (whatever the person they are struggling with), a person becomes fully aware of their thoughts and gain insight on their struggles. It becomes an interactive way and embodied approach which moves a client away from an abstract realm or thinking. In a similar manner, the *sahwira* becomes the embodiment of the deceased, who is facilitating or aiding the process of helping people to grieve, to get in touch with their emotions, thereby discouraging denial. Through the *sahwira*-embodied act, a person is given room to express desires, appreciation, resentment, regrets; whatever feelings and thoughts a person has internalised since the death. By bringing the life stories of the deceased into the funeral space, it encourages people to mourn. Mourning is essential since it is a natural way of achieving healing and validating the loss people are experiencing.

Sahwira as a joker-facilitator

As a joker/facilitator, the *sahwira* played a mediating role by expressing the will of the deceased. When a friend passes on, it is part of the responsibility of the *sahwira* to oversee the proceeding of the funeral. They were the major testament of the deceased's will, which was often verbal. Culture, as noted by Kershaw (1992), is saturated with discourses of power. The *sahwira* is presented not only as an authoritative figure, but one who seeks to balance out power relations and resolve tensions at the funeral site. By bearing the will of the deceased, the *sahwira* commands power and authority. (The challenges of a verbal will are part of a different discourse to be explored.) The *sahwira* figure is observed as one that shifts between role playing or performing the deceased and performing the *sahwira* roles (playing themselves) "out of character" or after de-rolling, hence becoming a half actor. In the instance where the *sahwira* de-roles, they become a joker-facilitator. Along with such character shifts, the power and authority of the *sahwira* also shifts from being highly powerful, when in character, to moderate authority, when becoming a joker. The aims of jokering are to arbitrate the will of the deceased, expressing the desires of the deceased, informing people where there is need for compensation, and assisting in the distribution of the estate.

The *sahwira* as a half actor is observed to perform the everyday life of the deceased and his own. Boal (1979) conceptualises how each person in life carries a mask made of habits of thoughts, language, and profession. All relations are therefore governed by these patterned habits. Goffman's (1956) conception of "performance" refers to all the activity of an individual which occurs during a period marked by his continuous presence before a particular set of observers and which has some influence on the observers. In like manner, the *sahwira* has a patterned behaviour when they are out of the funeral space, but when they get into the funeral space, they immediately take up the "mask" relevant to their roles. At the same time, the *sahwira* will shift from wearing the mask of the deceased (the half actor) to wearing the *sahwira* mask (as joker). It is these performative roles that allow the *sahwira* to testify to the life and will of the deceased.

At one funeral, the *sahwira* said, *"Dai Nyasha anga aripano izvezvi angadai akutoti handei kubhora."* (If Nyasha were here right now, she would has said let's go play soccer.) While wearing a football uniform (perhaps belonging to the deceased), the *sahwira* subsequently began a dance simulating a footballer kicking a ball. In this manner, we observe that the *sahwira*'s act has assumed the role of a joker and a facilitator. The joker is arbitrating the will and testament of the deceased, in the interest of the deceased's family. Ideally, this also serves to facilitate healing and restoration in the family of the deceased, since issues of inheritance are potentially contentious. It can be argued therefore that, through the *sahwira*'s role of joker-facilitator, the deceased, who is physically embodied and represented in the *sahwira*, is enabled to rework the past for the present and future. In other words, the *sahwira* character reconstructs the past, through the use of signs and conventions, for the purpose of sharing realistic memories of the deceased; and through this process thereby creating an ideology around the life of the deceased. On the other hand, the family can then transact meaning out of that performance and (re)negotiate their standing relationship with the deceased. In this manner, while the life of the deceased is being validated, the grief of the grieving person is also validated as a means to achieve healing.

Conclusion

This chapter has demonstrated how the transformation of the funeral home space makes room for the symbolic performance of the *sahwira*, with a fluid audience-performer relationship, thereby setting the context for people to share and witness the memories of the deceased. The process of sharing memories validates the life of the deceased as well as healing grief. The performance of the *sahwira* has also been described and analysed, not as a world of make believe; but rather, a presentation of everyday life, using everyday symbols and codes. The *sahwira* comes across as a dramatist, storyteller, and half actor; at certain times playing himself (or herself) as friend of the deceased, and also role playing the life stories of the deceased. In such an act, the *sahwira* assumes the character of the deceased and presents everyday scenarios which portray lived realities and shared memories. The role play by the *sahwira* has been shown as having symbolic elements that provide room for embodiment, sharing of memories, reflection on lived realities, and finally prompting the grieving towards transformation. This presumably has a cathartic effect on the grieving persons, such as Aristotle's catharsis in Greek tragedy. The funeral site can, therefore, be deemed as a place of tragedy in the Aristotelian sense; however, in the African worldview, it is a rite of passage which exudes transformative abilities. The pain of the bereaved is not just viewed as a loss, but as a necessary and progressive transition in life. Further, the *sahwira* institution offers a valuable model for the national healing process. It is characterised by non-censorship, truth telling, and commitment to relationships. It is a powerful resource that can be appropriated to promote national healing and integration.

References

Balme, C. 1999. *Decolonising the Stage*. Oxford: Clarendon Press.

Benyera, E. 2014. "Debating the Efficacy of Transitional Justice Mechanisms: The case of National Healing in Zimbabwe 1980–2011," PhD UNISA.

Boal, A. 1979. *Theatre of the Oppressed*. London: Pluto Press.

Bojuwoye, O. 2013. "Integrating Principles Underlying Ancestral Spirits Belief in Counselling and Psychotherapy. *IFE Psychologia* 21(1), 74–89.

Bourdillon, M. F. C. 1987. *The Shona People*. An Ethnography of the contemporary Shona. Gweru: Mambo Press.

Braund, M. 2015. "Drama and Learning Science. An Empty Space?" *British Educational Research Journal* 41(1), 102–121.

De Bruijn, M., R. van Dijk and D. Foeken. 2001. *Mobile Africa: Changing Patterns of Movement in Africa and Beyond*. Leiden: Brill.

Denzin, N. 2003. *Performance Ethnography: Critical Pedagogy and the Politics of Culture*. Thousand Oaks, CA: Sage.

Goffman, E. 1956. *The Presentation of Self in Everyday Life*. Edinburgh: University of Edinburgh. Social Sciences Research Centre.

Juma, J. O. 2011. "African Worldviews: Their Impact on Psychotherapy and Psychological Counselling," MA Dissertation, University of South Africa.

Kershaw, B. 1992. *The Politics of Performance*. Radical Theatre as Cultural Intervention. London and New York: Routledge.

Korpela, D. 2011. *The Nyau Masquerade: An Examination of HIV / AIDS, Power and Influence in Malawi*. Tampere: Tampere University Press.

Muchemwa, B. 2007. *Death and the Shona Christians: A Theological Analysis of the Catholic Burial Rite*. Harare: Catholic Pastoral Centre.

Muchinako, A. 2014. "Mental Illness and the Shona People of Zimbabwe, Some Key Issues," *International Journal of Advanced Research in Management and Social Sciences* 2(3), 161–172.

Mwandayi, C. 2011. *Death and After Rituals in the Eyes of the Shona*. Bamberg: University of Bamberg Press.

Ngugi, W. 1981. *Decolonising the Mind: The Politics of Language in African Literature*. Harare: ZPH.

Nyota, S. 2008. "The Communicative Impact of Shona Commercial Adverts," *NAWA Journal of Language and Communication*, 92–105.

Parker-Starbuck, J. and R. Mock. 2003. "Researching the Body in/as Performance," in B. Kershaw and H. Nicholson (eds.), *Research Methods in Theatre and Performance*. Edinburgh: Edinburgh University Press.

Rosenblatt, P. C. and B. R. Wallace. 2005. *African American Grief*. New York: Routledge.

Wrolson, J. 2009. "Re-Inventing Memory and Reforming Performances: A Genealogy of Panic Theatre in Zimbabwe," PhD University of Kansas.

10 Theatre, grassroots civility, and healing/reconciliation

A critique of *Heal the Wounds*

Nehemiah Chivandikwa, Kelvin Chikonzo,
and Tafadzwa Mlenga

Introduction

This chapter draws from *Heal the Wounds* by Stephen Chifunyise to examine how theatre design might be a site to foster grassroots/ society-centric civility on healing/reconciliation in political conflicts that result from the use of violence in political contestations. In essence, *Heal the Wounds* presents tensions in balancing between on the one hand, civility in dialoguing political conflicts/reconciliation, and issues of justice on the other. In this chapter, civility is understood in broad sociocultural and political contexts that include; equal dignity, justice, rights to disputation and free speech, and tolerance/respect in public political life. The foregoing aspects of civility are understood in relation to political contests/disputations and conflicts (Wagmore and Gorringe, 2019). More specifically, the chapter recognizes that civility does not only belong to elites in state and civil society organizations. The play under consideration presents civility from the perspectives of grassroots communities, as well as elite forms of civility. Political violence is a reflection of a crisis of incivility, because violence shows failure to manage modes of political contestations. In such a context, adversaries are treated as enemies (to be beaten or killed) rather than antagonists of the same collective political community (Mitchell, 2018). Extant works in Zimbabwe (e.g. Chikonzo, 2014; Chivandikwa, 2012; Mhako, 2014; Seda and Chivandikwa, 2016) are largely concerned with how theatre as an agent of elite civil society might reform the state and engender civility within the Zimbabwean political system. Sadly, in Zimbabwe, political contestations have at times involved uncivil practices such as vote buying, corruption, and political violence (Seda and Chivandikwa, 2016). However, this chapter examines *Heal the Wounds* (2009–2011) as a site for promoting grassroots or society-centric civility and healing. The study is guided by the following questions:

1 How and in what ways does the level of aestheticization in theatre design enhance or complicate the function of theatre as a site for advancing grassroots or communitarian civility and healing in Zimbabwe?

2 What opportunities and/or dangers are embedded in the use of theatre as site for dialogue on national healing and reconciliation in relation to political violence?

Recognising that theatre performances have both mimetic and analytical qualities (Wright, 2006), the chapter contends that theatre performances both reflect and (re)imagine civic engagement in ways that may positively inform desired civic interactions that may heal wounds emanating from political violence. The findings of the article suggest that given the right level of aesthetic investment, theatrical productions can create a public sphere that nurtures progressive grassroots civility that can complement/subvert existing state-centric forms of civic engagement and democratic practices in order to address political ills that saddle the Zimbabwean polity.

Heal the wounds: Context and overview

Whilst carrying out research on spaces of performance in Zimbabwe (see Mlenga et al., 2015), the researchers watched *Heal the Wounds* three times during the period in which it was being showcased.

The researchers mainly employed observations, personal interviews with the cast, director, playwright, and members of the audiences and video recordings of the play. Consequently, observation of the live event is the most crucial in examining performances, since a researcher watches as the interaction between the audience and performers unfolds. It is through this interaction that most of the reactions and responses can be perceived by the performers and audiences; for instance, giggling, laughing, shouting, crying, eating, drinking, commenting on what is happening, and so on. The researchers also observed post-performance discussion, taking note of the different comments and interpretations by the audience. Watching live performances has a high level of objectivity, since the observation is effectively external in a natural context.

Heal the Wounds was written by Stephen Chifunyise and directed by Daves Guzha (2009). Its plot focuses on the Zinyemba and Nyikavanhu families holding discussions on the best possible strategy that the Truth and Reconciliation Commission can adopt to ensure that it fulfils its mandate. Godknows Zinyemba, a counsellor in Harare who has been chosen to be in the National Healing and Reconciliation Committee, is married to Esnath Nyikavanhu. Esnath's brother, Adam – with whom Godknows has been at loggerheads because of their political differences – is now working together with him in this Committee. Headman Nyikavanhu has invited both his son and son-in-law to their rural home to discuss the issue of healing and reconciliation further. Godknows's father, Mr Zinyemba, is also part of the discussions.

The family's discussion exposes how the politicians have dictated the healing and reconciliation process, as well as the yawning gap between the politicians' proposed understanding of the healing and reconciliation process and that of the subaltern. The government, tradition, and church doctrine clash, resulting in a stalemate of ideas. Mr Zinyemba and Headman Nyikavanhu force their sons to write a list of possible ways of enabling healing and reconciliation. However, their sons destroy the list, as they believe it violates human rights and government policy. In the end, nothing is resolved. This ending of the play is an invitation to audiences to consider three fundamental principles. The first principle is that civility is not a preserve of political and legal elites (Wagmore and Gorringe, 2019). Secondly, the play suggests that in the Zimbabwean context, cultural civility is inseparable from political civility (see Mitchell, 2018). Third, official notions of civility can undermine justice for victims of political violence (see Benyera, 2015).

Realizing the complex sociocultural ideological conflicts in Zimbabwe, Chifunyise decided to use theatre as a platform for self-understanding and reflection on issues of healing and reconciliation in the country. Through this play, Chifunyise hoped to engage people on how best to compromise and meet at a "real" point of healing and reconciliation (Chifunyise, 2014 personal interview). The play explores complex socio-political issues that characterized the country's post-2008 elections. In March 2008, Zimbabweans went to the polls, which resulted in the Movement for Democratic Change (MDC-T) winning the majority seats in parliament and the senate. The presidential race was so closely tied that there was need for a re-run between Robert Mugabe of the Zimbabwe African National Union Patriotic Front (ZANU PF) and Morgan Tsvangirai of the Movement for Democratic Change (MDC). The journey to the re-run in June 2008 was characterized by political violence, with cases of murder, torture, beatings, rape, death threats, abductions, damage to property, the displacement of people, burning of houses, and intimidation of the citizens.

The "post" crisis was characterized by a policy vacuum about how the healing and reconciliation exercise was to be carried out (Thomson and Jazdowska, 2012; Mbire, 2011; Bratton, 2011; Makwerere and Mandonga, 2012). These scholars point out that even though the inclusive government created the organ for National Healing, Reconciliation, and Integration (ONHRI), there was rarely any action taken by this organ to address issues of healing and reconciliation. The shortcomings of the organ then provided an opportunity for grassroots models of community healing which, according to Thomson and Jazdowska (2012: 90) "represented a potential strategy capable of challenging the existing policy vacuum."

Society-centric/grassroots civility and theater in Zimbabwe

Chikonzo (2014), Seda and Chivandikwa (2016, 2013), Chivandikwa (2012), Mhako(2014), and Mlenga et al. (2015) suggest that as agents of civil society, theatre artists perceive that it is their duty to create conditions that can lead to the transformation of the state. Unlike the foregoing works, which critique state-centric plays like *Decades of Terror* (2007), *The Two Leaders I Know* (2007) *Good President* (2007), and *Final Push* (2006), the current study engages a play that has an orientation towards society-centric or grassroots/communitarian civility. A society-centric version of civil society questions "statism," (see Helliker, 2006, 2011, 2012) as it endeavours to build autonomous structures, "beyond the utilitarian logic of the state" (Helliker, 2006: 3). While in Zimbabwe it might be difficult to identify such autonomous spheres, we posit that some theatre productions wittingly or unwittingly advanced notions of civil society that are not directly linked to agendas of regime change or the reformation of the State. There are theatre productions that did not seek to lampoon state actors such as the president, ministers, and the military. According to Mhako (2014), these include plays like *Heal the Wound* (2009), *Rituals* (2010), and *Waiting for the Constitution* (2010). To the extent that these plays emerged out of the need to connect with wider audiences outside the logic of the state (Mhako, 2014), the chapter submits that they are oriented towards society-centric notions of civil society. An interesting complication about these plays is that they incorporate some premodern notions of grassroots/communitarian civility, bringing out an element of tension, since protest theatre is generally sponsored by neo-liberal capital. These nuances and complications will be interrogated in later sections of this chapter, where *Heal the Wounds* is discussed as a case study.

Design approach: local civil society and neoliberal ideology

Heal the Wounds represents a brave but complicated attempt to depart from liberal moorings that are attached to civility (see Wagmore and Gorringe, 2019). *Heal the Wounds* is a scripted play with design suggestions by the playwright, and these were modified by actors and directors, without a specific designer to design both the costume and the set. In other words, the play is a synthesis of realist Western aesthetics and indigenous collective approaches. This design approach reflects the tension between traditional/indigenous communitarian and neoliberal aesthetics. In short, then, the aesthetic "compromise" that is reflected in the design approach can be conceptualised as symbolic of the ideological compromises that theatre artists engage in – owing to the fact that, as an institution of civil society, theatre is largely funded from abroad.

In Zimbabwe, theatre design approaches are characterized by multitasking, emanating from a combination of ideological or deliberate need to subvert realist conventions or poverty. Ideological consciousness relates to the need to challenge Western aesthetics, which are largely realist and associated with neoliberal consciousness and aesthetic sensibilities. The major approach seems to be devising as opposed to scripted plays. *Heal the Wounds* is caught in between these two approaches. This chapter's interest lies in the play's association with neoliberal aesthetic approaches, which complicates its aspirations to articulate indigenous grassroots forms of civility.

Ironically, however, unlike some plays in Zimbabwe which adopt everyday objects as a survival strategy, *Heal the Wounds* had received substantial funding from HIVOS, an international non-governmental organization whose mandate is to promote humanistic values, equal opportunities for males and females, and encourage citizens to take part in decision-making processes that affect their well-being. This connection is important because it brings to the fore part of the tensions and contradictions that complicate the desire to deploy theatre to strengthen civil society in Zimbabwe. Given the unequal global power relations, is it possible to have a vibrant local and authentic civil society in Africa which is supported by Western donors? Here, we see how the connection between Western neoliberal organizations and the theatre institution in Zimbabwe, which has resulted in the state accusing theatre artists of being "actors" in the political sphere rather than the cultural sphere (see Chivandikwa, 2012). While this chapter does not want to uncritically embrace the concerns of the state, it interrogates some of the complexities emanating from donor funding that is linked to neoliberal capital. In most instances, protest theatre that engages the audiences on matters of democratisation has been accused of "fitting the bill" – that is being paid to use theatre to achieve the imperial agendas of Western donors at the expense of authentic empowerment and genuine civic engagement (Mhako, 2014).

Since many theatre artists survive on donor funding (Mhako, 2014), they often make ideological compromises when Western-based donor agencies fund local theatre productions. It is for this reason that some theatre critics have expressed the view that funded theatre can hardly be defined as grassroots initiatives or genuine social movements (see Mundrawala, 2009). More specifically, Scharinger (2013) contends that donor funding compromises the ability of theatre to contribute positively to peace, national healing and identity-construction in "Third World" countries. Donor funded theatre is thought to be compromised because it is "paid activism." Mundrawal's characterization of donor-funded theatre is particularly interesting, since he cites issues of commodification and dependence on market relationships.

In the previously mentioned context, Mundrawal posits that donor funding in Africa and Asia, depoliticises theatre. In Zimbabwean theatre, however, it has been noted that donor funding of theatre has an ambiguous/complex socio-political role, since the Zimbabwe political protest theatre space "has become simultaneously a site for domination and radicalism. It has politicised the spectators as it has been simultaneously depoliticised by neoliberal sensibilities" (Mlenga et al., 2015: 10). The previous observation means that the anti-state radicalism of political theatre in Zimbabwe in general is neutralised by the fact that the same theatre reproduces neoliberal economics and consumerisms (ibid.). In the next section, the chapter discusses how the neoliberal dimensions of *Heal the Wounds* reflects the tension between liberal forms of civil society and the communitarian values of civility

Representational costuming: tension between communitarian civility and liberal civility

This section demonstrates how theatre as agent of urban elite civility may unwittingly undermine rural forms of cultural civility in relation to respect and dignity of rural characters. The section will show how cultural civility is inseparable from public political civility. In this section, the chapter shows how the degree of attention paid to detail in costume design can lead to a situation in which theatrical codes communicate negative or unintended forms of civil interaction. While advocating for grassroots forms of dialogue on healing and reconciliation, initially, the play was mainly preformed among elite NGOS employees, intellectuals, and middle-class citizens, and it was not showcased among peasants and working class "ghetto" people in high-density areas, where ironically political violence was rampant. Realist neoliberal representation in costume design was tempered by exaggerating the everyday costumes that came from homes of performers. The chapter argues that this "mix" compromised and undermined grassroots sensibilities and ultimately grassroots forms of civility. In most cases, the audience ended up just laughing at the resultant caricatures. Representational costume design unwittingly caricatured rural people in ways which resonate with regrettable attitudes, misconceptions, and stereotypes on "uncivil" rural sociality among urban citizens – "converts" of neoliberal modernity.

To visually express Chifunyise's themes and motifs, the director of *Heal the Wounds* and the cast selected everyday clothes from their homes. As such, the costume used on stage retained the likeness to life. However, although the clothes adopted for use on stage had been taken from people's homes, various degrees of aestheticization were affected. The intention was to enable the audience to link each character with the different sociocultural beliefs and values being represented on stage (Guzha, 2009, personal interview). Headman Nyikavanhu and Zinyemba, for example, are elderly men who live in a rural village and represent "the people."

In the productions that the researchers watched, Zinyemba wore a multicoloured woollen hat, an old brown jacket, a green shirt, and multicoloured tie, grey trousers, and old dusty brown shoes. Tafadzwa Muzondo, who played Zinyemba, brought the multicoloured woollen hat, shirt, tie, and shoes from his old collection of clothes at home, and borrowed the old brown jacket and grey trousers from his nephew. The woollen hat was not worn in the usual way but pulled down to cover his ears. The shirt and trousers were slightly oversized, but the jacket was a right fit and its collar was slightly pulled up and the tie was wrongly positioned around the neck. Headman Nyikavanhu wore old, faded beige shorts, a long-sleeved, multicoloured striped shirt tucked into his shorts, brown socks, a faded brown cone-shaped hat, and black dusty shoes. Charles Matare, who played the part of Headman Nyikadzino, brought the faded brown shorts, stockings, and shoes from his old personal clothes. He borrowed the multicoloured shirt from his father's collection of old clothes and the cone-shaped hat from his father's friend. To aestheticize the everyday clothes, the performers wore them in an extraordinary way. One of the sleeves on Zinyemba's shirt was rolled up to his elbow while the other was worn full length. Moreover, his shirt was tucked into his shorts, whilst the stockings he was wearing were pulled up.

The manipulation of unrelated colours, textures, size, and the mass of the everyday clothes adopted as costume magnified/exaggerated characterization for both characters. The modification of the everyday clothes adopted as costumes for Zinyemba and Headman Nyikadzino exaggerated the way in which rural people dress in everyday life. The degree of aestheticization depicted the characters as simple-minded and backward – distorting the play's objective of empowering the grassroots to express their views on how best to achieve healing and reconciliation in Zimbabwe. Such caricature images of the "common" people can potentially cloud critical thinking and thus have a potentially disempowering effect on the emancipation of the common man. The resultant characterization antagonized and undermined rural forms of sociality.

Conversely, the everyday suits worn by middle-class characters such as Adam and Godknows on stage without any modification and exaggerations, became symbols of respectability, progressiveness, neoliberal modernity, and urbanity. Although the suits brought in for use as costume were intended to reveal the contrast in social status, they unwittingly celebrated the dominant class as superior, thus legitimizing their dominance.

Mrs Nyikadzino was also iconically costumed. She wore an Anglican Mothers Union uniform: A blue skirt, white shirt with a blue collar, a blue *doek*, and black tennis shoes. She also had a maroon *zambia* wrapped around her. Mrs Nyikadzino symbolically represented the Church (Chifunyise, 2014, personal interview). The Church, therefore, became a symbol of orderliness, peace, reconciliation, healing, and unity.

The representational costuming of Mrs Nyikadzino (played by Joyce Mpofu) constructed the Church as an "idealized" institution, endorsing it as the neutral platform for discussing the possible ways of achieving healing and reconciliation in Zimbabwe. The Anglican Church was amongst the first churches to be established in Africa during colonialism and had a great relationship with the authorities of Southern Rhodesia (Chennells, 1988). As such, the presentation of the Anglican uniform without any modifications associates the play with Western religious imperialism, since the Church's roots are in England. The costume visually presents Mrs Nyikadzino as an intermediary, as it is a symbolic outfit which signals assumptions that she is a bearer of truth, peace, and wisdom. During the entire play, she constantly intervenes when Headman Nyikadzino and Godknows have different views, calming them down and also making her "peaceful" suggestions.

Ironically, *Heal the Wounds* was performed at a time when there were deep tensions and conflicts within the Zimbabwean Anglican Church. Bishop Nolbert Kunonga, who had been asked to leave the Church, resorted to court action, and was given authority over the Church premises. This resulted in more in-fighting, and the forced removal of members who rebelled against Bishop Kunonga from the church premises. Bishop Kunonga was publicly involved in partisan politics that seemed to celebrate violence, while his rivals seemed to be conduits of Western neoliberal imperialism.

The chapter cites Bishop Kunonga as evidence that the Church itself has been compromised, and as such it is not neutral. In spite of existing imperfections within the churches, Mrs Nyikadzino who represents the Church's ideology in *Heal the Wounds* is visually presented as "pure." Clearly, here costume design uncritically celebrates Western religious values at the expense of indigenous forms of religious civility. The danger with this costume is that it could unwittingly reinforce notions of urban elite civility – and in this case, specifically dismissing the characters who have more substantive matters on civility, namely, that official and elite forms of civility can undermine justice for victims of political violence (see Mitchel, 2018; Benyera, 2015).

Although this was apparently unintended, the point still remains that lack of attention to detail in imaging and (re)-imagining social forces and characters in civic contexts can potentially distort and undermine possibilities of mutual civic engagement between potential partners. It is very difficult to imagine how civil culture can develop in Zimbabwe without a vibrant rural-based grassroots civil society. For this to happen, urban-based agencies of civil society need to create a space in which communitarian civilities are respected and nurtured. We argue here that notwithstanding the fact that the impact of performances on spectators cannot be easily predicted, such lack of attention to detail in design may perpetuate negative attitudes about rural sociality/civility. Further, rather implicitly and more broadly, this section has shown that as an agent of elite urban and official civility (Wagmore and Gorringe, 2019), theatre is not always consistently "civil" in regard to treating all political actors with equal dignity and respect.

However, while there were challenges in the realist costume design, the chapter argues that metaphoric set design valorised rural spatiality, and consequently, rural-based forms of civility in negotiating healing and reconciliation. The next section, therefore, focuses on how scenic design in *Heal the Wounds* promoted society-centric forms of civil society. The analysis is based on the notion that scenic design is a form of place-making where insurgent groups can create spatial sites of self-assertion and subversion.

Metaphoric set design: place-making and possibilities of society-centric civility in urban contexts

This section shows how set design valorised rural spatiality in ways that suggest that in rural Zimbabwe, the community, rather the individual, is the cite of civility, and how this spatiality in *Heal the Wounds*, prompted spectators to consider touring the play to rural communities. This in itself is a sign that, in the end, the play broadly functioned to challenge official forms of urban civility which in Zimbabwe, largely undermine justice for victims of state -related violence. To this extent, the play advances the notion that civility is a double-edged sword (Mitchell, 2018). Civic engagement occurs in specific geographical locations or places. Recent scholarship, however, shows that places have both physical and social dimensions, which are informed by and can simultaneously inform social consciousness and identity-constructions. Places, then, contain ideas and practices which can circulate to other geographical locations or places (Rios and Watkin, 2015). The concept of place-making has been developed to account for the complex relationship between place and social movements and socio-political consciousness. Place-making is the mapping, building, and inhabiting of a place in ways that can inform social movements or relationships that relate to identity-constructions (see Vasquez and Knott, 2014). This section, however, is more interested in the notion that place-making is an everyday human practice by which insurgent or marginalized social groups create social, political, or spiritual or aesthetic spaces in which to assert their identities or as a form of socio-political expression (Knap, 2014). Accordingly, theatre is a form of place-making because it can transform existing geographical places for cultural expression and community.

This section, therefore, examines how everyday objects adopted as set in *Heal the Wounds* negotiated and reflected the inclusive and consultative healing and reconciliation approach in this play. It interrogates how scenic design as an element of place-making transforms the urban space into a site that can accommodate rural-based communitarian elements of civility.

The everyday objects adopted as set properties in this particular play include three tree stumps, a wooden stool, a wooden chair, two banana trees, and a *rupasa* (traditional reed mat). *Heal the Wounds* made use of a plastic cup, a water glass, two *tsvimbos* (knobkerries), a pen and paper, a snuff box, a box with grocery items, and a *rusero* (winnowing basket).

The everyday objects adopted as stage properties in *Heal the Wounds* were arranged in an open space to resemble a rural courtyard. The full action takes place during the day, outdoors, in the middle of Headman Nyikavanhu's courtyard.

The courtyard had two banana trees at the far end of the stage. The trees were wrapped in a blue cloth, which was meant to cover their support and create the illusion that they had been planted on stage. In-between the stumps was a blue curtain that served as a door, marking the entrance into Headman Nyikavanhu's hut. There was a *rupasa* (reed mat) besides the blue curtain that served as a wall portion of the hut. In the middle of the stage was a tree supported by sacks containing soil, dirt, and small flower plants. The sacks were covered with brown cloth, probably to hide the tree's support material. Small amounts of soil were scattered around the tree at the centre stage. Three tree stumps, a wooden chair, and a wooden stool surrounded the tree at the centre. The stage properties were mainly brown and green in colour, depicting the African vegetation.

Overall, the stage properties had a great impact in establishing a rural locale, creating the mood and style of *Heal the Wounds*. The previously mentioned arrangement of the objects on stage was so beautifully done that as the audience sat, they could reconnect with African sociocultural values. On set, Mrs Nyikadzino holds a winnowing basket (*rusero*) with groundnuts in it. From time to time, she stops winnowing to eat a few groundnuts. Headman Nyikadzino, on the other hand, holds a cup of *maheu* (indigenous non-alcoholic brew) which he sips, pouring some on the stage floor, possibly to remove chaff that may have gotten into it. This creates a typical rural atmosphere, taking the audience through a rural experience through the interaction of objects, smells, sounds, and other elements, It is through the interaction of the everyday objects, bodies in space, smells, sounds, amongst other things, that such atmospheres are created in performances.

The stage properties thus helped to create an African ambiance, making theatre a site for the recreation and (re)-imagining of an African "past," and promoting the preservation and enrichment of African culture. In other words, the urban theatre space was replaced with "foreign" spatiality (see Rios and Watkins, 2015). This level of aesthetic transformation endowed theatre participants with new emotionality and ideological consciousness in ways that are not common in urban centres. The spectators could be seen talking, smiling, relaxed, and engaging in casual conversation that fostered relationships transcending the theatre venue. The spectators were more intimate, friendlier, and more convivial than they would normally be in other theatre contexts. For those spectators and artistes with a rural background, theatre was a form of creating a sense of place away from "home." Rural modes of sociality became a living reality, at least during the course of the performance. This is crucial because place-making has a double function: It develops consciousness of place as well as engendering a feeling of belonging in one's cultural mores (See Knap, 2014). In fact, this convivial atmosphere inspired some theatre practitioners who were part of the show's audience to organize theatre festivals on civic engagements in rural communities (Maphosa, 2014, personal interview). Here in the end, the play functioned to persuade audiences as members of urban elite civil society to recognize the need for collective civility. This means all communities are made of citizens of equal dignity, rights, and obligations to publicly express their views and suggestions. Hence the audiences agreed with the message of the play – to balance between on one hand, different forms of civilities, in relation to reconciliation, peace and healing and achieving justice for victims, and their right to publicly and privately seek compensation and repentance from perpetrators of violence, on the other. Evidently, the Zimbabwean state has failed to achieve this balance (see Benyera, 2015).

Conclusion

This chapter has demonstrated how theatre can reflect and (re)-imagine civic engagement in the Zimbabwean contexts. We hope to have demonstrated how the degree of attention to detail in design might impact (negatively or positively) on the ability of theatre performances to (re)-imagine civic engagement in ways that may deepen and enhance or weaken desired civil interactions in Zimbabwe. While acknowledging specific contradictions and complications that were noted, we argued that theatre can be a significant site from which civil society organizations may initiate processes that can create vibrant collective civil interactions that include both rural and urban communities in negotiating spaces for eradicating uncivil practices such as violence and the need to promote civil practices such as equal dignity, trust, and the complex task of respecting political opponents and the quest for healing and reconciliation, without compromising on issues of justice, right to express dissent, and seeking repentance from perpetrators of political violence.

References

Benyera, E. 2015. "Presenting *Ngozi* as an Important Consideration in Pursuing Transitional Justice for Victims: The Case of Moses Chokuda," *Gender and Behaviour* 13(2), 6166–6773.

Bratton, M. 2011. "Violence, Partisanship and Transitional Justice in Zimbabwe," *Journal of Modern African Studies*, 49(3):353-380.

Chennells, A. J. 1988. "Anglicans and Roman Catholics Before and After Independence," *Zambezia* xv(i), 75–85.

Chikonzo, K. 2014. "Identity and Democracy in Pro-democracy Protest Theatre in Zimbabwe: 1999-2012," D.Phil Thesis, Harare, University of Zimbabwe.

Chivandikwa, N. 2012. "Theatre and/as Insurrection in Zimbabwe," *Studies in Theatre and Performance* 32(1), 29–45.

Guzha, D. 2009. *Heal the Wounds*, Rooftop Promotions. Harare.

Helliker, K. 2006. "A Sociological Analysis of Intermediary Non Governmental Organisations and the Land Reform in Zimbabwe," Unpublished PhD Thesis, Rhodes University.

Helliker, K. 2011. "Civil Society and Emancipation in Zimbabwe," Paper Presented at the Critical Studies Seminar Series, Rhodes University, 25 May.

Helliker, K. 2012. "Debunking Civil Society in Zimbabwe and Most of the World," Paper Presented at the Critical Studies Seminar, Rhodes University, 5 October.

Knap, C.E. 2014. Planners as Supporters and Enablers of Diasporic Placemaking: Lessons from Chattanoga Tennessee, Cornel University, New York.

Makwerere, P. and E. Mandonga. 2012. "Rethinking the Traditional Institutions of Peace and Conflict Resolution in Post 2000 Zimbabwe," *International Journal of Social Science Tomorrow* 1(4), 1–8.

Mbire, M. 2011. *Seeking Reconciliation and National Healing in Zimbabwe: Case Study of Organ for National Healing, Reconciliation and Integration (ONHRI)*, Masters Dissertation, Hague: International Institute for Social Studies.

Mhako, D. 2014. "Identities of Women in Zimbabwean Protest Theatre," MPhil Thesis, University of Zimbabwe, Harare.

Mitchell, L. 2018. "Civility and Collective Action," *Anthropological Theory* 18(2), 217–247.

Mlenga, T., N. Chivandikwa, W. Bere and T. Mangosho. 2015. "Contemporary Theatre Spaces: Politico-Ideological Constructions in Zimbabwe: A Dialectical Approach," *Studies in Theatre and Performance* 35(3), 221–236.

Mundrwala, A. 2009. "Shifting Terrain: The Depoliticisation of Political Theatre in Pakistan," D.Phil Thesis, Sussex University.

Rios, M. and Watkins, J. 2015. Beyond Place: Translocal Placemaking of the Hmong Diaspora, Journal of Planning Education and Research, 35 (2), 209-219.

Scharinger, J. 2013. "Participatory Theatre, Is It Really? A Critical Examination of Practices in Timor Leste," *Australian Journal of East Asian Studies* 6(1), 102–119.

Seda, O. and N. Chivandikwa. 2013. "Theatre in Combat with Violence: The University of Zimbabwe Department of Theatre Arts and Amani Trust Popular Travelling Theatre Project on Political Violence and Torture – Some Basic and Non-Basic Contradictions," in H. Barnes (ed.), *Interrogating Drama and Theatre Research and Aesthetics Within an Interdisciplinary Context of HIV/Aids in Africa*. Amsterdam: Rodopi, 20–37.

Seda, O. and N. Chivandikwa. 2016. "Civil Society, Religion and Applied Theatre in a Kairotic Moment: Preliminary Reflections on a Project on Political Violence and Torture in Zimbabwe (2001–2002)," *Journal of Commonwealth Youth and Development* 14(2), 81–89.

Thomson, A. and N. Jazdowska. 2012. "Bringing in the Grassroots: Transitional Justice in Zimbabwe," *Conflict, Security and Development* 12(1), 15–24.

Vasqueze, M.A. and Knott, K. 2014. "Three Dimensions of Religious Placemaking in Diaspora." *Journal Network* 14 (3), 326-347.

Wagmore, S. and H. Gorringe. 2019. "Towards Civility: Citizenship, Publicness and Politics of Inclusive Democracy," *Journal of Asian Studies* 42(2), 301–309.

Wright, R. 2006. "Performing Citizenship Tensions in the Creation of the Screen," Unpublished DPhil Thesis, University of Georgia.

11 *Ngozi* spirits and healing the nation at the grassroots

Diana Jeater

Introduction

Healing the nation is not a new project for Zimbabwe. There have been many moments of national healing – most obviously, perhaps, in 1980, with then Prime Minister Robert Mugabe's conciliatory television address when he won the election; but also in 1987, with the Unity Accord; and again, in 2008, with the Global Political Agreement which was consummated in 2009 with the inception of the government of national unity (GNU) or the inclusive government. In between, there have been times of drought, political conflict, and economic crisis, all of which have led to calls for national healing. As an historian, I am interested in what "national healing" might mean and how it is differently understood in different historical conjunctures. Specifically, in this essay, I am interested in thinking about *ngozi* spirits, and how they are represented at this historical moment, in the conversation about healing. *Ngozi* spirits *force* people to reconcile, and raise interesting questions about whether coerced reconciliation can nonetheless lead to healing.

National healing is often thought of in terms of justice and unity: the nation will be healed when internal political, ethnic, or religious divisions are healed over. Normally, this requires some form of accounting and reparations for past wrongs. But as Ismael Muvingi, Associate Professor of Conflict Resolution and African Studies at Nova Southeastern University observed at the African Studies Association conference in Washington, D.C. in 2016, war is not over when *violence* is over, or even when some form of justice has been done. War and military horrors continue in people's minds long after the official end of hostilities, exacerbated for some by knowing too much about where the bodies are buried; and for others by not knowing enough (if anything) about where the remains of friends and family now lie. Healing, then, is also a process of addressing what remains in people's lives, and particularly in their hearts and minds, when the violence stops. There can be national unity, and even the active construction of peace, without healing. Healing also requires the resolution of trauma, which has often passed down across generations.

Secular and spiritual responses to national healing in post-1980 Zimbabwe

A key question, then, is what creates the conditions in which healing can take place? In the analyses of Zimbabwe in the 1980s and 1990s, there was a tendency amongst left-leaning academics, and those whom they advised, to say that national healing was about social and material matters. Peace could only come with the resolution of the sources of material and economic tension in society (Hayes, 1992). This argument was framed as a rebuttal to a prevalent form of liberal voluntarism – of asking people to be nice to one another – and it was important in drawing attention to real inequalities that were still to be addressed. It was neatly summarised in that quotation from Peter Tosh's song: "I don't want no peace. I want equal rights and justice."

However, this approach meant that peace and trauma healing were not adopted as central concerns by the new government. Instead, advised by a host of international agencies pouring into the new nation, the government's attention to the economy began to override a concern with either peace or justice. "Development" was to be the mantra to bring peace to the nation. Ministry after ministry added the "& Development" suffix to its name. The advantage of "development" as a goal, rather than "healing," was that it focused on the future, not on the past; it aligned with Mugabe's promise in April 1980 that everyone was now equally a citizen of Zimbabwe, united in a shared project; and it did not require old – and destabilising – injustices to be addressed.

Consequently, in the first two decades of Zimbabwe's government, there was no significant state-led conversation about "healing the nation." A discourse of "healing" would have required an acknowledgement of ongoing sores in need of a cure. Land redistribution was one such running sore; continuing economic dominance by the white community was another. In addition, there were economic and social issues around gender, sexuality, and generation that continued to foster tensions and violence in Zimbabwean society. And, very slowly, information about the Gukurahundi began to emerge in the public sphere, often presented (and misrepresented) in ways that nudged the long-standing political tensions between ZANU and ZAPU into ethnic tensions. Focusing on a national project of "development" allowed all these issues to be swept under the carpet, at least at the national level.

At the grass roots, however, people were still hurting. After the liberation war, researchers rapidly noted the emergence of spiritual rituals intended to heal the psychic damage caused by war. The churches offered exorcisms and rituals of spiritual renewal. Terence Ranger noted in 1992 that, "healing rituals developed in almost all Zimbabwean churches after the war" (Ranger, 1992: 705). Elsewhere, rituals rooted in indigenous spirit beliefs flourished. During the 1980s, Richard Werbner recorded the rise of *sangoma* rituals in urban Matabeleland that paid particular attention to messages from the dead, warning people against forgetting the past. Heike Schmidt noted *ngozi* and *chikomba* rituals in the Honde Valley, which drew attention to the forms of ongoing hurt

(Schmidt, 1997, 2013). The Catholic Commission for Justice and Peace testimony also noted ex-combatants troubled by *ngozi* spirits, who came to identify the families of those they had killed, to whom they should pay compensation (Catholic Commission for Justice (CCJP), Peace in Zimbabwe and Legal Resources Foundation (Zimbabwe), 1997). Pamela Reynolds discovered that many children were turning to traditional healers for help with postwar trauma and spiritual healing (Reynolds, 1990, 1996).

Ranger situated these rituals, both church and non-church, in a broader concern for national healing. It was not only troubled spirits of the dead, but the troubled spirit of the land in total, that had to be appeased – to be made peaceful:

> African Zimbabweans had a different relationship [from whites] to the land which they were fighting to claim as their own. One could fight for it, spill blood on it in a just cause, but thereafter both the fighter and the land itself must be cleansed. The customs and institutions . . . operating . . . to hold together rural African society, could be suspended during a guerrilla war but could not go on being suspended without dreadful cost to individuals and collectivities.
>
> (Ranger, 1992: 704)

In September 1992, there was an unofficial but widely-attended healing ceremony for the ZAPU war dead, at the Pupu shrine in Lupane, a site that also marks Lobengula's vanquishing of the Allan Wilson patrol in 1893. The ceremony became an event of national, as well as individual, spiritual healing, with interventions from mediums representing the voices of spirits commemorating the war dead going back even earlier than 1893. There were hopes that this would become an annual event, but despite the importance of the shrine in nationalist history, there was no further national spiritual healing there.

The state did not respond positively to these initiatives. While on the one hand there was a growing confidence in African culture, on the other hand there was a determination to be seen as a "modern" African state. Those demanding a public and national-level spiritual healing were at best disregarded, as at Pupu; and at worst, treated as hostile to the state. For example, Ambuya Sophia Tsvatayi Muchini, who established herself at Great Zimbabwe as a medium of Ambuya Nehanda in 1980, called for a national ceremony there to thank the ancestors for independence; and a separate ceremony to settle the spirits of the dead comrades and cleanse the surviving veterans. Her calls were ignored, her dwelling at Great Zimbabwe destroyed, and, as a result of the ensuing violent fracas, she and her underage children were all arrested and imprisoned for murder in 1981.

Moving towards African-based concepts of "national healing"

Undoubtedly, there is strong support globally for state-led, nationwide reconciliation and healing initiatives in African nations. But there are limits to how far these initiatives can use African healing systems. There are many indigenous mechanisms for community healing that long predate the European development of human rights and war crimes discourses (Mangena, 2015). Some of these indigenous mechanisms are "traditional" but not overtly spiritual. Some are about spiritual memorialisation, but not engagement with spirits as agents (Zambara, 2015). In general, however, attempts to seek a national *spiritual* reconciliation are problematic. They do not fit comfortably into ideas about post-conflict reconciliation, either within Zimbabwe or internationally. Spiritual rituals are not controlled centrally, which makes the state uneasy; and they violate ideas about "modern" forms of justice (Heal Zimbabwe Trust (HZT) & Zimbabwe Civic Education Trust (ZIMCET), 2016: iv; Karimanzira, 2013).

Indeed, the priority from global "post-conflict" experts, who are strongly influenced by Human Rights frameworks, often seems to be not so much "national healing," but rather some form of justice. The most highly-publicised examples of "culturally-African" state-led reconciliation programmes have been the Truth and Reconciliation Commission (TRC) in South Africa (1996–1999) and the *gacaca* community courts in Rwanda (2002–2012). The TRC was distinctively African in that it sought restorative rather than retributive justice. The *gacaca* courts took this a step further and used indigenous legal forums as well as indigenous jurisprudence. The TRC was a very centralised process, while the *gacaca* courts were devolved to a more local level. Both of these initiatives won international endorsement. However, neither engaged overtly with *spiritual* interpretations of harm or healing, despite these elements being so important to the people whose testimonies were being heard. (Krog et al., 2009, makes this case powerfully regarding the TRC.) In the eyes of the global NGOs, states and institutions that offer assistance (in funds and kind) for national reconciliation projects, spirit beliefs, and rituals are not the proper work of state governments.

In Zimbabwe, the 2013 constitution mandated a National Peace and Reconciliation Commission (NPRC). The title of the commission, "*peace* and reconciliation," was a significant change from the title of the *Organ on National Healing, Reconciliation and Integration*, a moribund body formed by the coalition government in February 2009. Nonetheless, the 2013 constitution lists "healing," and specifically "national healing," as the first two functions of the NPRC. So clearly Zimbabwe is in a new historical moment, a particular conjuncture, in which "national healing" has been recognised as a project that the state must define and facilitate. This is linked with, but should be conceptually distinct from, calls for truth commissions, national integration, or justice hearings.

Analysis of a conjuncture requires historical contextualising and an understanding of what is specific to this moment, even when it seems to resonate with similar situations in the past. What constitutes "healing" *at this moment*? What is "the nation" that needs healing? "The nation" can be understood in diverse ways. For international agencies, 'the nation' is often treated primarily as "the state." But the prevalence and persistence of discourses regarding ancestors, and unsettled spirits, suggests that "healing the nation" can perhaps be better understood as healing the *people* who constitute the body politic: the citizens, the residents, the *vana vevhu*, the children of the soil.

In other words, while there is a need for national-level initiatives, there is also a need for local acts of reconciliation and healing at the grassroots. Indeed, much of the violence associated with political struggles during the past two hundred years (stretching back to the times of Nguni invasions in the west and east) has been violence by neighbours against neighbours. National-level justice hearings can create community tensions that reopen, rather than heal, those wounds. Moreover, when state-led or national-level reconciliation hearings address community-level tensions, they treat them as a whole and do not encourage local acts of individual reconciliation between families and neighbours.

In the chiShona-speaking communities, local acts of reconciliation and healing often take the form of rituals to appease *ngozi*. Although *ngozi* spirits have routinely been described in ethnographic literature as "vengeance spirits," they are, rather, spirits that force reconciliation and compensation to take place. *Ngozi* intervene when an injustice or crime is not settled before the victim dies. Then the *ngozi* forces the family of the perpetrator to seek out, recompense and reconcile with the family of the victim. This is reconciliation without time limits: *Ngozi* will persecute the perpetrator's family indefinitely, across continents and generations, until justice is done through the payment of compensation and spiritual reconciliation between the families. The reparation and reconciliation heals broken relationships between individuals, families, and communities.

The ways in which *ngozi* cases have been understood and the rituals of reparation have changed over time and differ from place to place. The practices that healed in the past, such as *kuripa ngozi* (giving a wife as compensation) won't necessarily heal today, when both the meaning of marriage and the status of women has changed. Nonetheless, this does not make *ngozi* cases irrelevant to the present, an ahistorical myth. Rather, this is a system of community justice with a deep history and continuing influence. In that history, even if it is incorrect to describe them as vengeance spirits, *ngozi* are not nice spirits: they are angry and ruthless in their pursuit of justice and in enforcing reparation and reconciliation. Yet, as with all traditional systems, there is plenty of room for adaptation to contemporary conditions, without losing the fundamental principles of reparation, reconciliation, and healing (Vambe, 2009: 71). There are many reasons for paying serious attention to *ngozi* as a way to assist national healing at a local level today.

National healing beyond the state

One of the attractions of turning to *ngozi* to address longstanding hurts and injustices between families and neighbours is that it gives agency to all the relevant parties, in ways that state-led initiatives, influenced by European systems of justice and national reconciliation do not. As Everisto Benyera has observed, "transitional justice occurs in Zimbabwe without the involvement of the state" (Benyera, 2014a: 342). At the grassroots, there are fewer boundaries around the issues that can be raised for consideration in national healing. Official national healing initiatives are normally directed towards state-sponsored violence. *Ngozi* cases, however, can also encompass human rights abuses in civilian-on-civilian violence.

Moreover, *ngozi* reconciliation is not limited to addressing state-defined episodes of violence. *Ngozi* cases can, and often do, draw attention to cases going back decades and even centuries. They draw families into addressing many different forms of violence and injustice in the nation's past, all of which have been festering in the body politic, but many of which fall below the radar of national and international definitions of crises in need of "national healing."

Ngozi cases make a poor fit with concepts of Western justice, not least because they require a degree of belief from those involved in the process. As Fortune Sibanda puts it, "they can be undermined by the formal court system as lacking empirical evidence until the victim of murder 'fights his/her own war'" (Sibanda, 2016: 357). As with other grassroots and traditional legal systems, *ngozi* cases evade capture by the box-ticking categories of judicial bureaucracy. They do not create institutional paper trails, align with international human rights standards, or lend themselves to documentation (Heal Zimbabwe Trust (HZT) & Zimbabwe Civic Education Trust (ZIMCET), 2016: iv).

But *ngozi* systems have traction precisely because they operate outside state institutions. All those involved have to agree to the process before any healing can take place, and a traditional leader is often brought into the process to confirm that compensation will be paid. But there is no need to wait for a state official or NGO worker to pay attention to these grievances. Spiritual responses to national healing offer people at the grassroots an opportunity to take control of the healing process and initiate it for themselves (Benyera, 2014b).

The state is inherently flawed as a mechanism for delivering national healing and justice, when justice is conceptualised in terms of community, reparation, and spirits. European concepts of human and civil rights limit liability to individuals, whereas *ngozi* cases are both individual and corporate. European justice punishes offenders, rather than recompensing and reconciling families. It is punitive, not reparative. Imprisonment of war criminals does nothing to allay *ngozi* cases. Even public truth and reconciliation hearings do not address the need for reparation and spiritual reconciliation as part of the process. TRCs tend to require forgiveness, which is not the same thing as spiritual justice and reconciliation. *Ngozi* cases, by contrast, hold individuals responsible for their acts; but the communities of which the individual is an offshoot take collective responsibility for the reconciliation.

At the grass roots in Zimbabwe, then, there have been doubts about whether the National Peace and Reconciliation Commission understands the prevalence and significance of *ngozi* cases. As one person said to me: "Even the government knows that there are *ngozi*. But the person who has been given the task of National Reconciliation is sitting in the office. He doesn't want to go to Chipinge, he doesn't want to go to Domboshawa, to go and tell people that, 'okay, you've got *ngozi* in your family. Please unite as family members to solve this.' He's just typing on his laptop while sitting in an office in Belgravia" (Tapfuma, pers comm, 2016). National healing, as it is framed by constitutions, NGOs, the UN, and other mainstream organisations, touches only a small corner of the "nation" and its processes of "healing."

The state has been reluctant to engage with traditional, spirit-based mechanisms of national reconciliation and healing. Global models of justice, reconciliation, and national healing only permit certain types of rationality. Global ideas of citizenship, rights, and culpability limit the available points of empowerment in national healing. But the lived experiences of Zimbabweans suggests that effective national healing at the grassroots needs to be able to use multiple registers and to empower both perpetrators and victims to find healing as an expression of spiritual life that is both individual and corporate.

While trauma healing tends to focus on individuals, and state/NGO/human rights interventions tend to focus on communities, *ngozi* cases address individual, kin, and community as multiple levels of intervention and interaction (Vambe, 2009: 76; Karimanzira, 2013: 126–127). Because spirits are attached to individuals and kinship groups simultaneously, they allow a different way of conceptualising the social units where reparation, reconciliation, and healing take place. They require the individual offence to be acknowledged, but hold the larger community to account. Individuals cannot hide behind the collective, but neither can the collective wash its hands of culpability (Heal Zimbabwe Trust (HZT) & Zimbabwe Civic Education Trust (ZIMCET), 2016: 16).

Conclusion

As an historian, my interest is not only in understanding what *ngozi* meant in the past, but also what *ngozi* means in the present, and how ideas about *ngozi* are currently framed to address a specific moment in grassroots national healing now, in the 2010s. The secular "development moment" of the 1980s has been replaced by a more sceptical relationship with NGOs and a growing confidence in African culture. There is disillusion with both the state and the "West" as sites of justice, human rights, and national healing, alongside a massive turn towards "the spiritual" in the public sphere. The global academy is turning towards the decolonisation of its founding concepts, and African states are turning towards indigenous forms of national healing. In Zimbabwe, both the prophetic churches and the government (at least in the infamous 2007 "diesel *n'anga*" episode) are granting that spiritual forces may have material agency. In these contexts, *ngozi* forms of justice begin to find a place in the chiShona-speaking communities.

Moreover, *ngozi* cases address real concerns about how to implement national healing at a time when political conflict continues to simmer, when there is no trust in the impartiality of the state, and when fragile relationships between neighbours and within families could be ripped apart by focus on past episodes of violence, particularly if other episodes are not given equal priority. They are not bounded by state-defined limitations on what are relevant episodes or allowable evidence. They are not about politics, but about unresolved pain, which may be connected with political events but is not reducible to them.

Ngozi cases are not top-down, state-run, western-oriented justice; they are about finding ways to build resilience and deterrence in deeply damaged communities. *Ngozi* cases encompass processes of socialisation and resocialisation, as much as questions of reparation for injustice. Tabona Shoko argues that *ngozi* stories frame communal ethics in chiShona-speaking communities and make future violations less likely (Shoko, 2007: 42; also Heal Zimbabwe Trust (HZT) & Zimbabwe Civic Education Trust (ZIMCET), 2016: 16). In contemporary discourses, disrespecting one's parents is a cause of *ngozi*. Attention to patterns of socialisation and community controls can reveal how young men, in particular, become incorporated into violent enterprises (Beinart, 1992: 481). They acknowledge, as Western systems of jurisprudence do not, that individuals are embedded in communities and collective responsibility. By focusing on the suffering of perpetrators, rather than victims, *ngozi* cases emphasize that both victims and perpetrators are members of their community, and recognise the need to heal both.

For all these reasons, *ngozi* cases are also dangerous, unwieldy, and potentially unjust themselves. The challenge is not how to suppress them and replace them with more formal systems of national healing. It is how to turn this threat into an asset, and to help agencies to work with, not despite, *ngozi* beliefs. If external agencies take on this challenge, however, they should be wary of the dangers of Western taxonomizing and regularising/regulation, as happened with *gacaca* courts: "The mechanisms remain key in ensuring that justice is domestically rooted and owned by local communities for sustainability of peace and justice" (Heal Zimbabwe Trust (HZT) & Zimbabwe Civic Education Trust (ZIMCET), 2016: iv). It is precisely because spirits cannot be contained by laws and spirit beliefs are uniquely flexible as a foundation for justice that *ngozi* justice speaks to the present moment.

References

Beinart, William. 1992. "Political and Collective Violence in Southern African Historiography," *Journal of Southern African Studies* 18(3), 455–486.

Benyera, Everisto. 2014a. "Exploring Zimbabwe's Traditional Transitional Justice Mechanisms," *Journal of Social Sciences* 41(3), 335–344.

Benyera, Everisto. 2014b. "Debating the Efficacy of Transitional Justice Mechanisms: The Case of National Healing in Zimbabwe," PhD diss., University of South Africa (UNISA).

Catholic Commission for Justice (CCJP), Peace in Zimbabwe and Legal Resources Foundation (Zimbabwe). 1997. *Breaking the Silence, Building True Peace: A Report on the Disturbances in Matabeleland and the Midlands, 1980 to 1988*. Harare: Catholic Commission for Justice and Peace in Zimbabwe.

Hayes, Graham. 1992. "Violence, Research, and Intellectuals," *Transformation* 17, 74–86.

Heal Zimbabwe Trust (HZT) & Zimbabwe Civic Education Trust (ZIMCET). 2016. *Exploring Indigenous Transitional Justice Mechanisms in Zimbabwe*, Transitional Justice Policy Brief Series 1. Harare: Veritas.

Karimanzira, Edith. 2013. "A Conflict Within a Conflict: An Analysis of the Concept of Kuripa Ngozi with Girl Pledging in Conflict Transformation in the Zezuru Culture of Marondera District in Zimbabwe," MSc diss., Bindura University of Science Education.

Krog, Antjie, Mosisi Mpolweni, and Kopano Ratele. 2009. *There Was This Goat: Investigating the Truth Commission Testimony of Notrose Nobomvu Konile*. Pietermaritzburg: University of KwaZulu-Natal Press.

Mangena, Fainos. 2015. "Restorative Justice's Deep Roots in Africa," *South African Journal of Philosophy* 34(1), 1–12.

Ranger, Terence. 1992. "War, Violence and Healing in Zimbabwe," *Journal of Southern African Studies* 18(3), 698–707.

Reynolds, Pamela. 1990. "Children of Tribulation: The Need to Heal and the Means to Heal War Trauma," *Africa* 60(1), 1–38.

Reynolds, Pamela. 1996. *Traditional Healers and Childhood in Zimbabwe*. Athens: Ohio University Press.

Schmidt, Heike I. 1997. "Healing the Wounds of War: Memories of Violence and the Making of History in Zimbabwe's Most Recent Past," *Journal of Southern African Studies* 23(2), 301–310.

Schmidt, Heike I. 2013. *Colonialism and Violence in Zimbabwe: A History of Suffering*. Oxford: James Currey.

Shoko, Tabona. 2007. *Karanga Indigenous Religion in Zimbabwe: Health and Wellbeing*. Aldershot: Ashgate.

Sibanda, Fortune. 2016. "Avenging Spirits & the Vitality of African Traditional Law, Customs and Religion in Contemporary Zimbabwe," in Pieter Coertzen, M. Christian Green, Len Hansen (eds.), *Religious Freedom and Religious Pluralism in Africa: Prospects and Limitations*. Stellenbosch: African SUN Media.

Vambe, Beauty. 2009. "Crime and Deterrence in an Indigenous Law of Zimbabwe: The Case of Ngozi Myth," *IUP Journal of Commonwealth Literature* 1(2), 68–77.

Werbner, Richard P. 1991. *Tears of the Dead: The Social Biography of an African Family*. Edinburgh: Edinburgh University Press.

Zambara, Webster (Ed.) 2015. *Community Healing: A Training Manual for Zimbabwe*. Harare and Cape Town: Institute for Justice & Reconciliation/Peace Building Network Zimbabwe.

12 Media and healing in Zimbabwe

Millstone or milestone?

Stanley Tsarwe and Wellington Gadzikwa

Introduction

Zimbabweans have endured various phases of violence and injustices as the country moves along successive stages of the democratic transition (Benyera, 2014; Sachikonye, 2011). Article 26 of the African Charter also encourages governments to carry out an official inquiry into human rights abuses and to establish national institutions to protect human rights (Human Rights Watch, 1991: 1–4). While there is no particular prescription about the nature of the purported practical actions, there are many such actions, and these range from the establishment of special courts and/or together with Truth and Reconciliation Commissions (TRCs), the use of diplomacy, mediation by church groups and non-aligned groups (Svärd, 2010), as well as using the media to open multiple channels of dialogue with affected parties.

For example, in Rwanda, a popular radio programme called *Musekeweya* (New Dawn) helped supporting national healing in a population traumatised by the 1994 genocide through carefully crafted psychological communication messages that stoked ethnic conflict and hatred (Tanganika, 2013; Von Scheven, 2008). This Rwandan experience provides a classic case in Africa of how the media implemented a raft of mediation activities meant to heal communities of the post-conflict wounds and hatred. Combined with the popular *gacaca* courts,[1] these structures were widely acclaimed as ideal models for grassroots initiatives aimed at facilitating justice in a "bottom up" fashion. In Kenya's post-2007 violent elections that claimed thousands, media forms such as radio, television, newspapers, and pamphlets played a critical role in conflict prevention, and these have largely been seen as successful peace-building initiatives (Malakwen, 2014).

In Burundi, Studio Ijambo used radio to promote constructive dialogue between previously antagonistic groups, the Hutu and Tutsi ethnic groups, to promote dialogue, peace, and reconciliation. Its carefully crafted slogan "Dialogue for the Future," reflects an emphasis by the radio station to highlight areas of common ground, rather than sources of differences, among Burundians. The independent radio station produced about a hundred radio programmes per month in a continuous campaign to build peace (Malakwen, 2014;

Gilboa, 2002). There are, however, other strategies involving other strategies not necessarily involving the media. These include the Sierra Leone and South Africa's Truth and Reconciliation Commissions (Svärd, 2010) aimed at producing an impartial historical record of the conflict and atrocities committed against the civilian population by examining the history of the conflict through a victim-centred truth-seeking process (Sawyer and Kelsall, 2007).

We argue that in addition to the strategies listed previously, the media can also be key in linking various communities and stakeholders affected by conflict together in dialogue. We propose that peace journalism (Galtung, 1986) should now be foregrounded in the mainstream as a unique approach to peacebuilding in Africa.

A somewhat novel approach, peace journalism has been defined as a form of journalism that takes a moral standpoint wherein journalists offer solution-orientated, people-orientated, and truth-orientated reporting (Ottosen, 2010). Journalists can achieve this by making conflict transparent (as opposed to hiding it), and giving a voice to all parties affected by violent conflict so that they are "heard" without prejudice (Galtung, 1986). In addition, peace journalism focuses on the suffering – particularly on women, the aged, and children – and it names the evil on all sides of conflicting parties (ibid.). In a study on electoral violence in Zimbabwe, Tsarwe and Mare (forthcoming) deployed the notion of peace journalism as alternative to what they view as war journalism practices that seem to pervade Zimbabwean media particularly during elections. An opposite of peace journalism, war journalism focuses on masking war secrets, is violence-orientated, propaganda-orientated, elite-orientated, victory-orientated, and celebrates a winner takes all contest (as in sports journalism) (Ottosen, 2010; Galtung, 1986). While peace journalism may bring its own set of challenges in resource constrained settings such as Africa as it requires more training and research, we argue in this chapter that it could work as challenger ethos to mainstream journalism that seems to pay lip service to victims of violent conflict (Rodney-Gumede, 2015). As we argue in this chapter, media is an important resource for national healing and reconciliation in politically volatile societies such as Zimbabwe.

The different forms of conflict that Zimbabwe has experienced over the past decades require a media that – as highlighted in our definition of peace journalism earlier – takes a moral stand point to foreground past and present atrocities in the public sphere so that such topics are given more salience and cease to be regarded as taboo in Zimbabwe's largely restricted media environment. The media can bring divided communities together to openly express their concerns on how past atrocities need to be solved, as well as helping such communities rebuild a sense of shared community. It can provide a public platform for victims of political conflict to speak in their own voices on the complex array of moral, political, and legal issues that must be addressed so as to actualize the healing process.

But is the existence of media platforms alone enough to foster national debate and reconciliation? What media and what attributes of journalism can enable the growth of a meaningful healing agenda in Zimbabwe? Using Jurgen Habermas's (1989) notion of the political public sphere as concerned with "rational" public discourse that; in ideal terms, would be expected to yield consensus on public policy and matters affecting citizens, this chapter documents and analyses the conditions under which the Zimbabwean media has dealt with issues of national healing in the context of known historical atrocities such as the Gukurahundi massacres and the widespread political killings that characterise Zimbabwe's electoral history beginning in the 1980s. We argue that if the media takes the responsibility and initiative to discuss healing as a national agenda, there are prospects that potential future triggers of political violence can be nipped in the bud. Most importantly, emerging journalism forms such as Galtung's (1986) peace journalism may provide some answers to conflict reporting, even though – as argued earlier – peace journalism may potentially bring a set of unique problems due to its novelty in Africa as well as limited empirical cases of success. Basing on the construct's focus on making conflict transparent, while foregrounding the plight of victims/survivors – especially women, children, and the aged – the problem of "silenced" and marginalised victims in Zimbabwe may be addressed. In the section that follows, the chapter documents some of the major known cases of political violence in Zimbabwe.

Zimbabwe and the history of violence

Zimbabwe experienced numerous moments of violence dating back from pre- to post-independent contemporary Zimbabwe. Prior to colonialism in the 1890s, various Shona autochthons living in present day Zimbabwe were mostly hostile to each other, leading to regular episodes of belligerence (Benyera, 2014; Mazarire, 2010). The arrival from present day South Africa of the Ndebele under the leadership of Mzilikazi in 1834 only intensified rivalry in a society that was already conflict riddled (Benyera, 2014; Pikirayi, 2001). Post the 1980 independence, rivalry between Shona and Ndebele people was once more pronounced as the contestation over the control of the new government took an ethnic twist from 1980–1987 (Santos 2011). In independent Zimbabwe, subsequent political polls have been largely characterised by violence and electoral disputes (Tsarwe and Mare, 2019), further entrenching divisions in various communities around the country (Sachikonye, 2011).

According to Benyera (2014), most of the violent episodes experienced in Zimbabwe are known by their metonymic names such as *First Chimurenga* (War of Primary Resistance, 1896–1897), *Second Chimurenga* (War of Independence, 1965–1980), *Hondo Yeminda* (land reform programme 2000), *Gukurahundi* (genocidal attack perpetrated in the two regions of Matebeleland and Midlands, early 1980s), *Operation Mavhotera Papi?* (election related violence, meaning literally "where did you place your vote?" 2008) (see Ndlovu-Gatsheni, 2011; Diamond and Plattner, 2010: 346; Sadomba, 2011: 229).

These violent historical epochs have all been captured by the international media, and our assumption is that given the extent of these enduring politico-ethnic divisions, local Zimbabwean media has the responsibility to set an agenda for national reconciliation and healing within local public spheres. The assumptions made in this chapter are influenced by the agenda setting theory and its postulations that the media agenda can strongly influence public agenda, and hopefully, allow affected people to come together in open dialogue around unresolved historical violence such as the *Gukurahundi* massacres in Zimbabwe's Matabeleland and Midlands regions. In ideal democracies, the media can draw and sustain public attention to particular issues (Soroka et al., 2013) and as such, direct people's attention towards those issues with the hope of finding common understandings. That is, there is a strong relationship between elements made prominent in the media agenda and those that subsequently become prominent in the public's minds. The assumption is that the media has the responsibility not only to direct the public's agenda on issues needing policy attention, but also in explaining to the public the implications of government policy and on the other hand influencing policymakers on issues needing policy intervention and vice versa.

It is arguable that in the context of a prolonged sociopolitical tension in Zimbabwe, the country has not experienced an opportunity for meaningful healing from past violent atrocities, with evidence of widening tribal and political divergence manifesting during notable moments such as national elections (Eppel, 2006). When hints are made to publicly discuss political violence and national healing, these attempts either lack the commitment deserving matters of such magnitude or are mistimed and bear little relevance as topics of violence are mostly raised during political rallies. The effect is that communities with apparently different political and ideological positions continue to live in state of uneasiness while past atrocities remain masked in fragile silence (Masunungure and Bratton, 2008).

The public sphere theory and possibilities for discussing national healing

In classical social theory, the media provides a space for dialogue where citizens discuss matters affecting their lives, and in the process, opening up spaces for democratisation and nation-building. For example, through the notion of the public sphere – and even though this concept has successively been attacked for drawing exclusively on European bourgeois history while lacking empirical application outside of Europe – Jurgen Habermas (1989) argued that the modern media provides a space "where private people come together as a public" (p. 27) to address fundamental social, political, and economic problems. For this study, what is particularly important is the view that the public sphere is the vehicle through which public opinion and debate puts the state in touch with the needs of society (p. 31). As alluded to during discussions on peace journalism in earlier sections of this chapter, the idea is to have a media capable of unmasking and making transparent all matters in the public interest, including making it possible for victims of violence to openly express how they want past wrongs to be addressed in a participatory "bottom up" fashion.

In the section that follows, the study uses the agenda setting theory (Lippmann, 1922; McCombs and Shaw, 1972) to illuminate how the media can ideally provide deliberative leadership by placing national healing at the core of political agenda. By juxtaposing the public sphere theory and the agenda setting theory, we hope to show that in useful ways, these two theories can be articulated to advance arguments about the ideal ways that the media can take a leading role in critical national discourses.

Agenda setting theory: How the media can place national healing on political agenda

Because of their privileged position of narrating and analysing topical national issues, journalists can actively frame news in ways that shape our overall perception of sociopolitical and economic affairs of nations. By framing national healing as desirable for a healthy society, and by problematizing the successive emergence of violence during predictable political moments involving national polls, the media can put national healing as an urgent matter requiring commitment and allocation of resources by national political elites. Thus, relationships between the mass media, the public, and policymakers are at the centre of building democracies capable of responding to the real problems society face.

The agenda setting theory focuses on how the media makes salient arguments of particular issues affecting society and make suggestions on how such problems can be overcome. Again, and as alluded to by the peace journalism notions introduced earlier, the agenda setting theory's reference to "salience" (making issues noticeable or visible) can be opposed to "silence" (making things less noticeable or invisible). Peace journalism is a form of conflict reporting that seeks to make transparent crimes and atrocities affecting silenced victims with the view of allowing equitable redress. Thus unlike its arch-rival form described by Galtung (1986) as "war journalism" (a journalism characterised by war secrets), peace journalism strives to make war and crime secrets transparent and accessible for discussion by all affected parties. This way, the media agenda can set genuine democratic public agenda. Following Cohen's famous hypothesis that "the media may not be successful much of the time in telling people what to think, but stunningly successful in telling its readers how to think about" issues (1963: 13), the agenda setting role of the media demonstrates that increased issue salience by the media leads to increased issue salience for the public (Dearing, 1989). The assumption made by the agenda setting theory is that the media agenda has impact on the public agenda which – in true democracies – should necessarily translate to policymakers tapping into the same agenda to formulate policy and guidelines for administration. In the context of this study, we expect national healing to be a pertinent issue deserving media attention particularly in view of the psychological repercussions that violence is known to have on its victims. There is a body of scientific knowledge highlighting the social and psychological consequences of violence (for example see Dillenburger et al., 2007; Christie et al., 2001; Ruback and Thompson, 2001). Outside of candid discussion and lobbying for meaningful healing structures and processes, Zimbabwe faces prospects for a democracy masked in fragility, while the threat of widening social polarisation remains a reality.

However, it is imperative to append a cautionary note against an unchecked optimism on the power of media as an agent of healing processes, and indeed the ideals proffered by peace journalism. In numerous instances, the media itself has been accused of failing to perform the integrative role of bringing society to a common cause such as national healing, nor has it been known for consistently championing for peace. For example, research on the sociology of news and news values point to the media's predisposed affinity towards violence, drama, and deviance. That is, there is evidence that issues involving dramatic events, crime, or conflict receive increased potential for media attention (Shoemaker, 1991), than the boring, often lengthy, and slow-moving peace negotiation and reconciliation processes. Journalists and the media are attracted to the fast-moving pace of action and violence and as such are often given to captivating headlines that sell news. If the media is given to the caprices of action, conflict, and drama, it is less likely to genuinely champion for peace without necessarily disrupting the very foundation of news values where drama, intrigue, and oddity are central. Arguably, this study posits that the Zimbabwean media would not likely be immune to the lure of violence as research elsewhere has shown, but despite the seemingly intractable lure for conflict, a responsible journalism is possible.

Research questions and methods

This chapter answers the following research questions: (1) In moments of violence such as during national elections, has the Zimbabwean media framed violence as a crisis needing urgent national attention?, (2) What conditions are necessary for the media to lead an agenda-setting role on national healing? To access data on how the media treats violent during moments of conflict and if it attempts to set a conciliatory agenda, the study conducted key informant interviews with civil society representatives, media workers (editors and journalists), as well as selected heads of quasi-government bodies whose work is broadly within or affect the media and human rights.

Findings

Framing violence in conflict moments: Political polarisation pervades the media and society

One of the research question probes whether during moments of violence and conflict the Zimbabwean media has been able to put healing and reconciliation on its agenda. The general sentiments expressed during research interviews was that the intractable political polarisation in the country has inevitably resulted in a media that is polarised along party allegiances, making it unable to name evil perpetrated by the party it endears. We argue that such allegiances are tantamount to subtle and overt media capture, with the result that Zimbabwean media is incapable of providing a space for genuine public dialogue. The polarised nature of the Zimbabwean media along political lines has greatly undermined the role of the media in championing an agenda for promoting national healing especially during elections as the private and public media assume the role akin to extensions of commissariat departments of political parties. Instead of highlighting peace and national healing, media reportage has tended to inflame the already volatile political environment in a bid to show the extent to which either side of the political divide has engaged in political violence. Usually, these commiserating tendencies become heightened during elections as the media follow political parties into the trenches as they engage in hate mongering battles. Instead of de-escalating conflict by toning down on hate speech, Zimbabwean media become co-opted into violence-oriented forms of journalism by regurgitating hate speech and divisive language spread by politicians.

As noted in the 2004 Information and Media Panel of Inquiry (IMPI), polarisation of the media along political lines has greatly affected the operation of Zimbabwean media and continue to undermine the media's role as the fourth estate across all the news genres. During interviews, an editor from a privately owned newspaper posited that:

> In our case, the polarisation existing in our media is an offshoot of the polarisation in our national politics . . . (We) have divergence of political attitudes to ideological extremes; principally between ZANU PF and the Movement for Democratic Change.
>
> Movement for Democratic Change (MDC)

These sentiments agree with what most informants said concerning the ability of the media to set an agenda for reconciliation and national healing in Zimbabwe, arguing that they are part of the process that is exacerbating rather than reducing tension in society. Because of the political polarisation that has infiltrated in all permeated sections of society, the Zimbabwean media mirrors the deep divisions along political lines in the country.

Because of protracted years of political conflict Zimbabwe has never recovered from tensions that run along both tribal and political divides. Tribal and political divisions are the crevices along which political violence continue to recur during moments such as elections when ideological contest spills into predictable anger and hatred against perceived enemies. For example, during the 2018 Commission of Inquiry into the shooting and death of civilians on 1 August 2018 in the aftermath of the 2018 Harmonised Elections, those who took the podium to give evidence to the Commission of Inquiry were clearly blinded by political biases even when only facts about what happened on the day of the shooting where the basis of the inquiry.

The testimonies from witnesses followed political lines to the extent that all the evidence on the same incident produced completely different facts. Zimbabwe has thus gravitated into a politically fractured society and the increasing political and social polarisation is only reflective of past human rights abuses which have not been resolved for decades. Furthermore, the violent disruption of the 2018 Commission of Inquiry in Bulawayo (Zimbabwe's second largest located in a region where the 1980 Gukurahundi atrocities were committed) by activists who questioned the logic of setting up an inquiry over the death of six people while nothing was done to the thousands who were killed during Gukurahundi demonstrates the extent to which healing of past atrocities remains hanging precariously and unresolved.

During interviews conducted for this research, one media academic noted that Zimbabwean media is actually complicit in fuelling conflict instead of being a means to promote national healing. He argued that the media does this by amplifying differences, especially between ZANU PF and MDC and also by being co-opted into the intraparty conflicts within the two main political parties in the country (Interview with a media lecturer 13/06/17). Furthermore, in a bid to attract audiences, the media are prone to publishing and selling the story of the "worst perpetrator" in an expository nature. In a recent research paper on media and electoral violence in Zimbabwe, Tsarwe and Mare (forthcoming) argued that Zimbabwean journalists reported the 2008 violent election as a contest by concentrating on the weaknesses of the so-called "loser" while amplifying the strength of the so-called "winner," further normalising the "winner takes all" tendency in African electoral politics. More generally, there seem to be no attempt by Zimbabwean media to foreground party policy propositions – issues that are arguably at the heart of any electoral campaign.

Rural-urban divide: Media and politicians reinforce divisions

Zimbabwean politics have for decades survived on divisions of the electorate on rural-urban dichotomies, with the main political parties (ZANU PF and MDC) harvesting on the different political consciousness and orientations notable between the largely elite urban population and the relatively peasant communal farmers. Notably, the media is also complicity in escalating divisions along these deep-seated divisions.

Interestingly, however, while the Zimbabwean rural population may lack a clear understanding of modern statecraft as well as the functions of modern democracies (these rural communities are largely closed off from the outside world and lack exposure to international trends through competing media channels), they have a firsthand experiential knowledge of the past atrocities perpetrated by the colonial regime, and are prone to manipulation by modern politicians (particularly the ruling party politicians) into succumbing to propaganda around the need to protect the gains of a protracted struggle against the colonial regime. Politicians know very well the political gains arising from manipulating rural populations by invoking images of the liberation war atrocities and packaging these together with coercion and intimidation during elections. On the other hand, the urban population may be relatively knowledgeable about modern statecraft and the functions of modern day democracy due to their relative exposure to alternative international media, but lack first-hand experiences of the atrocities perpetrated during decades of colonial rule as experienced by their rural counterparts. These fundamental differences in political consciousness are a major political dividend used by major political parties to divide and create targeted campaign messages. Given these widened ideological differences, Zimbabwean media and journalists find themselves caught between these divisive politics.

Untenable conditions: Fear, despondence, and the hushed silence

One factor that also limits the ability of the media to set an agenda for national healing and reconciliation is the fear that pervades the Zimbabwean society after years of systematic violence. Most news sources and victims are not willing to open up due to fear of reprisals. While it is generally agreed that the media is the "voice" of the voiceless – in this case, a society repeatedly traumatised over prolonged periods of political instability beginning with the unpopular British colonial rule through to decades of violent and disputed elections – the media have become targeted for "speaking" on behalf of the voiceless. A journalist who covered issues of political violence in reprisals in rural areas explained during interviews that it was very difficult to interview victims of political violence due to fear of victimisation. Some of the victims actually opened up to the interviews after the journalist made them believe that he was a government official (Interview with freelance journalist 04/12/17). This demonstrates the tension that exists in the society, and this is exacerbated by the fact that in most cases the perpetrators of violence walk scot-free and law enforcements agents – who are naturally compromised politically – take no action.

An activist with a human rights civic organisation noted that the media sometimes is not doing enough as it unquestioningly reports issues to do with violence mainly from an official point of view and then assumes that unity among political leaders translates into national healing (Interview with human rights activist 06/06/17). What is needed to promote national healing is to create other platforms such as a community radio station where people are free to discuss the issues so that meaningful healing and reconciliation can take place. Meaningful reconciliation can only be promoted starting from a grassroots level in remote villages where most people have no "voice" or means with which to access the mediated public sphere. Unlike in other democracies, the media in Zimbabwe is still very far from providing a platform for reconciliation due to polarisation along political lines and the entrenchment of sensationalism in a desire to attract readership in a declining economy.

Although the media stands accused of not setting an agenda for national healing, the restrictive media environment has also been a millstone in that attempts to publish stories on past atrocities such as Gukurahundi have met with unspecified action, mostly from government security operatives. Such subjects are perceived as a threat to the existence of the political elites who have remained in power and are largely blamed for perpetrating the atrocities in the country's history. As has become known both in social and journalism circles, such subjects are viewed as anti-state sentiments or are interpreted as ideas meant to foster disunity in the country.

The Zimbabwean government has been able to silence and control the media from exposing sensitive issues and create an environment of impunity through what emerging researchers have called legal and extra-legal measures (Moyo, 2009). Zimbabwe's media laws have attracted criticism from activists and journalists for being notoriously restrictive, leaving very little space for journalists to discharge their duties without fearing arbitrary reprisals. Most importantly, Zimbabwean media laws force journalists to practice self-censorship, and this has the effect of discouraging investigative forms of journalisms where reporters are able to dig and expose sensitive issues, including atrocities that the state has perennially kept under wraps from public knowledge. A number of Zimbabwean journalists have been hauled before the courts under such charges as sedition, and while most of these charges have been dropped for lack of evidence, the chilling effect is that journalists stay clear of stories that may land them into unending legal battles. Notoriously restrictive and arbitrary media laws in Zimbabwe include the Access to Information and Protraction of Privacy Act (AIPPA), Public Order and Security Act (POSA), Censorship and Control of Entertainment Act (Chapter 78), the Broadcasting Services Act (BSA), and The Criminal Law (Codification and Reform) Act.

Conclusion

From the above discussion, it is clear that the deep-seated political polarisation which manifests itself in Zimbabwe's politics has inevitably infiltrated into media reportage. Zimbabwean media overtly reflect a bifurcation that characterises its politico-social environment. We argue that this has had a crippling effect on the role of the media in national healing as the government-owned media continue to clearly take a defensive stance on occasions when the government has been accused of failing to take corrective practical actions to curb political violence and hatred. On the other hand, the privately owned media has also become co-opted into political and ethnic skirmishes that further stoke polarisation and entrench deep hatred and tension in society. It appears that without genuine political will to comprehensively deal with past atrocities and human rights abuses by the government, as well as a genuine desire to liberalise and pluralise the media environment, the role of the media in such issues as healing and reconciliation may not be as effective.

In terms of promoting national healing in Zimbabwe, what is critical for the media is balancing the ugly past with the agenda of the new political dispensation that came in 2017 after the ouster of long-time ruler Robert Mugabe. Media can be critical in national healing through truth-telling, and this can serve as the bedrock of genuine social healing in societies experiencing violence and conflict. The media also need to be extremely delicate in its approach to national healing since it must report constructively with no subjectivities to avoid further polarisation in a society already fractured along political and tribal lines. The media should be truthful about past atrocities, while at the same time refraining from inciting retributive justice.

Lastly – and informing our suggestive and tentative solutions – more resources need to be invested in retraining of journalists in such specialised journalism forms related to peacebuilding. Earlier in this chapter, we introduced the notion of peace journalism as one possible means through which Zimbabwe can deal with violence and conflict, but most importantly, with healing and reconciliation in a context where matters related to political violence remain a taboo in national public discourses. For decades, past atrocities such as the Gukurahundi massacres as well as the now recurrent electoral violence have been denied genuine media coverage, with journalists seeking to foreground these issues being viewed as driven by rabble-rousing motives. Backed by the already existing constitutional provisions that created healing and reconstruction-related commissions, the media may have a real opportunity for generating the much-needed healing and reconciliation dialogue.

Note

1   This is a community justice system inspired by Rwandan tradition where "gacaca" can be loosely translated to "justice amongst the grass."

References

Benyera, E. 2014. "Debating the Efficacy of Transitional Justice Mechanisms: The Case of National Healing in Zimbabwe, 1980–2011," Submitted in Accordance with the Requirements for the Degree of Doctor of Literature and Philosophy in the Subject of African Politics at the University of South Africa.

Christie, D. J., R. V. Wagner and D. A. Winter (Eds.) 2001. *Peace, Conflict, and Violence: Peace Psychology for the 21st Century*. Englewood Cliffs, NJ: Prentice-Hall.

Cohen, Bernard. 1963. *The Press and Foreign Policy*. Princeton, NJ: Princeton University Press.

Dearing, James W. 1989. "Setting the Polling Agenda for the Issue of AIDS," *Public Opinion Quarterly* 53(3), 309–329.

Diamond, L. 2010. "Introduction," in L. Diamond and M. F. Plattner (eds.), *Democratization in Africa: Progress and Retreat*. Baltimore: The Johns Hopkins University Press, ix–xxviii.

Dillenburger, K., M. Fargas and R. Akhonzada. 2007. "Psychological Impact of Long-Term Political Violence: An Exploration of Community Service Users," *Traumatology* 13(2), 15–25.

Eppel, S. 2006. "Healing the Dead: Exhumations and Reburials as a Truth Telling and Peace Building Activity in Rural Zimbabwe," in T. Borer (ed.), *Truth Telling and Pacee Building in Pots Conflict Societies*. Notre Dame: University of Notre Dame Press.

Galtung, J. 1986. "On the Role of the Media in Worldwide Security and Peace," in T. Varis (ed.), *Peace and Communication*. Costa Rica: Universidad para la Paz.

Gilboa, E. 2002. *Media and Conflict: Framing Issues, Making Policy, Shaping Opinions*. Ardsley, NY: Transnational Publishers Inc.

Gunaratne, Shelton A. 2003. "Habermas, Public Sphere, and Communicative-Action Theory: Eurocentrism or Universalism?" A Paper Presented During the ANZCA03 Conference, Brisbane, July.

Habermas. Jurgen. 1989. *The Structural Transformation of the Public Sphere*. Cambridge: Polity Press.

Human Rights Watch. 1991. *Human Rights Watch World Report 1990 – El Salvador*, available at: https://www.refworld.org/docid/467fca32c.html [accessed on 29 October 2019].

Lippmann, Walter. 1922. *Public Opinion*. New York: Harcourt.

Malakwen, B. K. 2014. "Media Initiatives and the Promotion of Peaceful Coexistence Among Communities in Kenya," *International Journal of Humanities and Social Science* 4(11), 101–111.

Masunungure, E. and M. Bratton. 2008. "Zimbabwe's Long Agony," *Journal of Democracy* 19(4), 41–55.

Mazarire, G. 2010. "Reflections on Pre-Colonial Zimbabwe: c850-1880s," in B. Raftopoulos, A. Mlambo (eds), *Becoming Zimbabwe*. Avondale: Weaver Press, pp. 1–38.

McCombs, Maxwell and Donald Shaw. 1972. "The agenda-setting function of mass media." *Public Opinion Quarterly* 36(2), 176–187.

Moyo, Dumisani. 2009. "Citizen Journalism and the Parallel Market of Information in Zimbabwe's 2008 Election, " *Journalism Studies* 10(4): 551–567.

Ndlovu-Gatsheni, S. J. 2011. "The Construction and Decline of *Chimurenga* Monologue in Zimbabwe: A Study in Resilience of Ideology and Limits of Alternatives," Paper Presented Under Panel 109: Contestations Over Memory and Nationhood: Comparative Perspectives from East and Southern Africa at the 4th European Conference on African Studies (ECAS4) on the Theme: African Engagements: On Whose Terms? Held at Nordic Africa Institute, Uppsala, 15–18 June.

Ottosen, R. 2010. "The War in Afghanistan and Peace Journalism in Practice," *Media, War & Conflict* 3(3), 261–278.

Pikirayi, I. 2001. *The Zimbabwe Culture: Origins and Decline in Southern Zambezian States*. Walnut Creek, C: AltaMira Press.

Rodney-Gumede, Y. 2015. "Coverage of Marikana: War and Conflict and the Case for Peace Journalism," *Social Dynamics* 41(2), 359–374. doi:10.1080/02533952.2015.1060681.

Ruback, R. Barry and Martie P. Thompson. 2001. *Social and Psychological Consequences of Violent Victimization*. London: Sage.

Sachikonye, L. 2011. *When a State Turns on Its Citizens: 60 Years of Institutionalised Violence in Zimbabwe*. Harare: Jacana Media and Lobby Books.

Sadomba, Z. W. 2011. *War Veterans in Zimbabwe's Revolution: Challenging Neo-Colonialism, Settler and International Capital*. Harare: Weaver Press.

Santos, P. 2011. "Representing Conflict: An Analysis of The Chronicle's Coverage of the Gukurahundi Conflict in Zimbabwe Between 1983 and 1986." A Thesis in Fulfillment of the Degree Requirements for a Masters in Journalism and Media Studies Degree; Rhodes University, South Africa. Accessed from http://encore.seals.ac.za/iii/encore_ru/record/C—Rx1054028—Sphillip%20santos—P0%2C1—Orightresult—U—X2?lang=eng&suite=ru on 29 October 2019.

Sawyer, E. and T. Kelsall. 2007. "Truth vs Justice? Popular Views on the Truth and Reconciliation Commission and the Special Court of Sierra Leone," *The Online Journal of Peace and Conflict Resolution* 7(1), 36–68.

Shoemaker, P. J. 1991. *Communication Concepts 3: Gatekeeping.* Newbury Park, CA: Sage.

Shoemaker, P. J. 1999. "Media Gatekeeping," in M. B. Salwen and D. W. Stacks (eds.), *An Integrated Approach to Communication Theory and Research*, 79–91.

Soroka, S., S. Farnsworth, A. Lawlor and L. Young. 2013. "Mass Media and Policy-Making, Stuart Soroka, Stephen Farnsworth, Andrea Lawlor and Lori Young," in E. Araral, S. Fritzen, M. Howlett and M. R. Xun Wu (eds.), *Routledge Handbook of Public Policy.* London: Routledge.

Svärd, P. 2010. "The International Community and Post-War Reconciliation in Africa: A Case Study of the Sierra Leone Truth and Reconciliation Commission," *African Journal on Conflict Resolution* 10(1), 35–62.

Tanganika, Frank. 2013. "The Role of 'Musekeweya,' an Entertainment-Education Radio Soap Opera in the Promotion of Reconciliation in Rwanda," *Rwandan Journal of Education* 1(2), 55–68.

Tsarwe, S. and A. Mare. 2019. "Journalistic Framing of Electoral Conflict in a Politically Fragile Society: A Comparative Study of the Zimbabwean Weekly Press." *African Journalism Studies* 40(1), 19–35.

Von Scheven, F. 2008. "Rwanda Radio Soap Opera Casts a Healing Spell," *The New York Times.* www.nytimes.com/2008/01/04/technology/04iht-radio07.1.9024735.html (accessed on 19 June 2017).

Interviews

Interview with media leaders (06/13/17).
Interview with a freelance journalist (04/12//12).
Interview with human rights activist (06/06/12).

13 Remembering and healing post-colonial violence

An analysis of Christopher Mlalazi's *Running with Mother*

Josephine Muganiwa

Background

The chapter analyses Christopher Mlalazi's representation of the violence in Matabeleland in the early 1980s known as Gukurahundi in his novel *Running with Mother* (2012). The novel highlights the complexities arising out of the newly-formed state of Zimbabwe emerging from colonialism. The conflict is a result of these complexities, coupled with misunderstanding of the issues at hand. I argue that the same misunderstandings and polarisation prevail in present-day Zimbabwe and militate against healing and true reconciliation.

Introduction

Zimbabwe, as a nation, was born out of the armed struggle for independence from the Rhodesians who had declared independence from Britain in 1965. Central, then, are the political power struggles that shape the lives of the people in Zimbabwe regardless of personal political affiliation or indifference. Rafto-poulos (2004: x) notes that the Lancaster House settlement was determined by a series of national, regional, and economic forces that established the contours of the compromise that necessitated the policy of reconciliation announced by then Prime Minister Robert Mugabe in 1980. These forces have been well described by Ibbo Mandaza:

> Mugabe would have to begin the delicate task of nation-building in an atmosphere of intense suspicion and even hostility on the part of those he defeated at home; against the covert threats of military, political and economic destabilisation from South Africa; and with the pervasive threat of economic and political blackmail by the imperialist powers that had been the undertakers of the Lancaster House Agreement but were now seeking to keep the new state in line.
>
> (Mandaza, 1986: 42)

The quotation just mentioned shows that while the policy of reconciliation was publicly adopted and announced, its implementation was not an easy task due to the various power dynamics at play in the new state: Military, political, and economic. Priority was given to fostering economic ties at the expense of military and political reconciliation. That means that Zimbabwe's economy remained in the hands of minority whites and British companies which alienated the masses from the elite ruling class. The attempt to integrate the major political parties in the national army was marred by tribalism and led to the disturbances in Matabeleland (cf. CCJP report 1997; Alexander et al., 2000). Raftopoulos (2004: ix–x) argues:

> Thus, while the ruling party used the language of reconciliation to structure relations with the white elite and international capital, it deployed the discourse of unity to control and subordinate the major opposition party and the incipient civic forces.

What this suggests is that reconciliation was not genuine but a political gimmick to cull oppositional forces. Over the years more political parties and civic groupings were to become alienated from the state, making healing an imperative agenda if Zimbabwe is to succeed as a nation.

The *Oxford Universal Dictionary* (Onions, 1973: 877) defines the word "heal" as to make whole or sound, to cure a disease or wound. The figurative meaning is to save, purify, cleanse, repair, and amend in order to achieve well-being, safety, prosperity, and deliverance. This means that if Zimbabwe is to achieve national healing, there is need for the people that have been at the receiving end of violence and injustice to be restored to well-being. The relationship to the state that has been severed needs to be amended then we can talk of reconciliation.

While there are many incidents in Zimbabwe that point to the need for healing (MDC-ZANU conflict, Land Reform, Murambatsvina, Gender- based violations, including LGTB rights), this chapter is strictly on the depiction of Gukurahundi (violence in Matabeleland) in Mlalazi's novel, *Running with Mother*, and lessons that can be gleaned thereof in relation to national healing (see also the previous chapter by Muganiwa in this volume). The novel is Mlalazi's contribution to the debate on the meaning of the violence in Matabeleland and the way forward. Literature, by its very nature, is ideological and seeks to persuade readers to a certain way of perceiving reality. This chapter is, therefore, a literary analysis of the novel in the context of the national healing debate.

Gukurahundi contextualised in the Zimbabwean narrative

Before analysing the novel it is expedient that a brief background on the Matabeleland experience is given in order to contextualise Mlalazi's novel. It becomes clear what his narrative is alluding to, as literature works by presenting images that evoke meaning. White (1984) notes that all narratives are arbitrary and represent the author's views. Musvoto (2011) notes that such narratives are linked to the expression of power and identity as "discursive power is wielded by the dominant classes who authorize certain self-serving discourses and versions of history which dominate and even silence the narratives of the powerless social groups" (Musvoto, 2011: 181–182). State sanctioned sources have silenced narratives on *Gukurahundi*, except for cryptic statements such as defining it as a "moment of madness" or unfortunate (Eppel, 2004: 47). Barnes (2004) traces the source of the conflict in the manipulation of historical narrative by colonial historians whose texts were taught in schools:

> Portrayals of Shona-Ndebele relationships were manipulated during the colonial era in order to divide and rule . . . The colonially-propagated narrative was that, in the 19th century, defenceless Shona peoples were attacked by the fierce Ndebele warriors coming from the south, who fleeing the wrath of Shaka Zulu, crossed the Limpopo and proceeded to raid for cattle, women and land. Raids continued until the pioneer column arrived in the 1890s and put an end to this oppression. In the colonial version, then, the Shona are disorganised weaklings; the Ndebele are mindless militaristic bullies, while the enlightened white settlers and the British South Africa Company bring peace, order, God and the Union Jack.
>
> (Barnes, 2004: 142)

The Ndebeles are portrayed as the savage foreigner who victimises the Shona who are then rescued by the colonial powers. Hostility between the two ethnic groups is, thus, projected as natural. The same narratives were disseminated through Shona literature churned out by the Rhodesian Literature Bureau. Such narratives become the basis of later divisions along tribal lines promoted by those with discursive power, though it contradicted the truth on the ground. The following quotation best describes the situation;

> The rift in the nationalist movement was seized upon by the propagandists, who attempted to fit the split neatly into their "tribally"-divided model. In fact, the break away from the Zimbabwe African People's Union (ZAPU) in 1963 and the formation of the Zimbabwe African National Union (ZANU) was not a purely ethnic squabble, but a rejection of the conciliatory policies then endorsed by ZAPU's leadership. ZAPU was not a movement exclusively supported by Ndebele speakers, but included large numbers of people who spoke Shona dialects. ZAPU leader Joshua Nkomo was inaccurately stereotyped as Ndebele, although he is Kalanga – a Shona sub-group which has close cultural affinities with the Ndebele. Similarly, the Ndebele-speakers among ZANU's leaders and soldiers were also conveniently overlooked by analysts who saw only "tribally"-based divisions straining the Patriotic Front alliance.
>
> (Frederickse quoted in Barnes, 2004: 143)

Such narratives led to the collating of identity of dissidents as "Ndebeles" and the indiscriminate killing of people in Matabeleland and the Midlands by the

5th Brigade trained in North Korea specifically to deal with the security threat posed by dissidents and the South African based Super ZAPU. Barnes (2004: 144) notes that:

> The Gukurahundi, as it came to be known, was a time (1983–1987) of many atrocities committed against a largely unarmed and already war-weary rural population in the south and west. Although largely a silenced conflict in the country at the time, it has now been identified as a shameful national episode.

Mlalazi's characters are ordinary people who are apolitical in order to widen the debate beyond the political parties' paradigm. The Unity Accord of 1987 did not solve the problem for the general apolitical masses who lost relatives and homes during this conflict. This has led to the formation of the contemporary Mthwakazi party that advocates for the secession of Matabeleland and Midlands from Zimbabwe on the basis that they suffered Gukurahundi that the issues have not been resolved. Mlalazi's narrative also debunks the ethnic myth of Shona-Ndebele dichotomy in the representation of the Jamela family, comprising a Shona mother, Ndebele father, and "hybrid" Rudo who is comfortable with her dual heritage, making her a true representative of Zimbabwean identity. The family is used to critique the polarised nature of Zimbabwean society which militates against healing and reconciliation.

Summary of the novel

Running with Mother is a story of Rudo Jamela, a fourteen year old girl who suddenly finds herself amidst violence she does not understand on her way from school. She is saved from sexual violation by soldiers because she can speak Shona. She then meets her mother on the way who informs her that her father has been captured as he got off the bus from Bulawayo where he works. Aunt MaJamela comes back from the clinic and informs them that everyone has been captured by the soldiers just after she had left and hid in the bushes. The three of them discover that the rest of the Jamela family members have been burnt and stacked in Uncle Genesis's house. They hear a baby crying and manage to retrieve Gift from an underground safe under the charred bodies. From there they escape into Phezulu Mountain with the hope to make it to the city. It is this escape journey that is narrated from Rudo's point of view.

Setting of the novel

The novel is set in Saphela area, Kezi district of Matabeleland South Province in the early 1980s. The language spoken there is predominantly Ndebele. Captain Finish in the novel is surprised to find a Shona speaker in the area. The author mixes fictional names for the place settings with real location so as to give his story a historical feel. The accounts recorded in the CCJP/LRF (1997) report are mainly from Kezi district, Bhalagwe camp and the events in *Running with Mother* are an allusion to this experience. Lang (2000), writing on Holocaust, notes that any representation is a shadow of the real experience and only gives the perceptions and versions of the author on what happened. They are therefore useful in so far as they give insight into the phenomenon represented. Saphela means "we are finished" and speaks to the massive killings that take place in the area. Phezulu mountain is both a place of refuge and offers vantage view of the village and mine below. The narrator is able to watch and report on the violence she has escaped from the safe place in the mountain. During the liberation struggle, the same mountain had been used as a place of refuge by the guerrillas and also facilitated meetings with the villagers for dialogue and strategizing. In this regard the setting evokes a sense of *déjà vu* on experiencing military violence, but then questions the value of independence if black people have to hide from their own soldiers who are supposed to be protecting them.

Narrative technique

The novel employs a child narrator who is assumed to be innocent and hence gives a detailed account of what she sees and hears without editing what can implicate her. The reader is also thrown into the story without explanations and moves with the narrator so as to fully imbibe the horror and trauma of her experience. Rudo Jamela's normal routine is disturbed within a few minutes and her life is changed forever by events beyond her control. She is forced to witness adults that she has looked up (parents and teachers) to being stripped and humiliated, consequently failing to protect her or offer meaningful guidance because no one really knows what is happening. Clues are dropped along the way but always accompanied by a critique of the underlying assumptions in the form of questions. On hearing that her father has been captured by the soldiers, Rudo asks,

> "Did father commit a crime?"
> "No. The soldiers said they're just killing all the Ndebele people, maiwee zvangu! What will happen to people like us, who are married to Ndebele husbands, [what are we] going to do?"

> (p. 17)

Rudo knows that soldiers are supposed to protect the people of the land and deal with criminals. It therefore does not make sense to her why her father should be captured and prevented from joining his family. Mother expresses distress in that the killing of Ndebeles affects her personally and hence the soldiers' seeming mercy to her because she speaks Shona is no mercy at all. This also dispels the myth that only Ndebeles were affected by Gukurahundi in Matabeleland. That makes the problem a Zimbabwean one rather than an ethnic challenge. At this juncture in the story, it is not clear why Ndebeles are being targeted.

After discovering the charred remains of Uncle Genesis and Uncle Francis together with their families, Auntie laments;

> They are all dead. . . . What did they ever do to anybody? And to die like this? Burned alive! (. . .) Genesis and Francis never did anything to anybody. Never . . ." Auntie wailed, but her voice wasn't so loud. "They were not dissidents, just simple people looking after their families and their livestock.
>
> (p. 24)

Auntie drops the next clue and the reader gets to know that the soldiers are killing Ndebeles because they assume that all Ndebeles are dissidents. This is the second myth that Mlalazi's narrative seeks to debunk. The irony is that Uncle Genesis built a safe in his house after being robbed by the real dissidents, which means he needed protection from the soldiers rather than the persecution he receives. Apart from the injustice of their deaths, they are denied burial and their remains are eaten by jackals. Auntie says it is a terrible thing that displeases ancestors (p. 30). This is another sore point that requires healing as African spirituality demands proper burial rites for one to be able to join the ancestors.

As the family escapes to the mountains they come across decapitated bodies floating in the river and narrowly escape detection by the helicopter hovering over them and commanding everyone to go back to the camp at the primary school. The full import of the helicopter and the camp is revealed in the cave towards the end of the novel when the naked teachers join the Jamelas so as not to be detected by the soldiers in a helicopter. Mkandla says that the soldiers are making neighbours kill neighbours and "forcing men to rape their neighbours' wives with their children watching (p. 130)." This is inhuman treatment and ensures spiritual death before physical death. The bodies are dumped in mine shafts at Saphela mine (p131) which is further desecration of the land. Rudo observes her mother's reaction,

> "Oh my Lord!" Mother put her heard in her hands, as if this was the last piece of information was simply more than she could bear. "Whatever's happening?" she whispered. Soldiers? Behaving like this? And why is the government allowing it to happen?
>
> (p. 132)

The questions serve to show that the soldiers and government are abrogating their duty towards Zimbabwean citizens as they should never be partisan. Mother's questions trigger a debate on what is really happening, revealing the different positions adopted by Zimbabweans. Mkandla represents the ethnic view in his insistence that Shona people are killing Ndebeles with the "permission of the Prime Minister" (p. 132). He fails to separate the offices of government and soldiers from the ethnicity of the people holding office at the time represented by the Prime Minister and Captain Finish. Mkandla's perceptions also reflect his lived reality in that he says, "How can I relax when Shona soldiers are killing our defenceless families?" Mr Ndlovu's argument is too abstract for him in the face of his empirical experience. The challenge is to convince the Mkandlas of the efficacy of national governance when they have learnt to mistrust government forces through experience. Mkandla's anger militates against meaningful dialogue and he considers retaliation as a solution. Unfortunately two wrongs do not make a right as highlighted in Mugabe's reconciliation speech;

> It could never be a correct justification that because the Whites oppressed us yesterday when they had power, the Blacks must oppress them today because they have power. An evil remains an evil whether practiced by white against black or by black against white. Our majority rule would easily turn into inhuman rule if we oppressed, persecuted or harassed those who do not look or think like the majority of us.
>
> (Raftopoulos and Savage, 2004: x–xi)

The irony is that Matabeleland massacres were precisely a way of persecuting those who thought differently without resorting to dialogue in order to resolve the differences. Mkandla adopts the same attitude as he declares that he never wants to see a Shona person near him and orders Mother out of the cave regardless of the danger he knows lurks outside the cave. This is also regardless of the fact that he has benefited from the woman's kindness to cover his nakedness and shame. Where the soldiers have caused his pain, the Shona woman has contributed towards Mkandla's healing but his anger blinds him to this fact. He is also cowardly in that while he hides from the soldiers, he victimises a defenceless woman and, therefore, simply represents the same genocidal tendencies as Captain Finish (Muponde, 2015). This shows that while national healing is an agenda, there are many impediments to healing that need to be considered and eradicated for national healing to be effected.

The ultimate effect of the narrative technique is to show that the Matabeleland experience defies logic and is therefore senseless destruction. If healing is to take place, the affected people need answers to questions posed and that can only happen through dialogue as opposed to silence or accusations thrown about. The Rwandan *gacaca* model might be good to follow as it speaks directly to the rural folk's personal experience as opposed to adopted Western models of constitutions and political parties that have been manipulated and used against ordinary people.

The family motif

Central to Mlalazi's narrative is the family motif to represent the nation of Zimbabwe. A sociological definition of a family is an intimate domestic group of people related to one another by bonds of blood, sexual mating, or legal ties. The Constitution of Zimbabwe outlines the legal ties that make all Zimbabweans kin regardless of race, colour, or creed. The government is responsible for regulating these ties. In *Running with Mother*, the women are convinced that the soldiers are transgressing because the prime minister is outside the country. They find it hard to believe that he comes back and actually sends more soldiers to terrorise innocent villagers. Mlalazi uses the Jamela family to represent his vision for Zimbabwe.

The marriage between Jamela and Mamvura is a rejection of the Mkandla/ Finish ethnic centred identity that militates against an inclusive multicultural Zimbabwean identity. Marriage by its very nature entails compromise and sacrifice. Jamela learns to eat mice with his wife despite the fact that his people consider it a mark of the inferiority of Shona people. Their daughter is called Rudo which means love, signalling that love must be given precedence in their relationship. When Mamvura is spared and told to escape, she waits because she is concerned about the welfare of her husband and household. She ensures that all survivors are under her care and they strive to survive. Similarly, when Jamela escapes from Mbongolo Primary he first goes back home to check on his family leading to his recapture. Mkandla and Finish are self-centred and think in terms of personal capacity rather than what others around them need. Mlalazi seems to suggest that patriotism must be marked by love for humanity rather than ethnic divisions.

Mamvura adopts Gift as her own son and nurses him. Her belief in the Christian God helps her to value life as a gift and to be hopeful in gloomy circumstances. She believes God watches over them and guides them. Mlalazi may be alluding to the role of the church in national healing as the Christian God will transcend ancestral affiliations and render the colonial narrative of ethnic hostility invalid as all humanity becomes one family under God the Father. This is clearly reflected in Mamvura (mother)'s prayer;

> "*Mwari wedu*," mother started praying. "We thank you *Mwari wedu* for keeping your little baby alive in the middle of a fire, and without your kindness this would never have happened. We thank you *Mwari wedu* for being our father when we are in need, and we ask that you show us the way to safety so that our children can live and grow up to be adults also. We also pray to you *Mwari wedu* to look after all the dead and raise your hand against all those who have sinned against you today. We ask for protection in this dangerous time, *Mwari wedu*, in the name of the son and the Holy Spirit. Amen."
>
> (p. 28)

There is constant reference to *Mwari wedu* (our God) which is inclusive of the survivors, the dead, and the sinners. Mamvura surrenders her destiny to God in a way that takes away the anger and enables her to think rationally and extend kindness to those who need it in the time of crisis. Gift is a symbol of rebirth representing Zimbabwe. He survives the fire in the same way that the nation of Zimbabwe has survived the multiple challenges. The prayer applied to the nation implies that Zimbabwe should transcend current challenges to be a great mature (adult) nation. By surrendering the right to punish to God, Mamvura opens the pathway to dialogue as she seeks way to promote life in the present. Mlalazi might be calling to the aggrieved parties to let bygones be bygones and concentrate on building new lives.

In the novel, Mamvura does not insist on rights but seems to always turn the other cheek. When Mkandla chases her out of the cave, she moves out with her children without protesting. Auntie who tries to fight back ends up falling over the cliff and losing her memory. Mamvura continues to take care of her, implying the nation must take care of its citizens that are no longer functional due to trauma. Where rehabilitation is possible it must be effected. Auntie fights for her sister-in-law, showing that Mamvura's attitude towards her persecutors may lead them to repentance and reconciliation in the spirit of Mugabe's speech quoted previously. Mamvura provides refuge for Auntie from her abusive husband and her home becomes a place for healing. In the crisis, she refused to buy into the ethnic discourse of the soldiers and continues to provide and guide the family to safety. Auntie is convinced of the goodness of Mamvura's heart and apologises for her own earlier discrimination. In this, Mlalazi seems to suggest that those who know the wrong they have done must apologise to ensure proper national bonding. The two women are related by marriage (legal ties), but have to go the extra mile of interpersonal relationship (dialogue) for them to be truly family and share the same vision (raising children to adults).

The current nation state is a colonial heritage, but its boundaries and constitution are binding to all Zimbabwean citizens. All groups must make the effort to understand and cooperate with others for healing and future sustainable development.

Conclusion

Mlalazi's *Running with Mother*, written some 25 years after the conflict in Matabeleland, highlights the areas that need to be addressed in terms of healing of the community. It is a historical novel in as far as it represents events that happened in actual life and is set in the region where the events took place. The story highlights the plight of ordinary people so as to reflect the folly of political ideology that fails to mirror the reality of the people. The violence in Matabeleland was a result of political machinations based on ethnic rivalry and resulted in massive killings of innocent people. The wounds have not been addressed and there is need to do so if the nation of Zimbabwe is to move forward as a truly multicultural society as represented by the bilingual and multicultural Rudo in the novel and the Jamela family in general. The healing must be holistic to encompass the psycho-social, political, economic, and spiritual lives of the affected. Only then can the alienated be reconciled to the state as full citizens.

References

Alexander, J., J. McGregor and T. Ranger (Eds.) 2000. *Violence and Memory: One Hundred Years in the 'Dark Forests' of Matabeleland*. London: James Currey.

Barnes, T. 2004. "Reconciliation: Ethnicity and School History in Zimbabwe 1980–2002," in Brian Raftopoulos and Tyrone Savage (eds.), *ZIMBABWE: Injustice and Political Reconciliation*. Cape Town: Institute for Justice and Reconciliation, 140–159.

Catholic Commission for Justice and Peace in Zimbabwe/The Legal Resources Foundation. 1997. *Breaking the Silence, Building the Peace: A Report on the Disturbances in Matabeleland and the Midlands 1980–1988*. Harare: CCJP/LRF.

Eppel, S. 2004. "'Gukurahundi' The Need for Truth and Reparation," in Brian Raftopoulos and Tyrone Savage (eds.), *ZIMBABWE: Injustice and Political Reparations*. Cape Town: Institute for Justice and Reconciliation, 43–62.

Lang, B. 2000. *Holocaust Representation: Art Within the Limits of History and Ethics*. Baltimore and London: The Johns Hopkins University Press.

Mandaza, I. 1986. "Introduction: The Political Economy of Transition," in Ibbo Mandaza (ed.), *Zimbabwe: The Political Economy of Transition 1980–1986*. Dakar: CODESRIA.

Mlalazi, C. 2012. *Running with Mother*. Harare: Weaver Press.

Muponde, R. 2015. *Some Kinds of Childhood: Images of History and Resistance in Zimbabwean Literature*. Trenton, NJ: Africa World Press.

Musvoto, R. A. 2011. "Rethinking History and Identity in Zimbabwe," *UNISA Latin American Report* 27(1), 181–194.

Onions, C. T. 1973. *The Oxford Universal Dictionary Illustrated*. (Little William, Fowler H. W and Coulson, J.) (revised and edited). London: Oxford – Clarendon Press.

Raftopoulos, B. 2004. "Unreconciled Differences: The Limits of Reconciliation Politics in Zimbabwe" in Brian Raftopoulos and Tyrone Savage (eds), *ZIMBABWE: Injustice and Political Reconciliation*. Cape Town: Institute for Justice and Reconciliation.

Raftopoulos, B. and T. Savage (Eds.) 2004. *ZIMBABWE: Injustice and Political Reconciliation*. Cape Town: Institute for Justice and Reconciliation.

White, H. 1984. "The Question of Narrative in Contemporary Historical Theory," *History and Theory* 23(1), 1–33.

14 The beauty of forgiveness

Lessons for Zimbabwe in conflict-transformation and peace-building from Chimamanda Ngozi Adichie's *Purple Hibiscus* and *Half of a Yellow Sun*

Ruby Magosvongwe

No victor and no vanquished.

(Adichie, 2015: 535)

Introduction

Chimamanda Ngozi Adichie's selected novels subtly dismantle high-sounding motifs, in problematising human individual foibles using intra-family tension-ridden relationships in Nigeria's post-independence – a subtle recasting of Chinua Achebe's *The Trouble with Nigeria*. In intricate subtle ways, Adichie explores the interplay of individual psycho-emotional violence with the massive repercussions that play out in the "group consciousness of a people" (Armah, 2010: 81). She places at the centre of her fictional family tussles within larger Nigerian national struggles, calamities, sociocultural, and religio-historical wars. Echoing disillusionment about post-independence maladies in Achebe's *Anthills of the Savannah*, at the core of some of the struggles that Adichie explores are desires to restore and reinforce pride in African cosmologies, indomitable cultural values, dignity, and self-worth that have been dislodged by a conundrum of cancerous colonial and neocolonial legacies. Using her characters, Adichie exposes the labyrinthine dangers of bottled anger arising from a diminutive self-worth, ethnic intolerance, and egoistic self-aggrandisement masquerading as philanthropy and patriotism. Going by Adichie's borrowing and reproducing the historical broadcast by General Philip Effiong just before he surrendered to the Nigerian (Federal) Armed Forces, her selected novels signify a couplet dramatising historical realities of post-independence Nigeria that should not be separated from their social and historical settings. *Purple Hibiscus* and *Half of a Yellow Sun*, thus, provide a historiography that subtly theorises the bedrock of conflict at individual, family, community, and national levels in Nigeria's post-independence.

The conundrum is not peculiar to post-independence Nigeria. Zimbabwe in particular, is similarly gripped with violence induced by political, ethnic, and religious intolerance, thereby calling for urgent need for dialogue, healing, and reconciliation. Rearing an ugly head earlier in the early 1980s but culled and capped with the 1987 Unity Accord between ZAPU and ZANU, ushering in UNITY Day that is observed annually on 22nd December, intra-racial tensions and conflicts particularly deepened, becoming most acute after 2000 between the ruling ZANU PF Party and the opposition MDC Party. Thus, Zimbabweans' story, like the Biafra-Nigeria case study that Adichie captures in her fictional narratives, calls for careful treading if sustainable peace and futures for all are to be secured and guaranteed.

Setting the premise

Purple Hibiscus and *Half of a Yellow Sun* expose the "greedy little caste" (Thomas, 2007: 157) – intellectuals, political elites, leading business and religious leaders, as well as other community leaders – grappling and striving to attain the best in life, play out the drama in Adichie's exploration. This "caste" influences the image of Africa that the international community eventually "sees" and relates with – "mutilated" public and private spaces showing Africa being a menace to any order. "The underlying truth" (Versenyi, 1963: 153) cannot be divest from individual consciousness/self-awareness, self-efficacy/self-worth, self-dignity, historical and cultural awarenesss, and self-pride that should give people sure-footedness in dealings with self and others.

Adichie foregrounds an internally haemorrhaging society that should be agentive in its own mending and healing. This is why the present article uses Adichie's theorisation of "The Danger of a Single Story" and its introspective approach:

> Stories matter. Many stories matter. Stories have been used to dispossess and to malign, but stories can also be used to empower and to humanise. Stories can break the dignity of a people, but stories can also repair that broken dignity.
>
> (Adichie, October, 2009)

The cultural centre and perspective from which these stories are being interpreted matters. Theorisation can neither be innocent nor neutral (Armah, 2010; Vambe, 2005; Mazrui, 2002). How stories are read and/or interpreted is therefore crucial. Freire (1998: 232), argues: "[T]he reading of the world precedes the reading of the word." In other words, what agendas and which/whose epistemologies shape the word that eventually encapsulates the story that the world eventually reads?

The writer-cum-reader should therefore be a questioner, an ironist. Monolithic theorising of experiences risks destroying innovative and empathetic readings into rigid attitudes, experiences, and sociological conditions undergirding relations with self, others, and the world. Ironically Adichie embraces her invidious role as writer and critic: "They threaten all champions of control, they frighten usurpers of the right-to-freedom of the human spirit" (Achebe, 1987: 153).

Purple Hibiscus and *Half of a Yellow Sun*, therefore, brazenly and candidly explore respective individual and collective insecurities from a multiplicity of angles, in post-independence Nigeria, exposing the brokenness of individuals, families, and society. At the core of these fractured identities is failure and reluctance to deal with anger, bitterness, contempt, envy, fear, hatred, resentment, self-centredness, and diminutive self-efficacy emanating from life-sapping experiences undermining release and regeneration. More apparently in *Purple Hibiscus*, using the Catholic-trained Eugene, father, husband, church-server, and financier, Adichie foregrounds savagery mercy of "aggressive individualism and triumphalism over others" (Asante, 2007: 141) that ferments "chauvinistic rationalism" (Asante, 2007: 145) and competition against self and others. In turn, religious bigotry and fanaticism, elitism, regionalism, and nepotism foment strife, spiritual sterility, fractured social relationships, diminished self-efficacy, domestic violence, cultural intolerance, and crass materialism. These labyrinthine dangers obscure realities from which people must carve sustainable futures for the greater good.

Labyrinthine questions about identity: Who am I? Why and how are we here? What is our destiny?

While cognitive intelligence and physical development can be learnt, emotional and spiritual intelligence are acquired differently, inculcated to help develop the whole person, but from a particular identifiable cultural centre (Asante, 2003, 2007; Shujaa, 2003). Theorisation advancing continual negativity about the self's human worth, vision and destiny, remains anti-life. This is why the quandary to rediscover self and recover emotional healing in *Purple Hibiscus* and *Half of a Yellow Sun* underscores critical historical and socio-psycho-spiritual awareness: "Brother, what are we? What are we black men who are called French?" (Oyono, 1990: 4), rising from slumber of "false consciousness." Because of dangerously poor self-knowledge, Eugene in *Purple Hibiscus* rationalises physical and emotional abuse of self, wife, and children: "Everything I do for you, I do for your own good" (Adichie, 2012: 196). Gowon similarly pleads reconciliation at the end of the Biafran-Nigerian war: *"No victor, no vanquished"* (Adichie, 2007: 535).

Eugene in *Purple Hibiscus* uncritically pledges his entire brutalised life at the altar of white Catholicism, snubbing his African cultural roots and its spirituality. Eugene suffers multiple deaths outside his cultural identity before his natural demise. Philosophically and spiritually, Eugene fails to relate with self, others, and the environment. Appiah (2005: 138) argues: "One's culture constitutes/contributes to one's identity . . . Therefore slighting one's culture, persecuting it, holding it up for ridicule, slighting its value, affects members of that group, [especially the individual's potential to flower]." Appiah (2005: 139) further supports how cultural identities intrinsically reinforce positive self-efficacy, citing

Margalit and Raz who put forward that: "mere common sense show [that] individual dignity and self-respect require that the groups, membership of which
contributes to one's sense of identity, be generally respected and not be made
a subject of ridicule, hatred, discrimination, or persecution." This awareness is
inseparable from people's humanity (Ndebele, 2009). True to the spirit of self-
preservation, the narrator in the Prologue to *So the Path Does Not Die* (Hollist,
2012: v) observes:

> Only a fool ... cuts down the baobab in her/his village and replaces it with
> the one from a neighbouring village. If the tree does not die, the shade it
> casts changes and the village changes forever.

The beauty of forgiveness: conciliatory route to self-affirmation and harmony

The multiple interwoven experiences that Adichie explores challenge readers to self-examine. The society cannot be different and inescapable from the
individuals who make it. For example, individuals' intolerant, resentful, abusive, manipulating, and generally unforgiving attitudes play out in the broader
society. Hurting individuals make up hurting and sour families that constitute
hurting and bitter communities, countries, and nations. This conceptualisation
undergirds Adichie's interrogation of instabilities leading to the 1960s Nigeria-
Biafra war in *Half of a Yellow Sun*, similarly informing Eugene's corrosive bitterness in *Purple Hibiscus*.

Despite exposure to similar corrosive elements, people make conscious
choices as evidenced by the antithetical paths taken by Eugene and his only
sibling, Aunty Ifeoma. Eugene, psycho-spiritually incarcerated and haunted by
the fear of "Godlessness. Heathen worship. Hellfire" (p. 211), severely beats his
only daughter Kambili to the point of almost losing her life (p. 210–211), for
staying in the same room with a sinner whilst on a visit with Aunty Ifeoma at
Nsukka University, and traces of affection for the same late "heathen" yet affa-
ble grandfather, Papa Nnukwu:

> The stinging was raw now, even more like bites, because the metal landed
> on open skin on my side, my back, my legs. Kicking. Kicking. Kicking. . . .
> I could hear a swoosh in the air . . . More stings. More slaps. . . . I closed my
> eyes and slipped away into quiet.

(p. 211)

Eugene's brand of Catholicism is anti-life and anti-African. His overzealousness
and over-ambition to save his family from sin to a point of coercion is self-
negating. Eugene's depiction demystifies the horrors and violence of foreign
and borrowed religions that colonised subjects imbibe out of intimidation and
psychological blackmail. The inability to accept self on one's familiar cultural
turf and to let go of so-called inadequacies results in self-consuming anger that

replicates itself in the multilayered violence, driving away those dearest to the victim. Eugene is driven by the desire to be recognised, acknowledged and rewarded, self-effacing and leaving him in the space/place that is in-between mired in fear, uncertainty, anxiety, and bitterness. Eugene himself a victim, harbours misgivings about the punitive religion that he holds sacred, yet scared to let go of it, and cannot admit it. His nervous condition appears to be a common outcome of miseducation. Mungoshi's *Waiting for the Rain* (1975) similarly depicts cultural-cannibalism: "I was born here against my will. I should have been born elsewhere – of some other parents," showing the "abyss of dehumanisation" (Sithole, 2015: 2).

His handicapped psycho-emotional ego unleashes the pain and bitterness on those more vulnerable than him in that they depend entirely on him for protection. The result is an insensitive psychopath subjected to more fear at the thought of losing his only daughter after the grievous bodily injuries that he inflicts:

> Papa's face was close to mine . . . I could tell that his eyes were soft, that he was speaking and crying at the same time. "My precious daughter. Nothing will happen to you. My precious daughter." I was not sure if it was a dream.
>
> (*Purple Hibiscus*, p. 212)

Further, the culturally sterile Eugene negates and desecrates the very source of his own life, a point that Papa Nnukwu clearly isolates as his son's tragic undoing. Papa Nnukwu's caution to Father Amadi before the latter's departure for missionary service in Germany: "Never teach them to disregard their fathers." This point separates and destroys families – "a streak of madness," for "it is not just the naked men in the market who are mad" (*Purple Hibiscus*, p. 173). Thus, Adichie exposes the pestilence of silence over the dismembering of the African psyche. Papa Nnukwu, an ordinary "heathen," challenges religious bigotry that has socially wreaked havoc. Amnesiac of "the nightmare of history" (Muponde, 2015: 97), Eugene paradoxically disconnects himself from the only ready repository and culturally-endowed agent "and retrieval of communal memory" (Vambe, 2004: 72) – Papa Nnukwu. Responsibility to weave and walk the path that nurtures life, psycho-intellectual and spiritual freedom, rests with individuals.

Purple Hibiscus exposes Eugene's propensity for self-annihilation through self-hatred, self-denigration, victimhood, bitterness, self-righteousness, anger, and non-forgiveness masquerading as propriety. Eugene lays blame for his seething pain and emotional incarceration on the missionaries. Yet, the choice to let go of past hurts and present injurious pain cannot be extrinsically imposed. Letting go cannot be a result of brainwashing either. Adichie's Eugene epitomises psychological self-sacrifice at the altar of emotional imbecility and moral darkness colluding to negate the self. His missionary experiences also show that a determined assault on a people's culture, values, and life principles deals stultifying blows on one's cultural pride. Ironically, Eugene's missionary saviours are themselves barren demagogues with festering psycho-spiritual and emotional wounds.

Eugene's wife, consumed with self-hate for her inability to defend her children against their abusive father's violence, her silence and inability to talk about her pain, leads to her poisoning and killing Eugene: "I started putting poison in his tea before I came to Nsukka. Sisi got it for me; her uncle is a powerful witch doctor" (*Purple Hibiscus* p. 290). The bottled anger, pain, and resentment manifest differently in both husband and wife, but the ultimate result is arguably the same – self-destruction.

However, Adichie salvages the negativity underlining her narrative through the conclusion: "A different Silence – The Present." Jaja and Kambili, brother and sister, typify the present and future solution to marital and domestic violence. Jaja and Kambili refuse to be crippled by their parents' self-consuming anger. They refuse to imbibe, internalise, and harbour death in their hearts, consciously choosing to take authority and control by forgiving both their wounded and maimed parents. They refuse to be prisoners of "the silence of when Papa was alive" (p. 305). The new silence is not suffocating, it gives individuals room/space to self-introspect and make informed choices of who and what they want to become, including the actions they should take to be whom they want to be individually and as a family.

Jaja serves a prison term, claiming to have poisoned their father, serving a prison term that their mother should have served. He realises they cannot lose both parents to bitterness, self-defeat, self-hatred, and anger. Further, despite the emotional hurt and losses, Kambili fights together with her psychologically wounded mother for "innocent" Jaja's release from prison. They are both released from the silence of their father's religious fastidiousness, a "disabling nature of patriarchal history" (Muponde, 2015: 97). In their conscious release from normalising the vulnerability of the post-colonial subject, they take moral charge and refuse to internalise religious intolerance, including its labyrinthine disempowering dangers. Jaja and Kambili symbolically memorialise forgiveness – the ability to transcend hurts and embrace peace. Kambili attests:

> I have not told Jaja that I offer Masses for Papa every Sunday, that I want to see him in dreams, that I want it so much I sometimes make my own dreams, when I am neither asleep nor awake: I see Papa, he reaches out to hug me, I reach out, too.
>
> (*Purple Hibiscus* p. 305–306)

Non-violence, readiness to embrace the human soul, self-acceptance, and forgiveness, then, constitute the best catalyst towards bringing about healing and oneness, despite the labyrinthine hurts of past experiences. In consciously releasing others, Adichie's characters therapeutically release themselves to emotional wholeness. Versenyi (1963: 99) buttresses:

> to harm another, means to injure oneself, for a man has to live a communal life for his own benefit, and the better his neighbours are the better he himself will live . . . Who would voluntarily corrupt his own life? For that

is what harming others means . . . Therefore, the wise man, knowing what is good for him, will necessarily be just.

Building on restoration and renewal in *Purple Hibiscus*, Adichie's *Half of a Yellow Sun*'s twin sisters and only siblings, Kainene and Olanna, representing Biafra and Nigeria, finally confront the sterility ingrained in intolerance, envy, and jealousy that plunge them into unproductive violence and self-negation. The couples, Olanna and Odenigbo, Kainene and Richard, and Olanna and Kainene's parents, typify encapsulations of marital infidelity and marital forgiveness wrapped in one. Olanna and Kainene, initially torn apart by sibling rivalry, finally consciously bury their differences and fight to preserve each other's lives during the civil war. For both, prolonged periods of bitterness, coldness, and avoidance breed emotional and psychologically- distressing pain to the point of individual numbness. Adichie extends these misgivings to "the pitfalls of national consciousness" (Fanon, 1967) that plunge Biafra and Nigeria into the 1960s civil war whose total carnage on the individuals and families can neither be wholly appreciated nor adequately quantified. The labyrinthine effects of ethnic, tribal, religious, class, gender, and regional hatred are evident in the compounded Nigerian internal tensions, bloody conflict, and crises characterising the civil war between Biafrans and other Nigerian ethnic groups who feel threatened by the Biafrans' prominence in government.

The position is not one of minimising the detrimental legacies of colonialism and/or oppression and slavery. Such extreme human suffering is undeniable. The problem is what individuals should consciously do to break "conceptual incarceration" (Akbar, 2003: 133) that blights their potential to soar and experiment with other regenerative possibilities. *Half of a Yellow Sun* challenges the emotionally, ethnically, and psychologically bashed characters to transcend ashes of egotism, intolerance, victimhood, and self-effacing debasement and circumvent negativities of any debilitating psycho-social, economic, and political environment.

The capacity to self-define, self-name, self-examine, self-explain, self-describe, self-decide, and self-determine (Hudson-Weems, 2004, 2012) without necessarily bowing down to excessive external pressures allows for release from indoctrination that until now accounts for sterility, infantilism, and emasculation of individuals. Self-naming, self-describing, and self-defining (Morrison, 1987) using one's own cultural binoculars and critical historical knowledge enables a knowledge construction that expunges fear and self-debasement.

Mda (2009: 31) argues: "The constant looking over our collective shoulder in fear of racist judgement of our conduct and performance has stifled the self-examination and self-criticism that is essential for community development." *Half of a Yellow Sun* goes beyond infantile whining that is self-negating. Olanna and Kainene consciously take responsibility for their actions, so do the two generals of Biafra and Nigeria at the end of the novel. Adichie further develops the motif she introduces in *Purple Hibiscus* through Eugene and only sibling, Aunty Ifeoma whose commitment is "*To restore the dignity of man*"

(*Purple Hibiscus*, p. 132). Rather than heap accusations on others, she adopts an *action*-oriented approach in her dealings with her brother Eugene's family. Aunty Ifeoma pleads: "This cannot go on, *nwunye m* . . . When a house is on fire, you run out before the roof collapses on your head" (*Purple Hibiscus* p. 213). Aunty Ifeoma advocates peaceful retreat in order to reflect, then advance to restore diminished lives and family ties. Eugene lacked this freedom: "to muster the courage to exercise one's critical intelligence in order to understand and change one's self and circumstances" (West, 2008: viii).

Using the West African Sankofa philosophy (Temple, 2010), intelligent readings of Adichie point readers to critical self-knowledge and critical historical knowledge as prerequisites for genuine self-renewal. "It is not taboo to go back to fetch what you forgot" (Stewart, 2004: 3). Adichie thus, "in part, [tries] to find the aspirations of [her] society . . . new ways of seeking understanding in the light of traditional values as they are confronted with the impact of modern values . . . [aware that] their society was not mindless but frequently had a philosophy of great depth and value and above all they had dignity . . . [that] they must now regain" (Killam, 1973: xiii).

"Sometimes we are angry because of our own helplessness": *Purple Hibiscus*

Eugene is a pitiable figure. He cannot "separate his thought from European thought, so as to visualize a future that is not dominated by Europe" (Ani, 1994: 2). This cultural domination, "is more subtle and its effects long-lasting . . . [killing not only] the body but [. . .] the spirit" (Wa Thiongo, 2009: 57). Eugene sees Europe and its doctrines inseparable from Africa's civilisation – "Do our people have sense? Will you pinch the finger of the hand that feeds you?" (*Purple Hibiscus* p. 96). Whites set the standard, showing "the penetrative capabilities of Europeans" (Mazrui, 2002: 23): "You would never see white people doing that" (*Purple Hibiscus*, p. 104). One wonders then, the kind of "truth" that Eugene, the sole proprietor of the local *Standard* newspaper, dares tell about Nigerians. For his "diligent contributions" through the *Standard*, Eugene wins a peace award from *Amnesty World*. Through him, Adichie satirises the whole concept of memorial awards, subtly exposing Africa's cultural holocaust. Behind the award winner and austere husband, father, and fastidious church deacon is a vulnerable/fragile being constantly desiring acceptance and affirmation. For him, taking part in the traditional *mmuo* celebrations degrades and tarnishes his self-righteousness. Nonetheless, the real reason is that Eugene fears that these familial ties threaten to take away the only human beings who are closest to him, who always "empathise" and give him moral and spiritual support for all his endeavours. Without their support, "things were destined not to be the same" (p. 209): "Mama told Jaja and me often to remember to hug Papa tighter, to let him know we were there, because he was under so much pressure" (p. 208).

What does this say about the post-colonial figure? How much "post" is the post-colonial in him? Eugene's vulnerability is sharpened by his inability to question arising from a mutilated self-worth and diminished being. Eugene cannot endure the thought of "a heathen being, [his father], in the same house as his children" (p. 181) and upon Papa-Nnukwu's passing on, he declares: "I cannot participate in a pagan funeral" (p. 189). Eugene tearfully scalds his children's feet in boiling water in a bathtub for showing affection for their late grandfather. He claims: "Everything I do for you, I do for your own good" (p. 196):

> He poured the hot water on my feet, slowly, as if he were conducting an experiment and wanted to see what would happen. He was crying now, tears streaming down his face. . . . "That is what you do to yourself when you walk into sin. You burn your feet," he said.
>
> (p. 194)

Eugene's Catholicism cannot compare to life-supporting pagan values personified in Papa-Nnukwu – gentle, loving, caring, forgiving, sensitive, understanding, supportive, and tolerant – emphasising "responsibility rather than right" (Patrick and Bennett, 2011: 227). "As members, one of another, people are expected to be mutually caring and concerned, in other words, responsible for one another" (ibid.) so that social integration and greater cohesion can make life blossom, knowingly subscribing to being "pieces of each other" (Gwekwerere and Mheta, 2012: 196). To this end, Papa Nnukwu defies the defeatism, and lives his life to the full – a fulfilled life. Conversely, the staunch Eugene dies a brutalised and bastardised soul. One does not expect such sterility from a "civilising" religion.

Cesaire (1972: 43) attests to Western sterility exuding from transposed alien cultures we see manifesting in *Half of a Yellow Sun*'s 1960s Biafra-cum-Nigeria:

> I am talking about societies drained of their essence, cultures trampled underfoot, institutions undermined, land confiscated, regions smashed, magnificent artistic creations destroyed, extraordinary possibilities wiped out.

Renewal and restoration of human dignity in *Half of a Yellow Sun*

How much of the "post" is the being in the "post-colonial" is a question posed in the previous section discussing *Purple Hibiscus*'s Eugene. The present section focuses on *Half of a Yellow Sun* delving into self-annihilating non-forgiveness. Adichie explores private enclaves and personal narratives that memorialise the 1960s Biafran-Nigerian civil war – its sacrifices, losses, pains, hurt, disillusionment, and dehumanising effects. Self-preservation rooted in safeguarding respective ethnicities' land/soil and cultural heritage, trans-generationally (Magosvongwe, 2013: 264). Abrahams (2000: 375) rightly argues: "For Africans . . . land . . . mothers all who depend on it for life." Similar to Abrahams's conceptualisation, for Adichie identities are not conceptualised in terms of abstractness or disembodied ideologies. Belongingness and identifying with Biafra's or Nigeria's cause galvanise individuals and ethnicities to rally with the military leaders for preservation and self-defence during the 1960s civil war.

Adichie exposes the dangers of ethnic intolerance, and arrogance that plunge whole communities into self-inflicted bloody penury. The defenseless women and children are the most vulnerable, an aspect also dramatised in the Boko Haram purges that Hollist explores in his debut novel, *So the Path Does not Die* (2012). Achebe (1990: 43) argues: "What we need to do is to look back and try and find out where we went wrong." Blaming others postpones regeneration, Adichie judiciously enjoins the African in the post-colonial. "This mutual acceptance underscores our strength because we share in the joy and pain, the agony and victory of our collective people" (Asante, 2008: 4). Achebe (ibid.: 45) similarly enjoins: "The writer cannot expect to be excused from the task of re-education and regeneration that must be done. . . . For he is, after all . . . the sensitive point of his community." Small and little things matter. Sexual violations, infidelity, betrayal, and gross human rights violations start with "small" self-seeking individual slips whose blame can be easily passed on to the next person. For example, the injurious psychological pain that drives the tensions at Nsukka University begins first with self-betrayal on the domestic front. Odenigbo cheats on Olanna when he succumbs to his mother's machinations to ouster Olanna out of a marriage that has failed to give her a grandson to cover Odenigbo's "impotence." Odenigbo's Mama muses: "When this baby comes, I will have somebody to keep me company and my fellow women will no longer call me the mother of an impotent son" (*Half of a Yellow Sun* p. 298). Blinded by the self-seeking desire to cover individual shame and hurt, Mama is oblivious to the damage she causes her son's marriage. She pushes Amala onto the drunk Odenigbo resulting in an unwanted pregnancy, violently tearing the lynchpin of a joyous and successful marriage. Ugwu their helper is apprehensive: "Master's fear worried him" (p. 298). Mama's blackmail injects further pain: "You are refusing your child and not Amala" (p. 300). The drama and suffocating tension that follows is cataclysmic:

> Olanna's raised voice was audible enough. "It's *you* and not your mother. It happened because *you* let it happen! You must take responsibility!" . . .
>
> "I am not a philandering man, and you know that. This would not have happened if my mother didn't have a hand!" . . .
>
> "Did your mother pull out your [manhood] and insert it into Amala as well?" Olanna asked.
>
> (p. 301)

[T]umultuous crowding of pain and thoughts and anger (p. 290), make Olanna snap. She sleeps with Richard, her twin sister's "husband," whom she has no feelings for to avenge Odenigbo's "flagrant way he continued to sidestep responsibility and blame his mother" (p. 305). Compounded emotional pain, betrayal, and guilt separate her from her only sibling Kainene. Pain blinds her to the potential damage to her relationship with Kainene. "Kainene doesn't forgive easily" (p. 304). Kainene later confirms: "It would be forgivable if it were somebody else. Not my sister" (p. 322). "It is stupid to expect me to forgive this" (p. 323). Both Olanna and Kainene are conscious that in their bid to self-vindicate, individually they take responsibility for the choices they make – letting go or holding themselves emotional and psychological fugitives. Olanna decides to legally adopt Odenigbo's 'natural' daughter with Amala, Baby, whom both Mama and Amala reject from birth as an epitome of shame. In the end, Olanna and Kainene choose their commonalities over their differences, consciously refusing to be pawns in "outsiders" game. Ani (1980: 1) observes that

> until we learn that it serves our objectives to emphasize the similarities, *-the ties, the unifying principles, the common threads and themes that bind and identify us all as "African", we will continue to be politically and ideologically confused.

What happens on the individual/domestic front replicates itself more viciously on the national front. Adichie raises the tempo from the specific to broader more complex, sophisticated, and uncontrollable levels when she explores pitfalls of ethnic "cleansing," initially against the Igbo, and then across other ethnicities, and between the Hausa and non-Hausas, that spreads unabated as a result of ethnic and religious intolerance that cripple and destabilise Nigeria. The collegiality at Nsukka University collapses, leaving the community internally bleeding, with the Yoruba digging in to defend themselves and crafting a new symbol of identity: "a painting of half of a yellow sun – 'the Biafran Sun'"(p. 218). People scatter for safety to the four winds. Microcosmic of greater Nigeria, Nsukka's carnage is unquantifiable.

The world does not really care about individuals who have no regard for their own lives and care least about transformative regeneration. Ephraim (2003: 420) urges: "black people must make redemption the theme of their everyday existence." This is what Olanna consciously chooses by confessing her betrayal to Kainene and Odenigbo, thereby recovering her trounced self-confidence from further self-denigration, self-hate, self-negation, and self-destruction:

> Look at you. You're the kindest person I know. Look how beautiful you are. Why do you need so much outside of yourself? Why isn't what you are enough?
>
> (p. 290)

Simultaneously on the war-front, political rhetoric from commanders: "*I was told that Biafrans fought like heroes, but now I know that heroes fight like Biafrans*" (p. 394) "proof that Biafra would triumph" (p. 444), do not abate the calamities.

Radio Biafra continues shifting blame for the calamities – 'a country born from the ashes of injustice would limit its practice of injustice'" (p. 395):

> *These African states have fallen prey to the British-American imperialist conspiracy to use the committee's recommendations as a pretext for a massive arms support for their puppet and tottering neo-colonialist regime in Nigeria.*
>
> (p. 334)

A non-exhaustive catalogue of the cataclysmic cancers continues spiralling. Children are sexually violated at relief centres that should be their spiritual sanctuaries, subtly themselves becoming "cannibal" centres thriving on the defenceless youths. Biafra and Nigeria become deathbeds. The ending to the armed conflict in *Half of a Yellow Sun* is therefore refreshing. Adichie accurately recaptures one of post-independence Nigeria's landmark resolutions:

> *Throughout history, injured people have had to resort to arms in their self-defence where peaceful negotiations fail. We are no exception. We took up arms because of the sense of insecurity generated in our people by the massacres. We have fought in defence of that cause. . . .*
>
> *I am convinced that the suffering of our people must be brought to an immediate end. . . . I urge General Gowon, in the name of humanity, to order his troops to pause while an armistice is negotiated.*
>
> (pp. 514–515) (emphasis mine)

The common good exhorts leaders to stop the war. This is the re-education, the healing, that the "post" in the "post-colonial" should attain to self-chart sustainable and peaceable livelihoods. Self-superintending underpinned with forgiveness emerges the surest way to achieve genuine freedom and dignity.

Symbolically, Olanna and Kainene, like Biafra and Nigeria, are self-deflecting and self-destructive by fomenting non-forgiveness, ethnic intolerance, and bitter resentment. Olanna and Kainene end their rivalry after talking over and laughing about the folly of bitter anger and resentment. Biafra and Nigeria similarly come to the negotiation table and talk over their differences to promote human lives. Biafra's losses offer no gain to Nigeria. Similarly, Olanna's loss of Kainene renders her dysfunctional at losing her twin – different shades of the same person. For genuine self-recovery and renewal to take root, individuals should transcend self-seeking self-righteousness, and egotism. That Adichie uses the twins to self-describe, self-name, self-explain, self-narrate, and recognize the self-annihilating pitfalls of self-seeking ambition and hatred sugar-coated as patriotism, philanthropy genuinely brings regeneration.

Reflections and undertakings: Lessons for Zimbabwe

"Violence for whatever reason, . . . perpetuates . . . the cycle of dehumanisation, and differential human worth" (Magosvongwe, 2013: 266). Apparent at the core of Adichie's cited novels is the insistent persuasion to protect the fragile inner-self against imbibing cancerous self-righteous and self-aggrandising dogmas that are psycho-intellectually incubated and birthed for certain powerful persons' agendas, who themselves are driven by compensatory behaviour because of inherent deficiencies hidden from public scrutiny. The worst losers in the conflict between Biafra and Nigeria are their respective citizens, worst of all women and children who are vulnerable/defenseless/shelter-less and starving victims of the war-torn conflict. Political leaders of both Biafra and Nigeria realise that by perpetuating the conflict, they have both abrogated their primary mandate and responsibility to guarantee security, tranquillity, cohesion, and oneness of their people as they are driven mostly by malice and avarice-induced self-aggrandisement. They therefore become tools in their own self-destruction.

Memorialisation and re-memory, from critical knowledge of history and critical self-knowledge, answer to calls for self-introspection in order to survive and become. Without knowing who we are, what defines us, what the threats to our being are, including their source, and where we should go, informed choices remain a mirage. It does not come as a surprise that the salvation and renewal of the family and nation rests on the twin women symbolically representing Biafra and Nigeria, Kainene and Olanna in *Half of a Yellow Sun*, and Aunty Ifeoma and *nwunye m* in *Purple Hibiscus*, dealing a blow to gender dichotomies in Africa's post-independence. Women too have a critical political role in the healing and reconciliation processes beginning at the domestic level, radiating into the broader communities and society.

Like the twins, Kainene and Olanna, families and communities would become more exuberant, reinvigorated, and life-sustaining if individuals begin by embracing self-acceptance as well as taking pride in their cultural heritage and self-identity. Dichotomies created first on the family front are double-edged, first for ease of execution of tasks, but worse for fanning differences and mistrust to the detriment of the family cohort. Enemies camouflaged as friends capitalise on such differences to subtly manipulate members to fight one another, leaving the fighting parties weaker and more vulnerable. Once more vulnerable, both parties lose sense of freedom and objectivity, and become easy prey in life's perilous waters. A common African adage says, "when two brothers fight, it is the outsider who reaps the harvest." They are both archetypical losers.

Forgiveness becomes the most "foolish" approach. Yet, it remains the invaluable and priceless balm that individuals can ever administer on themselves, in their personal relationships, in the family, and communities at large. Why? Bitterness begets more bitterness thereby increasing the intensity of the cancerous damage that destroys the incumbent first as it keeps on spiralling to destroy others as is the case with the depictions in our selected fictional narratives. The beauty of forgiveness emanates from intrinsic loyalty and commitment to the fire of transformative change that is embedded in reciprocal relationships – *No victor and no vanquished* (Adichie, 2007/2015: 535).

Conclusion

Refuting "the dangers of a single story," *Purple Hibiscus* and *Half of a Yellow Sun*, laud a transcendental and triumphal vision. Practical wisdom and emotional intelligence demonstrate sensitivity to happiness undergirded by peaceable coexistence. Both novels interrogate possibilities that promote genuine reciprocal respect for every person's human worth, talent, expertise, and dignity for humanity's greater good. Zimbabwe needs to appreciate that rather than being divisive, differences must be taken, appreciated, viewed, and utilised in their complimentary capacity in order to make communities richer, healthier, and more successful as collaborations in wealth-creating projects increase rather than decrease visibility. Seeing that female characters initiate processes of forgiveness and reconstruction, thereby igniting reconstruction like Kainene and Olanna achieve in *Half of a Yellow sun*, Adichie deconstructs feminism as gendered discourse. In "no victor, no vanquished," Adichie glorifies reciprocity in peace-building and candidness that is principal to conflict-resolution. Coming together *"in the name of humanity"* (*Half of a Yellow Sun* p. 515) encapsulates transcendental triumphalism embedded in reciprocity as a sure way towards regeneration. Clear-minded forgiveness benefits both doer and recipient alike, but more importantly the forgiver. Nevertheless, what we witness in Adichie's novels is the importance of eloquence, ability to judge and be objective, and more importantly the need for one's reconnection with "memory" that is the antennae into the recesses of one's being. Without the reconnection, it becomes almost infeasible to chart the way to forgiveness because one cannot forgive that which they are oblivious of/about. Thus, Adichie provides the template for healing that Zimbabwe must embrace with enthusiasm.

References

Abrahams, P. 2000. *The Black Experience in the 20th Century*. Bloomington, IN: Indiana University Press.

Achebe, C. 1984. *The Trouble with Nigeria*. London: Heinemann.

Achebe, C. 1987. *Anthills of the Savannah*. London: Heinemann.

Achebe, C. 1990. *Hopes and Impediments*. Doubleday.

Adichie, C. N. 2015. *Half of a Yellow Sun*. New York: Anchor Books (originally published in 2007).

Adichie, C. N. 2009. "The Danger of a Single Story," October, Address and Interview. You-Tube.

Adichie, C. N. 2012. *Purple Hibiscus*. Chapel Hill, NC: First published 2012 by Algonquin Books of Chapel Hill.

Akbar, N. 2003. "Afrocentric Social Sciences for Human Liberation," in A. Mazama (ed.), *The Afrocentric Paradigm*. Trenton, NJ: Africa World Press, Inc., 131–143.

Ani, M. 1980. *Let the Circle Be Unbroken: The Implications of African Spirituality in the Diaspora*. Paris: Présence Africaine.

Ani, M. 1994. *Yurugu: An African-Centred Critique of European Cultural Thought and Behaviour*. Trenton, NJ: Africa World Press.

Appiah, K. A. 2005. *The Ethics of Identity*. Princeton, NJ: Princeton University Press.

Armah, A. K. 2010. *Remembering the Dismembered Continent*. Popenguine, Senegal: Per Ankh the African Publishing Co-operative.

Asante, M. K. 2003. "Locating a Text: Implications of Afrocentric Theory," in A. Mazama (ed.), *The Afrocentric Paradigm*. Trenton, NJ: Africa World Press, Inc., 235–244.

Asante, M. K. 2007. *An Afrocentric Manifesto: Toward an African Renaissance*. Cambridge, MA: Polity Press, 2007.

Asante, M. K. 2008. "New Leadership for a Resurgent Africa: Discovering Strength in African Values," Commencement Address at the University of the Witwatersrand, Johannesburg.

Cesaire, A. 1995. *Notebook of a Return to My Native Land*. Newcastle upon Tyne, UK: Bloodaxe Books Ltd.

Cesaire, A. 1972. *Discourse on Colonialism*. New York, NY: Monthly Review Press.

Ephraim, C. W. M. 2003. *The Pathology of Eurocentrism: The Burdens and Responsibilities of Being Black*. Asmara/Trenton, NJ: Africa World Press.

Fanon, F. 1967. *The Wretched of the Earth*. Harmondsworth, London: Penguin.

Freire, P. 1998. *Pedagogy of Hope: Reliving Pedagogy of the Oppressed*. New York, NY: The Continuum Publishing Company.

Gwekwerere, T. and G. Mheta. 2012. "The Afrotriumphalist Commitment to Life in Freedom and Dignity in Transatlantic African Literature," *South African Journal of African Languages* 32(2), 195–206.

Hollist, P. 2012. *So the Path Does Not Die*. Cameroon: Langaa Research & Publishing Common Initiative Group.

Hudson-Weems, C. 2004. *Africana Womanism: Reclaiming Ourselves*, 4th ed. Troy, MI: Bedford Publishers, Inc.

Hudson-Weems, C. 2012. "Ending De-Womanisation, De-Feminisation And De-Humanisation Via Self-Naming, Self-Definition And Genuine Sisterhood," in I. Muwati, Z. Mguni, T. Gwekwerere and R. Magosvongwe (eds.), *Rediscoursing African Womanhood in the Search for Sustainable Renaissance: Africana Womanism in Multi-disciplinary Approaches*. Harare, Zimbabwe: College Press Publishers, 1–7.

Killam, G. D. 1973. *African Writers on African Writing*. London: Heinemann, Putnam.

Magosvongwe, R. 2013. "Land and Identity in Zimbabwean Fictional Writings in English from 2000 to 2010: A Critical Analysis". Unpublished DPhil Thesis, University of Cape Town.

Magosvongwe, R. and A. Nyamende. 2015. "This Is Our Land: Land and Identity in Selected Zimbabwean Black- and White-Authored Fictional Narratives in English Published Between 2000 and 2010," *South African Journal of African Languages* 35(2), 237–248.

Mazrui, A. 2002. *Africa and Other Civilisations: Conquest and Counter-conquest*. Trenton, NJ: Africa World Press.

Mda, Z. 2009. "Biko's Children," in *The Steve Biko Memorial Lectures 2000–2008*. Johannesburg: The Steve Biko Foundation and Pan Macmillan South Africa, 21–40.

Morrison, T. 1987. *Beloved*. New York, NY: Penguin.

Mungoshi, C. 1975. *Waiting for the Rain*. Salisbury, London: Harare Publishing House.

Muponde, R. 2015. *Some Kinds of Childhood: Images of History and Resistance in Zimbabwean Literature*. Trenton, NJ: Africa World Press.

Ndebele, N. S. 2009. "'*Iph*' *Indlela*? Finding Our Way into the Future," in *The Steve Biko Memorial Lectures 2000–2008*. Johannesburg: The Steve Biko Foundation and Pan Macmillan South Africa, 5–20.

Oyono, F. 1990. *Houseboy*. London: Heinemann.

Patrick, J. and T. W. Bennett. 2011. "Ubuntu, the Ethics of Traditional Religion," in T. W. Bennett (ed.), *Traditional African Religions in South African Law*. Cape Town UCT Press, 223–242.

Shujaa, M. J. 2003. "Education and Schooling: You Can Have One Without the Other," in A. Mazama (ed.), *The Afrocentric Paradigm*. Trenton, NJ: Africa World Press, 245–264.

Sithole, T. 2015. "Aime Cesaire, Writing the (non)Human and the Ontoloigico-Existential Scandal," *Imbizo: International Journal of African Literary and Comparative Studies* 6(1), 1–26.

Stewart, J. B. 2004. *Flight: In Search of Vision*. Trenton, NJ: Africa World Press.

Temple, C. N. 2010. "The Emergence of Sankofa Practice in the United States: A Modern History," *Journal of Black Studies* 41(1), 127–150.

Thomas, G. 2007. *The Sexual Demon of Colonial Power: Pan-African Embodiment and Erotic Schemes of Empire*. Bloomington, IN: Indiana University Press.

Vambe, M. T. 2004. African Oral Story-Telling Tradition and the Zimbabwean. *Novel in English SubStance 117* 37(3), 37–72.

Vambe, M. T. 2005. "The Poverty of Theory in the Study of Zimbabwean Literature," in R. Muponde and R. Primorac (eds.), *Versions of Zimbabwe: New Approaches to Literature and Culture*. Harare: Weaver Press, 89–100.

Versenyi, L. 1963. *Socratic Humanism*. New York, NY: Yale University Press.

Wa Thiongo, N. 2009. "Recovering Our Memory: South Africa in the Black Imagination," in *The Steve Biko Memorial Lectures 2000–2008*. Johannesburg: The Steve Biko Foundation and Pan Macmillan South Africa, 51–72.

West, C. 2008. "Introduction". In R. Wright (ed.) *Black Power: Three Books from Exile: Black Power; The Color Curtain; and White Man Listen!* New York, NY: Harper Collins Publishers, vii–xiii.

15 The potential role of education in peacebuilding in Zimbabwe

Mediel Hove and Enock Ndawana

Introduction

Education refers to any act or practice that possesses an influential effect on the mind, personality, or physical ability of a person. Technically, education is perceived as a method by which society purposefully transmits its collected knowledge, skills, and values from one age group to another (Onen, 2017: 2). It is also deemed the engine that propels development. Many scholars believe that education is critical to the rebuilding process, peace, and stability after a conflict (Pigozzi, 1999; Bush and Saltarelli, 2000; Paulson, 2011). The growing significance of education in conflict resolution in the global arena was revealed in the 2011 Education for All (EFA) Global Monitoring Report, *The Hidden Crisis: Armed Conflict and Education*. It argues that armed conflict in the world's underprivileged countries was one of the chief obstacles threatening the EFA objectives. As a result, it implores the global community to reinforce the role of the education systems in averting conflicts and constructing peaceful social orders (UNESCO, 2011: 131–132). Education systems can possibly act as an influential force for peace, resolution, and prevention of conflicts by encouraging shared respect, acceptance, and acute thinking. Conversely, offering inadequate or imbalanced access and/or process and content of education can frequently cause violence (Hilker, 2011; Smith and Vaux, 2003). Denying access to education to large numbers of youth culminates in lack of opportunities, joblessness, and disillusionment and these can act as an influential conscripting ground for armed groups. Similarly, the usage of education systems to strengthen political domination and the relegation of sidelined groups and ethnic exclusion are a recipe for conflict (Brown, 2011).

Also, a growing number of case studies have singled out facets of education that have significance for conflict (Bush and Saltarelli, 2000; Smith and Vaux, 2003; Davies, 2010) and propose different reasons why we should be careful concerning how education is offered. In its conclusion, the 2011 EFA report notes that post-conflict rebuilding in education poses enormous challenges. Conversely, achievement in education may aid or strengthen the peace process, shape government acceptability, and restore a country on the path to recovery (UNESCO, 2011: 132). In the words of Kanyongo (2005: 67), "education in

Zimbabwe today aims at promoting national unity to contribute to national development particularly, economic development through the supply of trained and skilled teachers and staff."

Whilst there is growing literature discussing the impact of the Zimbabwean crisis on the provision of social services, which include education (Hove, 2012; Mlambo, 2013a; Nyazema, 2010), these works overlook discussing education's potential role in peacebuilding. This chapter attempts to address this lacuna. The existing literature on the impact of the Zimbabwean crisis on education largely underplays the fact that besides being seriously affected by the conflict, education in Zimbabwe was also part of the crisis. As a result, we argue that education should form the central part of the reformation, reconstruction, and peace-rebuilding efforts in Zimbabwe. This is because of the realisation that education is important for peacebuilding and development.

The values and goals of peace education

Peace education has many definitions. Harris (1990: 254) notes that "Education for peace assumes peace in education." Pupils can be educated on how to realise peace in the world, not merely by learning about subjects of war and peace, but by learning particular skills, manners, and personalities from the classroom milieu as well (Harris, 1990: 254–255, 2004: 5). This emphasises the importance of practice in promoting peace.

In addition, Harris and Synott (2002: 4) describe peace education as teaching experiences that extract from people their yearnings for peace and offer them nonviolent options for conflict management and the expertise for critical exploration of the structural activities that appropriate and generate unfairness and inequity. This view is encouraging because of its emphasis that conflict can be resolved through the engagement of nonviolent alternatives. Peace education has also been presented as signifying the process of encouraging the understanding, expertise, outlooks, and standards desired to bring about behaviour changes that will empower different groups of people, that is, children, youth, and adults to thwart both overt and covert conflict and violence; to peacefully address conflict; and to produce the settings encouraging to peace at different levels of human interaction in society (Fountain, 1999: 1).

Moreover, peace education is a process that aims to "empower people with the necessary skills, attitudes and knowledge in order to 'create a safe world and build a sustainable environment'" (Kruger, 2012: 20). It cultivates tolerance towards others and works to improve situations (Firer, 2008: 193). According to Harber and Sakade (2009: 174), peace education generally seeks to provide prospects to advance the expertise, understanding, and standards essential for the resolution of conflicts, communication, and collaboration regarding topics of war, violence, peace, conflict, and inequality. For Njoku and Anyanwu (2016: 52), peace education improves reflective, critical thinking, removing in the mind of individuals militarism, beliefs of prejudices, and all kinds of evil penchants while instilling in them the culture of peace indispensable for harmonious living and peaceful coexistence. It challenges all kinds of domination and conformity. The growth and realisation of peace and harmony create a win–win situation between or among the conflicting parties which include nation-states and racial or religious groups. Through humanising development of teaching and learning, peace educators attain and enable human development. The peace education facilitators strive to frustrate the dehumanisation generated by poverty, prejudice, discrimination, rape, violence, and war. This indicates that peace education has a role in encouraging unity and development.

Inculcating a culture of peace among the people of the world is another important goal of peace education. According to Maiyo et al. (2012: 31), it is solely via peace education that peace can be entrenched in the human mind as a remedy to war. This is more critical in light of the fact that in Africa and other continents there are many conflicts both structural and overt, where other countries are experiencing post-conflict, reconciliation process, and/or sociopolitical and economic uncertainty. In such instances the importance of inculcating a culture of peace need not be overemphasised. This is so because "to prevent our violence-ridden history repeating itself, the values of peace, non-violence, tolerance, human rights and democracy will have to be inculcated in every woman and man – young and old, children and adults alike" (Navarro-Castro and Nario-Galace, 2008: vii). Accordingly,

> The flourishing of a culture of peace will generate the mindset in us that is a prerequisite for the transition from force to reason, from conflict and violence to dialogue and peace. Culture of peace will provide the bedrock of support to a stable, progressing and prospering world for all.
> (Navarro-Castro and Nario-Galace, 2008: vii)

As a result, a culture of peace should substitute the culture of violence if humanity is to survive.

Peace education addresses various issues and the type of violence at hand determines the goal of peace education to be attained. Bar-Tal (2002: 28) has observed that "the programs of education for peace in different states differ considerably in terms of ideology, objectives, emphasis, curricula, contents, and practices." For Zimbabwe peace education's ideology, goals, emphasis, curricula, contents, and practices should also be decided on the basis of the problems the country has faced. These include ethnic and racial exclusion and tensions, unequal development, and the use of education as a tool of rooting the dominant political culture and ideology of the nation's ruling elites.

The Zimbabwean crisis and its effects on education provision

The Zimbabwean crisis, whose beginning period and causes are intensely contested amongst scholars, was responsible for the notable decline in the provision of primary, secondary, and tertiary education between 2000 and 2008.

Extensive literature analysing the background of the Zimbabwean crisis exist (Bond and Manyanya, 2002; Dansereau and Zamponi, 2005; Chimhowu, 2009) and that being the case, we just provide an overview in this chapter. A combination of economic, political, and social factors culminated in the disintegration of the provision of education. Political causes and dimensions of the crisis appeared to be equally important factors that contributed to the collapse of the country's education system. The political crisis has been repeatedly cited as the central cause of the Zimbabwean crisis that triggered the economic and social dimensions, including the fast track land reform programme (FTLRP) (Murisa, 2010: 3).

The remarkable and commendable strides Zimbabwe had made in education similar to other sectors during the first decade after independence sharply deteriorated to shocking levels. The post-independence Zimbabwean government had invested considerably in education with the aim of increasing participation at all levels (primary, secondary, and tertiary) because it viewed education as essential and critical for the country's socio-economic development. Amongst other things, the achievements include the expansion of education provision, removal of bottlenecks as well as other discriminatory practices such as access and quality in education perpetrated by the colonial government. Resources were channelled towards provision of education in formerly deprived communities (Jenjekwa, 2013: 554). New schools were constructed (about 613 government schools (primary and secondary) were built in rural areas and 117 in urban areas two years after independence) (Pape, 1998: 256). School enrolment extraordinarily increased largely due to the abolishment of primary school fees, affordable secondary school fees (Pape, 1998: 256–257), removal of age limitations to enter Grade One, and introduction of automatic progression to secondary school after completing Grade Seven regardless of the results (Nhundu, 1992: 81). In addition, teacher training, technical colleges, agricultural colleges, polytechnics, or nursing training colleges were built and two separate ministries of education were established, provision of learning and teaching materials and broader curriculum that included arts, practical and science subjects were offered by different schools depending on the availability of resources for Ordinary Level (Kanyongo, 2005). Zimbabwe achieved a 100% primary to secondary school transition rate (Nhundu, 1992: 80–81) and 92% literacy rate during the end of the first post-independence decade (Shizha and Kariwo, 2011: ix). These developments were due to the government's allocation of not less than 18% of the total national budget to education (Nyazema, 2010: 256).

However, the crisis had a foremost negative impact on the education system. Mlambo (2013a: 370) notes that the economic meltdown led to "low enrolment rates, declining attendance and completion rates, low transition rate to secondary schools and inadequate learning spaces, teachers and learning materials." In 2007 nearly 50% of those who completed Grade Seven failed to go to secondary school and the quality of education at all levels significantly declined because of the non-availability of textbooks, among other supplies and learning materials (Association for the Development of Africa, 2013: 27).

School attendance fell severely from about 85% in late 2007 to a mere 20% by the end of 2008 (Mlambo, 2013a: 372–373). Thus, the education system in Zimbabwe was by 2009 a "national disaster" because it operated at minimal capacity at the height of the conflict in 2008 (Mlambo, 2013a: 357, 374). We focus on 2008 as the cut-off year because the economic crisis which was a culmination of many negative developments including deindustrialisation and unemployment, mismanagement of funds, printing money to deal with budget deficits, and the resultant inflation was at its peak that year (Besada and Moyo, 2008: 14). By the time the Government of National Unity got into office in 2009, nearly one quarter of primary school children (100,000 children out of about 400,000) were not finishing Grade Seven, and an additional 70,000 did not proceed to secondary school (Chimhowu, 2009: 5). For that reason, about 170,000 children every year did not complete nine years of education that is fundamental to fully partake in socio-economic and political development (Chimhowu, 2009: 5). These direct and indirect impacts of the Zimbabwean crisis on the provision of education are critical for building the basis for arguing for the potential role of education in peacebuilding and development in the country.

The violence that targeted teachers for allegedly supporting the opposition since 2000 was significant. About 70,000 trained teachers left the country since 2000, going mainly to South Africa (Pswarayi and Reeler, 2012: 6). In 2007, about 25,000 teachers emigrated to South Africa, Namibia, and Botswana (Mlambo, 2013a: 372–373). According to Ranga (2015), besides social and economic drivers, the role played by the political conflict in Zimbabwe in the migration of teachers to South Africa need not be downplayed.

At tertiary institutions, the situation was also bad. The need for increased enrolment in tertiary institutions amid the economic crisis, particularly universities, created special problems which comprised under-funding, unqualified teaching staff, and insufficient library and teaching resources (Mlambo, 2013a: 361). In 2004 the main challenges facing the higher education sector were infrastructure development, equipping the growing number of tertiary institutions, motivation and remuneration for teaching staff, and staff shortages due to brain drain (SARUA, 2009: 5). The situation at the UZ affected other institutions of higher learning in the country, both private and public given that it is the major source of their academics (Chivore, 2006: 242–243). According to Mlambo (2013a, 370), senior and experienced academics left the country for greener pastures due to low salaries, increasing political intolerance, interference in university matters by government, the curtailment of academic freedom, and the reduction to a sorry state of the formerly popular higher education system. The academics left in part because of the worsening of their already poor working conditions and unavailability of transport and accommodation (SARUA, 2009: 5). Resultantly, a substantial decline in enrolments in vocational training centres and higher and tertiary institutions were recorded between 2007 and 2009 (Government of Zimbabwe/United Nations Country Team, 2010: 48). According to Nyazema (2010: 255), all state universities in

Zimbabwe during the economic and political crises years operated below 50% of their academic establishment.

Further, the government also faced challenges in funding any of its programmes meant to help students financially; for instance, the Cadetship Support Scheme (CSS) because of the then prevailing hyperinflation environment and general lack of resources (Mpofu et al., 2013: 328). The failure by government to pay for the cadetship programme affected both the institutions and the students. The institutions were plunged into serious cash flow challenges, while the students faced various challenges from the tertiary institutions as authorities demanded full payment of fees for one to be registered and to graduate (Madzonga, 2015). While the CSS continued to be the sole government student funding beyond 2008, it was eventually halted because of lack of funds and a huge debt to the tertiary institutions. By 2015 government was virtually not supporting students in higher education in any way (Madzonga, 2015). Unsurprisingly, with little or no government funding and the country's economy in total chaos, underfunding became the major problem facing Zimbabwean tertiary institutions (Mpofu et al., 2013: 328).

Education as a tool of ZANU-PF dominant political culture and ideology

In this section we highlight how the Zimbabwean education system, despite being threatened by the crisis, was also manipulated by the ruling party for the furtherance of its political interests in the name of instilling values of patriotism. The negative consequences this had on education are presented in anticipation that the concerned parties to the Zimbabwean conflict may be encouraged to design and implement policies to review the whole education spectrum in a drive to weed out the destructive and incisive contents. This will in the long run make education in the country a vehicle for sustainable peace, as well as socio-economic and political development.

History in Zimbabwe since 1980 has been interpreted and used for different intentions by different conflicting groups. As Ndlovu (2009: 67–68) observes, history is the academic discipline extremely susceptible to the cause of nation building and political elite interests hence prone to manipulation in hegemonic projects by political regimes as its role from the viewpoint of social constructivism is to cultivate social, cultural, and political values in society. ZANU-PF has used history to justify and sideline its opponents. The Zimbabwean government has engaged history to find legitimacy thereby making ZANU-PF the dominant political party responsible for shaping a sense of nationhood with an ideology rooted in the 1960s liberation war (Second Chimurenga), the First Chimurenga 1896–1897, and the third Chimurenga which began in 2000 (Ranger, 2004: 219). Accordingly, the works which present and glorify this continuity were used by ZANU-PF in its promotion of patriotic history (Barnes, 2007: 633). These works portray the Chimurenga (war of resistance) as demonstrating the agency of Africans united by the spirit of patriotism to dislodge colonialism but at the same time they are silent about the struggles within the liberation movement (Nyamunda, 2014: 74). This erroneously reduced Zimbabwean history to a sequence of wars of resistance and ZANU-PF's coming to power as a liberation movement marked the end of a process if not history (Phimister, 2012: 27–28).

While the teaching of history at secondary schools since 1980 demonstrates the pursuit of patriotic history by the Zimbabwean state, it became more acute after 2002. Barnes (2004: 144–145) notes that between 1980 and 1990 the secondary schools retained the pre-1980 Rhodesian syllabus used since the 1970s with few books focusing on Africa recommended. The nationalist syllabus replaced the Rhodesian syllabus and was used starting in 1991 and ending in 2002. The new history of Zimbabwe was told in a racially polarising account, filled with authoritative notions of ethnic inclusion and racial exclusion. However, the nationalist syllabus was credited for its promotion of diverse history teaching methodology "involving problem-posing, problem-solving, role play, written exercises and discussions" and by encouraging critical thinking it was an antithesis to the Rhodesian syllabus which emphasised rote-learning (Barnes, 2004: 146).

In addition to the new syllabus, new textbooks for teaching history were released and the books were unsophisticated in the way they presented the white Rhodesians as homogeneous both culturally and politically, and bent on maintaining colonial rule. The one-dimensional treatment did not escape Africans who were also presented as unbroken in their ethnicity and thus failing to appreciate African ethnicity. However, the texts tried their best to counter the divide and rule narrative of the colonial era dating back to the original settlement of the Ndebele in Zimbabwe in the nineteenth century (Barnes, 2004: 149–153). According to Moyo (2014: 11), the nationalist syllabus was intended to be in line with the replacement of capitalism with socialism as per state ideology hence the state's attempt to promote it in writing, language, and teaching of history uncritically celebrating the history of the nation. Apparently, the nationalist syllabus failed to promote racial harmony and understanding and despite the recommended books' quashing of colonial representation of the ruthless Ndebele victimising the Shona, the syllabus and the texts did not address the Gukurahundi and its socio-economic and justice problems. Overall, the nationalist syllabus and the texts published in its support failed to do much to promote national healing, reconciliation, and justice essential for peacebuilding.

The period after 2002 registered the radical modification of the nationalist syllabus which culminated in a syllabus that glorified ZANU-PF and requesting students and teachers to have pride in the party's role during the war of liberation. As Minister of Education, Sport, Arts, and Culture (2001–2009), Aeneas Chigwedere ensured that patriotic history texts were distributed to schools since 2001, instead of those sponsored by his predecessor in collaboration with the United Nations Educational Scientific and Cultural Organisation (UNESCO) and Danish International Development Agency (DANIDA). These books were written in series by many Zimbabwean teachers from education colleges on *Education for Human Rights and Democracy* but remained in warehouses despite the huge resources in money and time spent to produce them. The books were good and included history textbooks for Forms 1 and 2 and Ordinary level presenting

> universal history at its best, containing a great deal of comparative material on Nazi Germany and Soviet Russia; on slavery in Ancient Egypt and the Americas; on colonial repression and nationalist aspirations for liberty; on the slow emergence of international conventions on human rights.
>
> (Ranger, 2004: 225)

The history syllabus after 2002 failed to provide opportunities for nation building and reconciliation which is inclusive and necessary for peacebuilding. Therefore, history teaching in Zimbabwe over the years evolved to now resemble the colonial period scenario and a regression of both the nation-state and progressive teaching of history informed by patriotism. Resultantly, Zimbabwe became a good example to cite highlighting the dangers of the narrow use of the history curriculum with narrow definitions and exclusive political nation-building process (Ndlovu, 2009: 70). As Mlambo (2013b: 63) notes, Zimbabwe is yet to transform itself from being a geographical expression to become a true nation with an ordinary identity, values, and vision for the future. Without doubt, the weaknesses in the Zimbabwean history curriculum had negative impact on development and peacebuilding.

In pursuit of patriotic history, a National Strategic Studies (NASS) course was introduced and made compulsory to all tertiary-level students in 2003. Most students supported the MDC against ZANU-PF, thus, colleges and universities were accused of converting into "anti-Government factories" and university history was suspected in the countryside (Solidarity Peace Trust, 2003: 3).

Engaging education for peacebuilding

In this section, we grapple with some of the issues the Zimbabwean formal peace education curriculum content must reflect. This is done cognisant of the fact that there are challenges in teaching peace education in a racially/ethnically diverse society that has had a long history of racial/ethnic tensions. Besides, we are mindful that peace education may face problems in a context of economic challenges and inequalities.

In rebuilding education in Zimbabwe, peace education must be introduced at all levels of the educational spectrum. We are advocating for both the inclusion of the principles of peace education to every existing subject or education programme in the country apart from specific peace education modules or programmes at the tertiary level. It should be a learning outcome-based curriculum including values of peace, social justice, solidarity, conflict resolution, principles of negotiation and mediation, and the practice of nonviolence taking cognisance of the levels. In addition, concepts of national healing, racial/ethnic inclusion, reconciliation, and integration need to be part of the peace education curriculum in a drive to promote values and behaviour to reunite Zimbabweans and in the long run, encourage a culture of peace.

The methodology should, among other things, entail well-trained teaching staff, tailor-made courses, manuals and educational materials, and new tools in education all intended to encourage a deeper understanding of the root causes of conflict. This is because education "helps shape attitudes, behaviour and social structures" and can be a root source of conflict in a similar way as it can also be an influential tool of peacebuilding. For example, the education sector can promote peace through "addressing inequalities, overcoming prejudices and fostering new values and institutions" (Tschirgi, 2011: 4). Thus, the school and classroom settings need to be reoriented towards the values of peace, inculcating a social climate that addresses inequality that comes with education. In this regard, the classroom should offer teachers and students alike prospects to examine their own and others' prejudices, ruminate multiple perceptions and, interrogate the sources of information. The language of instruction need to be guided by the numerous recently recognised official languages in the country's 2013 constitution beyond the few previously used (English, Shona, and Ndebele) depending on the region and level, with English becoming the language of instruction from secondary school onwards.[1] This is necessary to avoid the omission of some mother-tongues of minority groups (numerically, but not in terms of rights) for the furtherance of those of majority groups which in the process engender conflict.

Besides shaping society, education helps in developing skills. The Zimbabwean case also requires prioritising "training and research in sustainable development; and skills for peaceful inter-human relations, good governance, the prevention of conflict and peacebuilding" (Kotite, 2012: 10). This is essential both for development and peacebuilding purposes. In this regard,

> the process and content of education, which create or reinforce social, political and environmental narratives that can have a powerful influence on an individual's beliefs, attitudes and behavior . . . has an important role to play in maintaining or building peace as well as fostering sustainable interactions with the natural environment.
>
> (Winthrop and Matsui, 2013: 4)

Consequently, it is instructive for Zimbabwe to embrace Ramirez-Barat and Duthie's (2015: 1) observation that the precise legacies of oppressive policies and human rights violations in the political culture of a country can be sufficiently dealt with in a number of ways, including education. This includes having the provision of education going beyond traditional processes like the physical refurbishment of schools, the reincorporation of children into the education system, but to also have a school core curriculum that upholds worldwide values of acceptance and social unity.

Zimbabwean educational policies should be bent on lessening the conditions contributing to the emergence of conflict. Indeed,

> curriculum decisions are not just about content and organising teaching/ learning of subject matter but careful considerations of philosophical, psychological and sociological issues. Research shows that without a thorough consideration of these fundamental principles, the designed curriculum may fail to address the needs of the society.
>
> (Makura and Makura, 2012: 509)

The inclusion of human rights in both Zimbabwean history and NASS will help inculcate an appreciation of respect and dignity of the other person. The importance of recognising these is hinged on the appreciation of diversity in both opinion and attitude and may be a good step towards harmony and coexistence. As Gallagher (2010) observed,

> a coexistence approach [that] acknowledges the importance of social cohesion and the need to build a sense of common citizenship; and . . . this sense of commonality is not pre-ordained and immutable, but is constantly evolving and subject to critical reflection and dialogue.
>
> (Gallagher, 2010)

This is critical to support socially cohesive societies. This is vital, cognisant of the dangers of misusing history and NASS education in Zimbabwe which culminated in the conditioning of many young people to only have unwavering support for the leadership of Mugabe and his party and visceral hostility to any other political contender (Solidarity Peace Trust, 2003: 10–20).

The content of history and NASS subjects must be revised to reflect realities and complexities about the role played by different groups in the struggle to bring independence to the country. There is need for a history that is detached from simply extolling the role of Mugabe and ZANU-PF (those in leadership positions) at the expense of others who failed to make it notwithstanding that they also played an equally important role. Against the evidence of university history being suspected in the countryside and the propagation of patriotic history at various levels, there is a need for agreement among stakeholders to weed out both this widespread mistrust and disarray in education. This means the agreement among the stakeholders will bring about trust and may be a starting point to adopt strategies to achieve harmonisation of interests and development of positive expectations that can contribute to sustainable trust and peace. Using education for legitimacy purposes through conscious manipulation, as ZANU-PF under Mugabe has done (Jansen, 1990), is doomed. It should be shunned because "delivering education in a way that fuels animosity, irresponsible behavior and corruption can have detrimental effects on a state's ability to develop human, social and political capital, all of which have significant social and ultimately financial costs" (Winthrop and Matsui, 2013: 4).

Conclusion

Overall, stakeholders in Zimbabwe must be mindful of the fact that for education to play a meaningful role in peacebuilding and economic development, it needs to be seriously modified at all levels. The current challenges in Zimbabwe entail that education also has to provide manpower with the technical skills and entrepreneurial knowledge required to address the twenty-first century challenges, including unemployment. More so, quality education nurtures "skills development – such as literacy, numeracy and critical thinking – [which] play an important role in economic growth and poverty alleviation, which is crucial for development" (Winthrop and Matsui, 2013: 4). The attainment of better education without opportunities for employment does not contribute to economic development in any way. Rather, it is a recipe for instability. As a result, reviewing the country's economic policies to make them attractive to investors in order to open up employment opportunities will also help to avert the lack of development and instability created by the dangerous combination of education and unemployment. This is because contrary to the view

> that well painted school buildings, large numbers of teachers and high statistical enrolment figures in schools are the marks of quality and yet quality education hinges even on elements like the nature of the curriculum, instructional technology, school management, professional expertise of teachers and support staff and the general motivation of teachers.
>
> (Jenjekwa, 2013: 554)

Note

1 According to Section 6 of the Zimbabwean Constitution (2013: 17), there are 16 official languages – namely, Chewa, Chibarwe, English, Kalanga, Koisan, Nambya, Ndau, Ndebele, Shangani, Shona, sign language, Sotho, Tonga, Tswana, Venda, and Xhosa.

References

Association for the Development of Africa. 2013. *Education in Reconstruction: Zimbabwe.* http://reliefweb.int/report/zimbabwe/education-reconstruction-zimbabwe (accessed on 22 May 2017).

Barnes, T. 2004. "Reconciliation, Ethnicity and School History in Zimbabwe 1980–2002," in B. Raftopoulos and T. Savage (eds.), *Zimbabwe: Injustice and Political Reconciliation.* Cape Town: Institute of Reconciliation and Justice, 140–159.

Barnes, T. 2007. "'History Has to Play Its Role': Constructions of Race and Reconciliation in Secondary School Historiography in Zimbabwe, 1980–2002," *Journal of Southern African Studies* 33(3), 633–651.

Bar-Tal, D. 2002. "The Elusive Nature of Peace Education," in G. Solomon and B. Nevo (eds.), *Peace Education: The Concept, Principles and Practices in the World.* Mahwah, NJ: Lawrence Erlbaum, 27–36.

Besada, H. and N. Moyo. 2008. *Zimbabwe in Crisis: Mugabe's Policies and Failures.* Waterloo: The Centre for International Governance Innovation.

Bond, P. and M. Manyanya. 2002. *Zimbabwe's Plunge: Exhausted Nationalism, Neoliberalism and the Search for Social Justice*, 1st ed. Pietermaritzburg: University of Natal Press.

Brown, G. K. 2011. "The Influence of Education on Violent Conflict and Peace: Inequality, Opportunity and the Management of Diversity," *Prospects* 41(2), 191–204.

Bush, K. D. and D. Saltarelli. 2000. *The Two Faces of Education in Ethnic Conflict: Towards a Peacebuilding Education for Children*. Rome: UNICEF.

Chimhowu, A. 2009. *Moving Forward in Zimbabwe: Reducing Poverty and Promoting Growth*. Manchester: The Brooks World Poverty Institute.

Chivore, B. R. S. 2006. "Private Higher Education in Zimbabwe," in N. V. Varghese (ed.), *Growth and Expansion of Higher Education in Africa*. Paris: International Institute for Educational Planning (IIEP), 231–248.

Constitution of Zimbabwe Amendment (No. 20), Act 2013. Harare: Government Printer.

Dansereau, S. and M. Zamponi. 2005. *Zimbabwe, the Political Economy of Decline*. Discussion Paper no.27, Nordiska Africa Institute, Uppsala.

Davies, L. 2010. "The Difference Faces of Education in Conflict," *Development* 53(4), 491–497.

Firer, R. 2008. "Virtual Peace Education," *Journal of Peace Education* 5(2), 193–207.

Fountain, S. 1999. *Peace Education in UNICEF*, UNICEF Staff Working Papers PD-ED-99/003. New York: UNICEF.

Gallagher, T. 2010. *Complementary Approaches to Coexistence Work: Key Issues in Coexistence and Education*. Massachusetts: Coexistence International.

Government of Zimbabwe/ United Nations Country Team. 2010. *Country Analysis Report for Zimbabwe*. www.undg.org/docs/12/23/Zimbabwe-Country-Analysis-2010-Report-05-09-11.pdf (accessed on 9 May 2017).

Harber, C. and N. Sakade. 2009. "Schooling for Violence and Peace: How Does Peace Education Differ from 'Normal' Schooling?" *Journal of Peace Education* 6(2), 171–187.

Harris, I. M. 1990. "Principles of Peace Pedagogy," *Peace & Change* 15(3), 254–271.

Harris, I. M. 2004. "Peace Education Theory," *Journal of Peace Education* 1(1), 5–20.

Harris, I. M. and J. Synott. 2002. "Peace Education for a New Century," *Social Alternatives* 21(1), 3–6.

Hilker, L. M. 2011. "The Role of Education in Driving Conflict and Building Peace: The Case of Rwanda," *Prospects* 41, 267–282.

Hove, M. 2012. "The Debates and Impact of Sanctions: The Zimbabwean Experience," *International Journal of Business and Social Science* 3(5), 72–84.

Jansen, J. D. 1990. "Curriculum Policy as Compensatory Legitimation? A View from the Periphery," *Oxford Educational Review* 16(1), 29–38.

Jenjekwa, V. 2013. "Education Provision in Zimbabwe: The Return of the Ghost of Stratification and Its Implications to Quality and Access in Education," *International Journal of English and Education* 2(3), 554–566.

Kanyongo, G. Y. 2005. "Zimbabwe's Public Education System Reforms: Successes and Challenges," *International Education Journal* 6(1), 65–74.

Kotite, P. 2012. *Education for Conflict Prevention and Peacebuilding: Meeting the Global Challenges of the 21st Century*. Paris: UNESCO.

Kruger, F. 2012. "The Role of TESOL in Educating for Peace," *Journal of Peace Education* 9(1), 17–30.

Madzonga, D. 2015. "The Plight of a Zimbabwean Student in 2015," *Zimbabwe Situation*, 27 February. www.zimbabwesituation.com/news/zimsit-m-the-plight-of-a-zimbabwean-student-in-2015-country-reports-publications-konrad-adenauer-stiftung-foundation-zimbabwe-konrad-adenauer-stiftung/ (accessed on 12 June 2017).

Maiyo, K. J., G. Ngao, D. Mulwa and P. Mugambi. 2012. "Peace Education for Sustainable Peace and Development: A Case of Kenya," *Journal of Peace, Gender and Development* 2(2), 28–33.

Makura, O. and A. H. Makura. 2012. "Rethinking the Definition and Value of the Curriculum Concept: The Zimbabwe Experience," *Anthropologist* 14(6), 509–515.

Mlambo, A. S. 2013a. "From Education and Health for All by 2000 to the Collapse of the Social Services Sector in Zimbabwe, 1980–2008," *Journal of Developing Societies* 29(4), 355–378.

Mlambo, A. S. 2013b. "Becoming Zimbabwe or Becoming Zimbabwean: Identity, Nationalism and State Building," *Africa Spectrum* 48(1), 49–70.

Moyo, N. 2014. "Nationalist Historiography, Nation-State Making and Secondary School History: Curriculum Policy in Zimbabwe 1980–2010," *Nordidactica-Journal of Humanities and Social Science Education* 2, 1–21.

Mpofu, J., S. Chimhenga and O. Mafa. 2013. "Funding Higher Education in Zimbabwe: Experience, Challenges and Opportunities of the Cadetship Scheme," in D. Teferra (ed.), *Funding Higher Education in Sub-Saharan Africa.* London: Palgrave Macmillan, 327–350.

Murisa, T. 2010. "Social Development in Zimbabwe," Discussion Paper Prepared for the Development Foundation for Zimbabwe. www.dfzim.com/wp-content/downloads/Social_Development_in_Zimbabwe_by_Dr_T_Murisa.pdf (accessed on 12 June 2017).

Navarro-Castro, L. and J. Nario-Galace. 2008. *Peace Education: A Pathway to a Culture of Peace.* Quezon City: Centre for Peace Education.

Ndlovu, M. 2009. "History Curriculum, Nation-Building and the Promotion of Common Values in Africa: A Comparative Analysis Zimbabwe and South Africa," *Yesterday and Today* 4, 67–76.

Nhundu, T. 1992. "A Decade of Educational Expansion in Zimbabwe: Causes, Consequences and Policy Contradictions," *The Journal of Negro Education* 61(1), 78–98.

Njoku, A. and C. A. Anyanwu. 2016. "Peace Education for Unity and Development," *World Scientific News* 26, 50–56.

Nyamunda, T. 2014. "Insights into Independent Zimbabwe: Some Historiographical Reflections," *Strategic Review of Southern Africa* 36(1), 72–89.

Nyazema, N. Z. 2010. "The Zimbabwe Conflict and the Provision of Social Services: Health and Education," *Journal of Developing Societies* 26(2), 233–261.

Onen, A. T. 2017. "Fighting Genocide Ideology in Post-Genocide Rwanda: The Contribution of Education," *International Journal of Science Arts and Commerce* 2(1), 1–10.

Pape, J. 1998. "Changing Education for Majority Rule in Zimbabwe and South Africa," *Comparative Education Review* 42(3), 253–266.

Paulson, J. (Ed.) 2011. *Education, Conflict and Development.* Oxford: Symposium Books.

Phimister, Ian. 2012. "Narratives of Progress: Zimbabwean Historiography and the End of History," *Journal of Contemporary African Studies* 30(1), 27–34.

Pigozzi, M. J. 1999. *Education in Emergencies and for Reconstruction: A Developmental Approach.* New York: UNICEF.

Pswarayi, L. and T. Reeler. 2012. "Fragility and Education in Zimbabwe: Assessing the Impact of Violence on Education. http://protectingeducation.org/sites/default/files/documents/fragile_state_and education_in_zimbabwe_december_2012.pdf (accessed on 12 May 2017).

Ramirez-Barat, C. and R. Duthie. 2015. *Education and Transitional Justice: Opportunities and Challenges for Peacebuilding.* Netherlands: International Center for Transitional Justice.

Ranga, D. 2015. "The Role of Politics in the Migration of Zimbabwean Teachers to South Africa," *Development Southern Africa* 32(2), 258–273.

Ranger, T. 2004. "Nationalist Historiography, Patriotic History and the History of the Nation: The Struggle Over the Past in Zimbabwe," *Journal of Southern African Studies* 30(2), 215–234.

Shizha, E. and M. T. Kariwo. 2011. *Education and Development in Zimbabwe: A Social, Political and Economic Analysis*. Rotterdam: Sense Publishers.

Smith, A. and T. Vaux. 2003. *Education, Conflict, and International Development*. London: Department of International Development.

Solidarity Peace Trust. 2003. "National Youth Service Training. 'Shaping Youths in a Truly Zimbabwean Manner': An Overview of Youth Militia Training and Activities in Zimbabwe," www.solidaritypeacetrust.org/download/report-files/youth_militia.pdf (accessed on 4 April 2017).

Southern African Regional Universities Association (SARUA). 2009. "Towards a Common Future: Higher Education in the SADC Region: Regional Country Profiles," Prepared to Accompany Report Titled "Towards a Common Future' Higher Education and SADC Regional Development." www.sarua.org/files/countryreports/Country_Report_Zimbabwe.pdf (accessed on 22 May 2017).

Tschirgi, N. 2011. "Conflict, Education and Peacebuilding: Converging Perspectives," *Conflict and Education: An Interdisciplinary Journal* 1(1), 1–5.

United Nations Educational Scientific Cultural Organisation (UNESCO). 2011. *The Hidden Crisis: Armed Conflict and Education: Education for All Global Monitoring Report*. Paris: UNESCO.

Winthrop, R. and E. Matsui. 2013. *A New Agenda for Education in Fragile States*. Brookings: Center for Universal Education.

16 "The Bruised and Troubled Nation"

Pentecostals, reconciliation, and development in Zimbabwe

Kudzai Biri

Introduction

This chapter examines the approach taken by Pentecostals in an attempt to mediate peace, forgiveness, and reconciliation in Zimbabwe. The hate, the wounds, and the grievances that many Zimbabweans harbour and the scars that they bear from the crisis and violence are deep-seated challenges that the church grapples with. Individuals and groups suffered due to different reasons. These included: ethnic identity and physical location (Gukurahundi: Sifting the chaff in reference to residents of the Matabeleland and Midlands provinces), race: During the "Third Chimurenga" to redress the economic imbalance between the black majority and the white minority in land occupation and ownership, others exploitation and harassment on the basis of political affiliation and greed of both religious and political leaders. Affiliation to opposition parties, especially the Movement for Democratic Change (MDC) led by the late Morgan Tsvangirai brought untold suffering to members. Some were exiled if they were not killed, maimed, or lost property. Given the wide array of challenges and problems, Zimbabweans are wounded, bruised, and a troubled nation. In order to appreciate the significance of the crisis, one can draw attention to the millions of Zimbabweans who have been forced to leave the country in search of better opportunities in other countries. The millions in diaspora through push factors mainly economic and political reasons are a testimony of the situation within Zimbabwe that has persisted for decades. The resentment that characterises different groups of people must not to be underestimated. What traditions and cultures do Zimbabweans rely on to redress the situation? It is within the climate of hate, unforgiving spirit, and the quest for healing that Pentecostal theology of forgiveness emerges within the matrix of an envisioned and imagined national agenda of rebuilding and developing Zimbabwe.

In this chapter the quest for development in Zimbabwe does not only refer to economic production for the betterment for the people's lives. In the context of the crisis in Zimbabwe, it also embodies the need for acknowledgement, responsibility, and accountability that can enable forgiveness, a healing process, and reconciliation. The crimes and atrocities that were committed against individuals hinder their emotional and spiritual development. It has to be pointed out that the violence and different forms of resentment vary and have had the effects in varying degrees. For example, the evils of Gukurahundi saw deaths, maiming of masses, and trauma. Verbal abuse of ethnic groups, races, and parties are also areas that require attention. Hate speech in political rallies by politicians and also by the former first lady Grace Mugabe are examples that cannot be swept under the carpet. The gravity of violence and the effects determine the level that masses call for justice to prevail. Also, the perceived perpetrators of violence (the political elite of the ruling regime) initiated forgiveness and reconciliation without admitting their crimes and tell the nation to forget the past and move forward. This is the context in which the Pentecostals come in with their message of forgiveness and reconciliation. While all these require healing, but the processes differ greatly. Hence it is the argument of this chapter that the entry of Pentecostals into the politics of forgiveness and reconciliation through generic sermons appears to turn a blind eye on the nature of crimes committed. Thus, while trying to address existential issues at stake on the one hand, they have espoused a very weak political theology on the other. It is important to briefly give a glimpse of the political developments in Zimbabwe that led to violence.

The political climate during the election period

David Kaulemu (2009) has described the culture of political violence in Zimbabwe especially the 2008 presidential elections, when it was clear to Mugabe that he could not compete against the more popular Morgan Tsvangirai of MDC. He says;

> Most of the historical violent campaigns have been moralised. They are seen as morally justified as ways of getting rid of, evil, dirty, ignorance, primitive culture and many other evils . . . exclusivist politics was at the heart of Murambatsvina political project, and the Fast track Land Reform Programme which culminated in the electoral violence of 2008.

On another note, Kaulemu (2009: 5) furnishes us with sensitive developments that saw the destruction of houses and business premises of people who were largely believed by the ruling elite to support Tsvangirai (the then leader of the main opposition party, the Movement for Democratic Change);

> some people have been regarded as chaff (Gukurahundi) and others "dirt" ("Murambatsvina") that culminated in the destruction of the so called illegal houses and loss of lives and jobs).

Hammar and Raftopolouos (2003: 28) echo the same sentiments as Kaulemu by specifically pointing to the ruling ZANU PF's responsibility in initiating and unleashing violence. This is not to deny that opposition parties did the same but in most cases they were reacting to provocation. Hammar and Raftopolouos (2003: 28) noted; "anyone seen as opposing the regime becomes an enemy, subject to violent attack and beyond any protection by the state is seen as an enemy." This was the prevailing situation in Zimbabwe that left the majority of people vulnerable, defenceless, and living in fear of victimisation, torture, disappearance, and death. Robert Mugabe played the card of hypocrisy, denouncing violence while his party continued to organise violent attacks on the opposition. It is in this context that the masses clamoured for the intervention of international bodies to restore the rule of law which was, however, futile because Mugabe had adopted a tough anti-Western stance and looked East for trade relationships.

Lack of a unifying national narrative

It has to be pointed out that political leaders continued to squander resources in Zimbabwe. In particular is the Chiadzwa diamonds that the nation was looking forward to. It was envisaged that they would rescue the collapsing economy. Thus there was dominant political rhetoric and lack of a unifying practical national narrative that fosters development. The political leaders continued to wine and dine, harping about protecting the legacy of the liberation struggle. They positioned themselves as the sole beneficiaries of that revolution by squandering state resources. Sanctions from the West became a scapegoat for the economic meltdown. The quest and contestation for power among both political parties has witnessed personal selfish agenda being perpetuated instead of a national narrative that envisages a vision for unifying and rebuilding the "bruised nation." This disunity has led to co-option of some religious leaders into the structures of the ruling structures through patronage networking. Some of these religious leaders could not critique the government's injustices. Instead, they became the mouthpiece of some politicians in telling the nation to forget the past and move forward. However, this is not to overlook the call for social justice, shunning violence, and the call for responsibility by the Catholic Commission for Justice and Peace (CCJP) and the Zimbabwe Catholic Bishops Conference (ZCBC). There was no space for citizens to vent out their anger as it should have been read as part of the healing processes. Those who dared raise issues of injustices have been labelled enemies of the state or puppets of the West, that have an agenda of destroying the hard-won independence. It has to be mentioned that most of the crimes were perpetrated by ZANU PF youths. Kaulemu (2009) says;

> It is clear that the moral vision of the ZANU led political project does not take moral responsibility for the people with different backgrounds, history and orientation from ZANU PF's. Under the ZANU PF government, non – party members have found it difficult to access national resources such as food in times of drought, freedom of assembly and association, access to land resources such as food, business opportunities and the right to think and express their thoughts without looking over their shoulder.

In the light of this statement, it cannot be disputed that advocating peace, forgiveness, and reconciliation is an uphill task. The sermons on forgiveness fall within Pentecostal political theology. Before examining the Pentecostal approach to reconciliation, there is need to establish the traditional worldview on wrongdoing and reconciliation in order to have a base of the cultural milieu and to critique the strength and weaknesses of Pentecostal theology.

Traditional understanding of forgiveness and reconciliation

The African people, generalisable to the Shona of Zimbabwe (the statistically and politically dominant ethnic group), had ways of settling wrongs and encouraging reconciliation. The traditional thrust emphasises dialogue and engagement and it is deeply entrenched among the Shona whenever there was violence and murder. The chapter gives attention to murder because of the perceived sacrality of life and the grievousness of murder which seem to have overlooked in the crisis moments during the Mugabe era. Mangena (2012: 25) points out the communal character of retributive punishment on murder. It emphasises the communal responsibility of murder by virtue of kinship ties (*dzinza*). Even the innocent people who did not commit the crime suffer by virtue of blood ties.

The Shona proverb *mushonga wengozi kuripa* (the only way to appease avenging spirit is through paying a fine) is significant (see the chapter by Jeater in this volume). However, in post-colonial Zimbabwe, we witnessed the resilience of traditional forms of appeasing wrongdoing and the suffering of the extended family, if proper rituals are not carried out for retributive justice. This raises questions on absolute claims of complete loss of ontological ultimacy. *Ngozi* (justice seeking spirit) teaches the murderer and the family to practice restorative justice and teaches wrongdoers how it feels to be treated in certain ways that violate a person's natural right to life. Bourdillon (1976) points to the forms of justice that are carried out. If it is murder, a large herd of cattle has to be paid to the wronged family and also a virgin girl accompanies the large herds of cattle. What is significant in this process to the chapter is not the token of the virgin girl because of post-colonial human rights discourses that are pro-women. However, it is the process of acknowledgement and settling the wrong that is significant as a sign of remorse, redressing, forgiveness, and reconciliation. How then do Pentecostals relate with this traditional culture as they attempt to mediate forgiveness and reconciliation in Zimbabwe?

The quest to rebuild Zimbabwe

Pentecostals should be applauded for preaching forgiveness and reconciliation in Zimbabwe. The call for unity is noble in a country torn apart on political, religious, tribal, racial, and economic grounds. Pentecostals have emphasised the need to rebuild Zimbabwe and restore the legacy that the nation had before the Mugabe regime ransacked the national coffers and compromised the socio-economic and political fabric of the nation. Pentecostals emphasise the need to rebuild Zimbabwe. They propound a noble agenda of unity and empowering the black race. Kalu (2008) aptly describes the Pentecostal dominant theology on development in Nigeria, but generalisable and applicable to the Zimbabwean context. Pentecostals preach the need for unity that transcends the colonial national boundaries and all differences. They call for all the citizens to participate in building and developing their nations. This begins with dealing with the "bruised self" that has gone through different challenges in life and extends to dealing with the issues of the nation as a concerned citizen. This teaching is very noble in as far as the Pentecostals emphasise the significance of their prospective countries and Africa at large. The ethos of accountability and responsibility is also very important in Pentecostal discourses of nation building. The important question to establish is whether or not the Pentecostals emphasise responsibility and accountability in post-violent periods as they teach on forgiveness and reconciliation.

Deployment of the Bible

Pentecostals rely heavily on the Bible. They teach that it is a must to forgive (Matthew 22: 21ff). Hence regardless of wrongs and crimes committed against the individual, forgiving the perpetrator is a must. This teaching has raised a lot of debate in light of the developments that took place in Zimbabwe. First, politicians had to move around in churches urging people to forgive those who had wronged them. An example is the late Vice President Nkomo who came to ZAOGA on their 50th Grand Jubilee anniversary in 2011 (Biri, 2013). He announced that, they were hoping that ZAOGA as one of the oldest and largest Pentecostal churches would take the lead to preach forgiveness and reconciliation. Who did what during the violent elections and what form of restorative justice was required? This is one of the pressing questions that people with scars have continuously raised. Because of the violent nature of events in Africa, the All Africa Conference of Churches (AACC) has often raised the need for perpetrators of violence to own their wrongs and crimes to enable a genuine process of forgiveness, healing, and reconciliation. This, therefore, points to the need for a dialogue forum, in the manner of the South African Truth and Reconciliation Commission that strove to bring matters to light and to bring restorative justice.

The deployment of scriptures without paying attention to the dynamics of the forms of violence appears to have wounded the wounded even more. Also, it shows direct glossing of a weighty matter within both the political and Pentecostal fraternity, just to just wake up and tell people to forget the past. Yet, the general feeling was that the perpetrators of violence (politicians from different political parties) did not qualify to preach peace without acknowledging their own wrongdoing. Second, it was more of a demand approach from perpetrators of violence instead of probing cases of violence in order to bring to book the culprits. The context of forgiveness in the Bible has to be understood; the one to forgive and the one to be forgiven and on what. But in the Zimbabwean context, perpetrators are known although they did not want to be accountable. Hence, this renders the deployment of scriptures futile.

For example, one of the top ZAOGA pastors at the Grange worship centre on 05–05–2016 implored the church to pray for the government because they were trying their best amidst economic hardships to pay civil servants. The researcher questioned the appraisal of the government because it was in the midst of the outcry by Zimbabweans following the missing fifteen billion dollars from the mining sector and corruption by the political elite. Most Zimbabweans were bitter because it was well known that it was the political elite that had misused the funds. Yet the excuse that was given for the economic meltdown was by arguing that the sanctions by the Western countries were responsible. Tudor Bismarck of Life Ministries International should be acknowledged for his consistently preaching an anti-Mugabe gospel in which he emphasised the hypocrisy of politicians and denounced their violence.[12] He emphasises the need for accountability, development, and unity of all Zimbabweans. Yet, other Pentecostal leaders appear to be on the side of the regime that had been responsible for the suffering of the majority of citizens.

Evidence of some Pentecostal leaders attending the lavish meetings, bashes, and state during which they donated huge sums of money raised eyebrows. Some critical citizens, including other Pentecostals, felt that the church had been compromised. When the Pentecostal fraternity is torn apart by contestation, the Christian body divided. The situation becomes worse when they are denouncing each other. Members of the community ask: Who then mediates the project of forgiveness and reconciliation? Such a question is an awakening call for the religious leaders to unite and push the vision and agenda to rebuild Zimbabwe.

The church remains the strategic institution to mediate forgiveness, peace, and reconciliation and pioneer development in Zimbabwe. However, in Zimbabwe, it Ezekiel Guti of ZAOGA has been sensitive to the traditional ways of forgiveness and reconciliation. In his teaching on *ngozi*, he advocates the Christian ethic of admitting wrong or committed sins (Biri, 2013). It opens the avenue for resuscitating the ritual of appeasing avenging spirits following suppression in the church. What is important in Guti's teaching is a call to admit crimes that one commits which enables restorative justice and then reconciliation. Marleen De Witte (2012: 171) has insights that accurately describe Guti's teaching on forgiveness and reconciliation. She argues that neo-traditionalism is a reformulation of "tradition" of what existed before, a conscious renewal and revival of what is considered to be tradition; "Neo-traditional religious movements strive for the rehabilitation for the indigenous religious traditions in new forms that are relevant to the present and the future." Guti has advocated paying a fine to the wronged family, which is totally overlooked in other Pentecostal discourses.

Evaluating the Pentecostal attitude

It has been pointed out by Mugambi (2002) that there is need for engaging African indigenous spiritualties in order to effectively deal with issues that are intriguing. The major challenge is that African traditional religions and culture are demonised by the Pentecostals. Yet, people's orientation betrays a strong lurking belief in indigenous spiritualties in relation to reconciliation and forgiveness. The concept of redressing the wrongs committed or perpetrated by an offender remains one of the challenging areas for Pentecostals to engage. While these indigenous spiritualties continue to lurk, Pentecostals appear to ignore them and emphasise that forgiveness is a must. Drawing the teaching of Jesus teaching his disciples, Pentecostals insist that forgiveness is unconditional. They say that the teachings of Jesus indicate that one must be prepared to forgive always and under every circumstance.

Another set-back is that Pentecostals have been compared to the Zimbabwe Catholics Bishops Conference (ZCBC), who have been consistent critics of the socio-economic and political injustices perpetrated by the Mugabe regime. Most of them were silent when they were expected to denounce the evils of Mugabe regime as the former First lady, a professed Pentecostal, heavily utilised Pentecostal women's gatherings to perpetuate ZANU PF agenda. Many people felt betrayed by Pentecostals who failed to be a voice for the voiceless, but quickly preached the message of forgiveness and reconciliation. Politicians had to force people at Pentecostal gatherings to tell them to forgive. Yet many people felt that these political leaders were perpetrators of violence and were forcing people to forgive and reconcile by burying the past or were instructing church leaders to preach forgiveness and reconciliation. The important question that the masses in Zimbabwe wanted and still want is the perpetrators of violence to take responsibility and acknowledge their wrong doing of corruption, mass murder, political torture and mass killings during the Gukurahundi.

The persistence of the clamour for ZANU PF leadership to acknowledge Gukurahundi is a sure sign of how the Zimbabwe masses remain trapped in traditional forms of reconciliation and not simply forgiving the enemy as preached by the Pentecostals. The traditional way of redressing, forgiving, and reconciling is through bringing the culprit to book and mapping the way forward; retributive justice (Mangena, 2012). One of the challenges faced by the new President Emmerson Mnangagwa is the pressure that he has to acknowledge and apologise on Gukurahundi. He has to address the critique that his new regime is "old wine in new wineskins," therefore associated with the brutality of the Mugabe regime as a former leader in Mugabe's cabinet and perceived as one of active players during Gukurahundi.

Pentecostals demonise and dismiss avenging spirits as demonic powers (Biri, 2013). Psalms 117: 17, "the dead know nothing" is often quoted. Yet, the first murder story in the Bible, Genesis 4 of Cain and Abel is important. The shed blood (not spirit) of Abel calls for vengeance (Gaster, 1969). Pentecostals are silent over such verses in their sermons on forgiveness and reconciliation. Although they are often regarded as people who heavily rely on scriptures, it appears they selectively choose scriptures to suit their agenda. In this discourse of reconciliation, the chapter argues that lack of critical stance against perpetrators of violence by Pentecostals against the ruling regime is another form of patronising with the political elite. Hence, they are also usurped of their prophetic voice for the voiceless. It is in this regard that the chapter recognises the CCJP and the ZCBC for an open and outstanding critique against the Mugabe regime, spelling out the injustices clearly.

The Pentecostals do not pay attention to the traditional dynamics of reconciliation. Apart from dismissing the belief in the avenging spirits, the Pentecostal teachings in general overlook the disintegrating relations for, instance, family relations, labour relations, race, ethnic, and political relations. Therefore, I argue that some of the sermons are a form of verbal violence against the "wounded and the bruised." However, the strength of the Pentecostal message lies in its emphasis of the virtue of solidarity, the need to forgive and develop Zimbabwe.

The chapter argues that there is need for social justice in Pentecostal sermons, calling the perpetrators of violence to account as a first step towards forgiving and reconciliation. Instead of imposing and forcing forgiveness on people who have a quest to be heard, people wounded and bruised and worse, who had never had the chances for telling their hidden narratives of pain as part of the healing process, Pentecostals must prioritise truth telling.

Reconciliation requires the perpetrators to feel remorse over their evil actions. However, in Zimbabwe, ZANU PF appears to be perennial perpetrators of violence hence the message of forgiving is questioned because they continue to unleash violence. It remains to be seen if the new president, Emmerson Mnangagwa is serious about changing the culture of violence in his party. Kaulemu (2009) rightly points to a deep-seated culture of political violence in Zimbabwe. It is within this climate that Pentecostal leaders should denounce violence vehemently as the basis for preaching reconciliation. Their messages, however, make sense in a context of the quest for development and rebuilding the destroyed pillars of Zimbabwe's socio-economic and political fabric. But it is the "fatigue" of Pentecostal gospel that makes their message of reconciliation ineffective. The failure to espouse the gospel clearly within the context of cultural conditions and force the state to "redeem its promises of democracy" that are required for forgiveness and reconciliation renders their message ineffective, for there continues to be unabated anger and grudges even within the "new" Mnangagwa regime. The messages that circulate on the social media calling for political leaders to address atrocities committed against communities in the Matabeleland and Midlands provinces are a testimony of the anger that people have emanating from Gukurahundi, decades after the crimes were committed. Hence the claim in this chapter is that the Pentecostals have failed to come up with a "redemptive and empowering theology" on forgiveness and reconciliation in spite of the noble agenda to promote forgiveness, healing, and reconciliation.

Conclusion

Pentecostals in Zimbabwe have focused on forgiveness and reconciliation in the post-conflict era. The message of forgiveness and reconciliation is needed in a crisis-hit Zimbabwe where many people harbour resentment against each other, political parties, ethnic groups, races, and the government. However, there appears to be a lack of serious engagement with the dimensions of forgiveness and reconciliation to effectively deal with the issues to promote an enabling environment to promote healing and development. It is important for Pentecostals to re-engage the cultural sentiments on forgiveness as a lasting solution for Zimbabwe as the nation seeks to deal with the past and move forward.

Notes

1 This paper acknowledges the diversities within the Pentecostal community and cannot claim universality on sermons. Hence, the sermonic discourses that are cited are based on general sermons that run through.
2 For ethical considerations, names of some leaders are not mentioned.

Sources

Biri, K. 2013. "African Pentecostalism and Cultural Resilience: The Case of the Zimbabwe Assemblies of God Africa," Unpublished DPhil, Department of Religious Studies, Classics and Philosophy, University of Zimbabwe.

Bourdillon, M. F. C. 1976. *The Shona Peoples: An Ethnography of the Shona Speaking Peoples of Zimbabwe*. Gweru: Mambo Press.

De Witte, M. 2012. "Neo Traditional Religions," in E. Bongmba (ed.), *The Wiley Blackwell Companion to African Religions*. West Sussex: Wiley Blackwell Publishers, 171–183.

Gaster, T. H. 1969. *Myth, Legend and Custer in the Old Testament, a Comparative Study with Chapters from Sir J. G. Frazer's Folklore in the Old Testament*. London: Gerald Duckworth.

Hammar, A. and B. Raftopoulos. 2003. "Zimbabwe's Unfinished Business: Re-thinking Land, State and Nation," in A. Hammar, B. Raftopoulos and S. Jensen (eds.), *Zimbabwe's Unfinished Business: Re-Thinking Land, State and the Nation in the Context of Crisis*. Harare: Weaver Press.

Kalu, O. 2008. *African Pentecostalism: An Introduction*. Oxford: Oxford Union Press.

Kaulem, U. D. (Ed.) 2007. *Imagining Citizenship in Zimbabwe*. Harare: KAS.

Kaulem, D. U. 2009. *Ending Violence in Zimbabwe*. Harare: KAS.

Mangena, F. 2012. *On Ubuntu and Retributive Punishment in Korekore-Nyombwe Culture: Emerging Ethical perspectives*. Harare: Best Practices Books.

Mugambi, J. N. K. 2002. *Christianity and African Culture*. Nairobi: Acton.

17 Zimbabwean theology and religious studies promoting national healing and reconciliation

Towards curriculum transformation[1]

Ezra Chitando and Nisbert T. Taringa

Introduction

The test of twenty-first century education leans heavily on the extent to which teaching, learning, and research it utilises upholds inspired contextual teaching, learning, and research. This direction, in which education at its highest level must take, must be well suited for service learning. There is need for socially embedded teaching, learning, and research; what one may refer to as public intellectualism. This requires identifying a particular issue, problem, or dilemma in the world/society, then looking for teaching content to systematically analyse and interpret so that the analysis sheds light on the issue or open paths for possible social transformation. This entails engaging in teaching that is concerned with contextual knowledge, interactively constructed, action oriented, and imbued with certain values.

Emerging critiques of African theology and religious studies (Chitando, 2010; Amanze, 2012) have drawn attention to the need to ensure that these disciplines address the existential realities that millions of Africans wrestle with. The major criticism is that these disciplines have tended to focus on themes that are prominent in Western theology and religious studies at the expense of addressing the lived realities of the learners and members of the community that the graduates will serve. As a result, African theology and religious studies have not focused on African realities, challenges, and experiences in a more systematic and transformative way.

Cognisant of these critiques, this chapter seeks to explore the role of Zimbabwean theology and religious studies in contributing towards national healing and reconciliation. The chapter maintains that Zimbabwean theology and religious studies can provide a firm basis for national development by engaging in conflict transformation. This can be achieved if the curriculum of Zimbabwean theology and religious studies includes a focus on national healing and reconciliation. As Gathogo (2012) has highlighted, there is a growing interest in healing and reconciliation in many parts of Africa. However, Zimbabwean churches have not built on their comparative advantage to implement sustainable programmes on national healing. Thus, "Religious leaders have not so far robustly deployed their national healing aptitude in any systematic way. They need to step up, as do the leaders of educational institutions" (Bratton and Masunungure, 2018: 15).

Acknowledging the role of religion in healing and reconciliation has become particularly urgent due to the global focus on religion and violence. The current tendency to associate religion with violence overlooks the ambivalence of religion, namely, the idea that religion can promote either peace or violence (Appleby, 2000). Such a position has become popular due to the growing interest in the idea of "religious violence" (Cavanaugh, 2009). However, in reality there is never "religious violence," but only certain groups with political agendas who appropriate religion in pursuit of their goals. It is, therefore, crucial for theology and religious studies to expose the manipulation of religion and promote security (Ushe, 2015). Further, it is critical to appreciate the impact of reconciliation on individuals, families and communities. Religion plays a major role in facilitating reconciliation. But, what is reconciliation?:

> Reconciliation means the restoration of the bonds of friendship and affection between people who are divided by strife, enmity, or even crime. It means a transformation of relationships, which are normally linked to a change in feelings, attitudes and opinions. Therefore, the culture of suspicion, fear, mistrust and violence must be broken down, and opportunities for individuals to hear and to be heard should be provided. Furthermore, healing and reconciliation need to go hand in hand, especially when the ethnic groups that have been involved in the conflict against each other must continue to live together. Thus, for reconciliation to take place and result in lasting peace, both victims and perpetrators need to be healed.
>
> (Banyanga and Björkqvist, 2017: 9)

The importance of reconciliation has been recognised in various disciplines, including in international relations. In their edited volume, *Apology and Reconciliation in International Relations: The Importance of Being Sorry*, Daas et al. (2016) demonstrate the value of saying sorry in international relations. This chapter appreciates the growing appreciation of the value of reconciliation by focusing on how Zimbabwean theology and religious studies could equip learners with knowledge and skills to facilitate healing and reconciliation in the country.

The first section of this chapter reviews some of the key literature on religion/theology and peace in selected countries in Africa. The second section focuses on how some researchers in theology and religious studies in Zimbabwe have included the focus on healing and reconciliation. The third section outlines themes in healing and reconciliation that can be included more purposefully in the teaching of these disciplines in Zimbabwe. In conclusion, the chapter argues that Zimbabwean theology and religious studies must promote the focus on healing and reconciliation in order to contribute towards development (Ilo, 2014). Zimbabwean theology and religious studies can be resources in the quest for development by ensuring social cohesion and integration. This will galvanise communities to invest in productivity and overcome negative tensions. Thus:

> Instead of continuing as mere recipients or conduits for development aid, the church in Africa needs to bring itself into the centre-stage of the development agenda of the continent as part of its cultural mandate to ensure in its membership hard work, discipline, saving and a culture of investment towards the future.
>
> (Hiagbe, 2015: 177)

Religion/theology and reconciliation in Africa: An overview

In order to put the role of theology and religious studies in Zimbabwe in promoting national healing and reconciliation into its proper perspective, it is important to summarise efforts that have been undertaken elsewhere in Africa. The interface between religion/theology and peace in Africa has attracted considerable scholarly attention. It is not possible to do justice to the review of the literature within the context of this chapter. Instead, we adopt a selective stance and concentrate on a few case studies and scholars from different regions in Africa in order to demonstrate the emerging trends and patterns in this discourse. We remain alive to the typology of the four areas where reconciliation has to happen, as formulated by Cecilia Clegg, namely, political reconciliation, societal reconciliation, interpersonal reconciliation, and personal reconciliation (cited in Vaule, 2015: 47–48).

For the case studies, we select case studies from Southern, East, and West Africa. Thus, we summarise reflections on the Truth and Reconciliation Commission (TRC) of South Africa, the Rwandan genocide and the conflict in Nigeria. While we recognise the specific nature of each conflict, we are persuaded that it remains possible to identify the emerging trends and patterns across the different contexts. We have left out some significant religious players in the conflict transformation process in Africa, such as the Interreligious Councils of Sierra Leone and Uganda due to space considerations.

The Truth and Reconciliation Commission of South Africa

South Africa's TRC has enjoyed considerable reflection. In fact, it has often been praised for its emphasis on forgiveness ahead of retribution. The TRC of South Africa has been celebrated for its role in bringing victims and perpetrators of violence in the same space to dialogue. It has enabled victims to have their pain acknowledged, while also allowing perpetrators to ask for forgiveness from their victims. In particular, Desmond Tutu, the celebrated church leader and theologian, who was also the chairperson of the TRC, promoted a version of healing and reconciliation that was informed by his religious convictions. The TRC has been held up as an example of a successful national healing process and has been recommended for adoption in other contexts of conflict. Gibson (2005) makes the following observation:

> Indeed, the world has acknowledged the success of South Africa's TRC through the numerous attempts to replicate its truth and reconciliation process in other troubled areas of the globe. Truth commissions modeled on the South African experience have proliferated, and one of the leaders of South Africa's experiment has created a major institute in New York to assist countries in developing plans for reconciliation in the world's many festering hot spots. Perhaps the judgment that the TRC succeeded is based on nothing more than the simple (and simplistic) observation that South Africa appears to have made a successful, relatively peaceful, and quite unexpected transition from the apartheid dictatorship to a reasonably democratic and stable regime. Some surely attribute South Africa's transformation to its truth and reconciliation process. If a TRC "worked" in South Africa, perhaps it can work elsewhere.
>
> (Gibson, 2005: 344)

Despite its global appeal, the TRC in South Africa has been criticised by a number of theologians. For example, the South African black theologian, Maluleke (2001), charged that the power structures favouring whites over blacks still remained intact. Similarly, another black theologian, Boesak (2008), utilises the biblical story of Zacchaeus (Luke 19: 1–10) to highlight the point that the TRC did not take the issue of tying reconciliation to justice seriously. Overall, it is important to note that the South African TRC has been touted as a model for promoting peace and healing in the country. Further, the distinctively theological and religious orientation of the TRC must be acknowledged.

Religion and the genocide in Rwanda

Religious bodies and religious ideas have also been appropriated in other African settings beyond South Africa. The genocide in Rwanda in 1994 highlighted the ambivalence of religion. Gatwa (2005) has examined the extent to which churches were implicated in the genocide. Whereas the general expectation is that religion will always promote peace and healing, some Christians and Muslims were actively involved in the genocide. However, Muslims appear to have fared better than Christians (Benda, 2012). That religion was implicated in the genocide was particularly devastating, as people of faith were expected to promote life under whatever situation. Thus:

> Organizers of the genocide exploited the historic concept of sanctuary to lure tens of thousands of Tutsi into church buildings with false promises of

protection; then Hutu militia and soldiers systematically slaughtered the unfortunate people who had sought refuge, firing guns and tossing grenades into the crowds gathered in church sanctuaries and school buildings, and methodically finishing off survivors with machetes, pruning hooks, and knives.

(Longman, 2010: 4–5)

As the foregoing citation shows, many people were killed as they sought refuge in religious institutions, with some religious leaders being actively involved in promoting the genocide. Religion was experiencing a very dramatic, "systems failure." Instead of promoting life, religion was sponsoring death. Thus, "It was not uncommon for a death squad in local communities to include prominent lay church people, priests, or other church employees, and at times church personnel themselves would lead the killers to the people seeking refuge in churches" (Schliesser, 2018: 3).

Despite the "theology of genocide" having influenced Rwanda's religious approach to the 1994 crisis, Schliesser (2018) argues that there has emerged a "theology of reconciliation" in Rwanda. This theology seeks to equip communities of faith to play a leading role in facilitating healing and reconciliation. It is clear, therefore, that religion is like the proverbial "double-edged sword." While it was implicated in the genocide, religion is now playing a major role in conflict transformation. This means that it is not possible for one to give a blanket assessment of the role of religion in Rwanda. There are moments when religion plays a positive role, and moments when religion plays a negative role. Orobator (2018: 81) categorises these as *prophetic practice* and *pathological performance* respectively (italics original).

Religion and terror in Nigeria

From East Africa, it is important to consider the role of religion in reconciliation in Nigeria, West Africa. A longer narrative is required to do justice to this theme. In this overview, we draw attention to the key themes. First, it is clear that the appropriation of religion in violence in Nigeria implies that religion has a major role to play in facilitating reconciliation in this vast country. Thus, ecumenical Christian bodies such as the Christian Association of Nigeria (CAN) have sought to promote peace and dialogue in the wake of religious violence in the country (Ilo, 2014). Second, there is a realisation that interfaith dialogue can contribute towards peace in Nigeria. Olupona, who has emerged as one of the leading scholars of religion in Africa, edited the volume, *Religion and Peace in Multi-Faith Nigeria* (Olupona, 1992). Scholars of religion, peace advocates, and government security officials all concur that interfaith dialogue is critical if peace is to be achieved in Nigeria. Thus:

In this direction, interfaith dialogue amongst religious, traditional and community stakeholders has been the focus of ongoing collaboration between the United Nations Development Programme (UNDP) Abuja office and the Institute for Peace and Conflict Resolution (IPCR). Since 2013, these two organizations have brought religious, traditional and community stakeholders together periodically to discuss modalities for initiating and promoting interfaith dialogue among diverse ethnic, religious and communal groups, especially in conflict areas such as the middle belt, north central zone and north east zone. The initiative has also included providing knowledge, skills and technical resources to empower stakeholders to undertake and promote various interfaith dialogue and cooperation programmes.

(Ahmed-Hameed, 2015: 87)

Overall, the role of religion in conflict transformation in Africa is attracting scholarly interest. Across the different regions of the continent, religious groups are making significant strides in promoting peace, healing, and integration. On their part, researchers are avoiding romantic approaches to the role of religion in conflict transformation in Africa. They have drawn attention to both the positive and negative contributions of religion. In the following section, we reflect on how Zimbabwean theology and religious studies can equip graduates to become more strategically placed to contribute towards national healing in the country.

Teaching theology and religious studies in Zimbabwe to promote national healing and reconciliation: Outlining the context

Cognisant of the critical role of religion in promoting reconciliation in different parts of the Africa, there is an urgent need to reflect on how Zimbabwean theology and religious studies could play a similar role. To achieve, this, however, requires curriculum transformation. Although Zimbabwean theology and religious studies have sought to address issues that emerge from the community (Chitando et al., 2014), they have not paid attention to the theme of healing and reconciliation in a more direct and sustained way. However, as we illustrate in this section, some valuable reflections have been provided on the role of churches in promoting healing and reconciliation in the country.

In order to promote a focus on healing and reconciliation in Zimbabwean theology and religious studies, there is need to ensure that staff and students are aware of the major issues and themes relating to the major challenges in the country's history. One of the major themes is violence. The history of the country is characterised by violence at different historical epochs, particularly in relation to colonial conquest and the struggle for liberation. Works by Sachikonye (2011) and Kaulemu (2011) have explored the impact of violence on the national consciousness. Therefore, staff and students in theology and religious studies need to be aware of the extent to which violence has affected individuals, communities, and the nation. As we shall argue later, this theme of violence in the national history is critical in order for one to understand the

Gukurahundi of the early 1980s when thousands of people were killed in the Matabeleland and Midlands provinces of Zimbabwe.

Theology and religious studies courses in Zimbabwe must be revamped in order to reflect the national quest for healing and reconciliation. However, there is need to understand the major issues that have affected the nation that inform the urgency of healing and reconciliation. We have already referred to the pressing issue of Gukurahundi in the foregoing paragraph. Other issues relate to Operation Murambatsvina/Clean Up/Restore Order in 2005 where hundreds of thousands were displaced and structures were destroyed, conflicts resulting from the fast-track land resettlement programme of the early 2000s, political violence relating to the 2008 elections, and other elections and other conflicts.

The curriculum must equip lecturers and students to gain a better appreciation of the different issues that have given rise to the need for healing and reconciliation. Further, there must be an investment in clarifying the role of religion in this quest. Although there is scope for further reflection and refinement, it is gratifying to note that some researchers have invested in trying to understand the meaning of reconciliation and the role of the church. For example, Muchena (2004) provides a detailed analysis of the strengths and weaknesses of the churches as they seek to mediate in the Zimbabwean crisis. On the other hand, Machingura (2010) has explored the multiple meanings of reconciliation in Zimbabwe through the prism of Matthew.

Chitando and Togarasei (2010) have sought to highlight the role of the church in national healing and integration. Approaching the theme of national healing from an African womanist perspective, Manyonganise (2015) has challenged churches to be on high alert in order to do justice to women's experience of violence. Mbire (2011) assesses the contribution of the Organ on National Healing, Reconciliation, and Integration (ONHRI), while Dombo (2014) has reflected on churches and national healing in Zimbabwe by examining the strengths and weaknesses of the church in promoting reconciliation. Munemo and Nciizah (2014) examine the contribution of churches to the peace and reconciliation process during the period of the Government of National Unity (2009–2013). Recognising the potential of religion to contribute to reconciliation, Tarusarira and Ganiel (2012) have sought to highlight how it can be a resource in national healing in Zimbabwe.

Addressing reconciliation in Zimbabwean theology and religious studies: Outlining key topics

In this section, we seek to outline some of the key topics that could be included in courses on religion and reconciliation in Zimbabwe. After introducing the course objectives, the course can begin by clarifying why people fight, or, reflecting on why healing and reconciliation become necessary in any given context. In this section, the course can explore historical, ethnic, political, economic, social, and other forms of exclusion (real or imagined) that often provide the context in which tension and violence emerge. At this stage, it is important to adopt a phenomenological, sociological, or descriptive approach, without rushing to bring in religion as a factor. Most scholars of religion face the challenge of wanting to see religion everywhere. Appreciating the role of inequality (real or imagined) as a factor in understanding why people fight is critical. Issues of memory, identity, exclusion, and perception of injustice are key to interpreting violence and creating pathways to peace (United Nations and World Bank, 2018).

With the students having been acquainted with reasons why tension and violence emerge, the course can proceed to discuss the concept of reconciliation. There are numerous approaches that can be used to introduce the theme of reconciliation to students. These include the linguistic, historical, comparative, psychological, theological, and other approaches. All these should highlight the complexity of the concept of reconciliation. In order to provoke in-depth reflection, the lecturer should not be constrained by the "chalk and talk" method of delivery, where they are the ultimate authority. Instead, they must invite students to make presentations and to share their ideas on reconciliation. It is under this theme that the issue of definition must be addressed. Although there are many definitions of reconciliation, the following definition by John Paul Lederach, one of the leading authorities on conflict transformation, is quite helpful. He writes:

> Reconciliation, in essence, represents a place, the point of encounter where concerns about both the past and the future can meet. Reconciliation-as-encounter suggests that space for the acknowledging of the past and envisioning the future is the necessary ingredient for reframing the present. For this to happen, people must find ways to encounter themselves and their enemies, their hopes and their fears.
>
> (Lederach, 1997: 27)

Alongside the previous definition by Lederach, it is quite helpful to reflect on some metaphors and concepts that have been used to make sense of reconciliation, especially from within African theology and religious studies. One major image which has been utilised is that reconciliation is a journey. For example, Charles Villa-Vicencio (2009), who played a prominent role in South Africa's TRC with Desmond Tutu, used the idea of a journey in his thoughts on political reconciliation in Africa. Emmanuel Katongole (2017) deploys the same image in his theological reflections on reconciliation in Africa, with case studies from East Africa. Another emerging idea is the "healing of memories." It has been used by Michael Lapsley (2012) in his workshops with victims and survivors of violence in Africa and other parts of the world.

After exploring the intricacies associated with reconciliation, the course can shift attention to the theme of religion and reconciliation. Once again, there are multiple perspectives that could be adopted. However, under this theme the course facilitator can focus on the idea that religion has the capacity to cause violence or promote peace. As noted in the introductory section, this notion has been articulated very effectively by Appleby (2000).

In this section, the course can focus on reflecting on the role religious leaders in promoting healing and reconciliation in different parts of the world. For example, religious leaders from different religions contributed to reconciliation in South Africa (Chapman and Spong, 2003). The course coordinator could also include reflections on the role of religion in the promotion of reconciliation in such diverse contexts as Northern Ireland, Israel/Palestine, Iran, Saudi Arabia, Macedonia, and Indonesia (Smock, 2006). Further, the contribution of ecumenical bodies such as the World Council of Churches (WCC) and the All Africa Conference of Churches (AACC) can be discussed in this section.

After the more general discussion in the earlier sections, the course can proceed to case studies. It would be strategic to cover Southern (South Africa), East (Rwanda), and West Africa (Nigeria) and focus on the case studies that we reviewed in the preceding sections. For Southern Africa, the TRC in South Africa is an important case study. Students can be equipped to understand how religious leaders played a major role in healing and reconciliation in the TRC. For example, it is important to appreciate the contribution of Desmond Tutu to the TRC. Thus, "Without notable religious figures like Desmond Tutu, the TRC would never have come about; without the high religiosity of South Africa, the TRC would likely not have achieved the success with which it is often credited" (Berkley Center for Religion, Peace, and World Affairs, 2013: 7).

Rwanda provides an intriguing case of the "ambivalence of the Sacred," whereby religion was both heavily implicated in the genocide and is now actively involved in promoting reconciliation and national healing. Bazuin (2013) has elaborated on the changes in religious affiliation due to individuals trying to come to terms with genocide, as well as the activities of different denominations that seek to promote healing and reconciliation in Rwanda. In this section, students should be able to debate the approach by political leaders, such as the president, Paul Kagame, to healing and reconciliation in the country. There is an emphasis on a shared, national identity, while rejecting ethnic identity.

In the Nigerian case study, the role of both Christian and Muslim leaders in challenging violence by religious extremists needs to be underscored. In a context characterised by Boko Haram and its use of terror, some Christian and Muslim leaders have emerged to denounce violence and to promote reconciliation. Crucially, the narrative of Christians and Muslims being perpetually locked in mortal combat in Nigeria needs to be challenged. Apart from the violence in the northern part of the country (and even there, stories of peaceful co-existence abound), in other parts of the country, Christians and Muslims enjoy cordial relations (Toki et al., 2015: 107).

From these case studies, the students should be able to highlight trends and patterns regarding the interface between religion and reconciliation in parts of Africa. They should be in position to identify the strengths that the faith community brings to the practice of reconciliation. At the same time, they should be able to bring out some of the challenges that religious people face when they seek to promote healing and reconciliation. Students can also create profiles of the types of conflicts that they discern from the different case studies.

Having attended to the conceptual and historical issues relating to religion and reconciliation and having examined selected case studies from different parts of the continent, the course can shift attention to Zimbabwe. There would be need to restate reasons why people have fought in Zimbabwe. Here, the course would need to pay attention to studies on the history of violence in the country. As we outlined in the discussion on the previous context, the course facilitator would need to highlight the extent to which the history of Zimbabwe has been characterized by different forms of violence across time.

In particular, however, there is need to draw attention to the violence of colonialism, the violent nature of the 1970s liberation struggle, and the violence in the Midlands and Matabeleland provinces (Gukurahundi) of the early to mid-1980s. Other instances of violence in the post-colonial period, including violence associated with elections (especially the 2008 election), Operation *Murambatsvina*/Restore Order in 2005 and others also need to be covered. Reflecting on how historical, political, ideological, ethnic, and other factors had a bearing on these forms of violence will enable students to have a clearer appreciating of these events. Machakanja (2010) provides valuable insights into the prospects and challenges of national healing and reconciliation in Zimbabwe.

The discussion on violence in Zimbabwe can be followed by an analysis of the role of the churches in addressing violence in the country. This could be done by following the traditional grouping of the different categories of churches. For example, an analysis of the responses of the Catholic Church, Protestant churches, African Independent/Initiated/Instituted churches (Dodo and Dodo, 2014), and Pentecostal churches (see the chapter by Biri in this volume) to violence would be quite informative. However, it is important to acknowledge the internal diversity that is masked by each one of the categories of previously named churches. Therefore, it is important to pursue how different denominations and personalities within these denominations have addressed the diverse forms of violence in Zimbabwe. As we outlined earlier, considerable literature has been produced in this area. Further, it is helpful to analyse the contribution of faith-based organisations such as the Ecumenical Church Leaders Forum and Grace to Heal that have sought to contribute to national healing and reconciliation in the country.

From the engagement with Christianity, the course can shift attention to the role of African Traditional Religions and *Ubuntu/Hunhu* in promoting healing and reconciliation. This is to counterbalance the contention that it is only Christianity which has the resources to contribute to healing and reconciliation. Since a discussion on *Ubuntu/Hunhu* and reconciliation could constitute a complete course in its own right, in this section, we will draw attention to some of the key issues. Some of the major considerations relate to defining *Ubuntu/hunhu* and relating it to healing and reconciliation (Tutu, 1999: 31; Metz, 2018). It must be underscored that *Ubuntu/Hunhu* provides valuable insights into how indigenous values can be utilised to promote national healing and reconciliation. Without romanticising this concept, it is possible to utilise *Ubuntu/Hunhu* to generate sustainable peace in communities (Mangena, 2012; Heal Zimbabwe Trust and Zimbabwe Civic Education Trust, 2016). The course can reflect on how *Ubuntu/Hunhu* handles issues relating to reconciliation and truth telling, justice, forgiveness, and other related concepts. For example, Benyera (2015) reflected on the concept of *ngozi* (justice-seeking spirit) (see also the chapter by Jeater in this volume) and how it can be regarded as an expression of transitional justice in Zimbabwe.

One of the most critical issues in healing and reconciliation relates to women's experience of violence. Although religion and gender has been mainstreamed in most departments of theology/philosophy and religious studies in Zimbabwe, it remains vital to ensure that students are sensitised to the gender dimension to religion and reconciliation. The course needs to tackle this from two related angles, namely, women as survivors of violence and women as agents of healing and reconciliation. Manyonganise (2015) has examined how current programmes on healing and reconciliation in Zimbabwe tend to leave out women. Writing from within the context of Nigeria, Onah et al. (2017) have underscored the urgency of prioritising women's experiences in contexts of ethno-religious conflicts. They highlight how gender inequality is deepened in the wake of violence, worsening women's poverty.

One of the last themes to be covered by the course relates to the emergence of theologies of reconciliation in Africa (and how they are incipient in Zimbabwean theology and religious studies). In this section, the course can interact with some of the significant voices on healing and reconciliation in Africa. These could include reflecting on publications, by, among others, Emmanuel Katongole, Desmond Tutu, Charles Villa-Vicencio, Tinyiko S. Maluleke, Joram Tarusarira, and others. As one would observe, these are African male theologians. Thus, it is strategic to examine how the Circle of Concerned African Women Theologians has handled issues of trauma and healing in their writings. Reflections by Molly Manyonganise and others who are focusing more specifically on theologies of healing are particularly helpful in formulating African theologies of reconciliation. Interfaith theologies of reconciliation, including the dialogue between Christian and Muslim approaches, could be addressed in this section. Further, the role and place of Ubuntu in African theologies of reconciliation will need further elaboration.

Conclusion

Zimbabwean theology and religious studies must invest in teaching and researching in the field of healing, reconciliation, and integration. In this chapter, we have undertaken an overview of developments in the field of churches and reconciliation in the different regions of Africa. We also reviewed how Zimbabwean scholars have approached the theme. We outlined the key themes to be covered in the proposed course, highlighting some of the major ideas and scholars. We are convinced that students who take up the course on national healing and reconciliation in Zimbabwe will emerge as critical resources in the quest for development. They will acquire the requisite skills and competencies necessary to transform their communities into healed and reconciled centres for development.

Note

1 The authors would like to express their appreciation to the Nagel Institute for support in the context of a research project on the churches and Gukurahundi in Zimbabwe.

Bibliography

Ahmed-Hammed, Aliyu. 2015. "Interfaith Dialogue: Preventing Extremism and Interreligious Conflict in Northern Nigeria," *International Journal of Humanities and Social Science Invention* 4(11), 82–89.

Amanze, James. 2012. "The Voicelessness of Theology and Religious Studies in Contemporary Africa: Who Is to Blame and What Has to Be Done? Setting the Scene," *Missionalia* 40(3), 189–204.

Appleby, R. Scott. 2000. *Ambivalence of the Sacred: Religion, Violence, and Reconciliation*. Oxford: Rowman and Littlefield.

Banyanga, Jean d'Amour and Kaj Björkqvist. 2017. "The Dual Role of Religion Regarding the Rwandan 1994 Genocide: Both Instigator and Healer," *Pyrex Journal of African Studies and Development* 3(1), 1–12.

Bazuin, Joshua T. 2013. "Religion in the Remaking of Rwanda after the Genocide," A Dissertation Submitted to the Faculty of the Graduate School of Vanderbilt University in Partial Fulfillment of the Requirements for the Degree of DOCTOR OF PHILOSOPHY in Community Research and Action May 2013, Nashville, TN.

Benda, Richard M. 2012. "The Test of Faith: Christians and Muslims in the Rwandan Genocide," A Thesis Submitted to the University of Manchester for the Degree of Doctor of Philosophy in the Faculty of Humanities.

Benyera, Everisto. 2015. "Presenting Ngozi as an Important Consideration in in Pursuing Transitional Justice for Victims: The Case of Moses Chokuda," *Gender & Behaviour* 13(2), 6760–6733.

Berkley Center for Religion, Peace and World Affairs. Georgetown University. 2013. *South Africa: The Religious Foundation of the Truth and Reconciliation Commission*. Washington, DC: Berkley Center for Religion, Peace, and World Affairs.

Boesak, Allan. 2008. "And Zacchaeus Remained in the Tree: Reconciliation and Justice and the Truth and Reconciliation Commission," *Verbum et Ecclesia* 28(3), 636–654.

Bratton, M. and E. V. Masunungure. 2018. *Heal the Beloved Country: Zimbabwe's Polarized Electorate*. Afrobarometer Policy Paper No. 49.

Cavanaugh, William T. 2009. *The Myth of Religious Violence: Secular Ideology and the Roots of Modern Conflict*. Oxford: Oxford University Press.

Chapman, Audrey R. and Bernard Spong (Eds.) 2003. *Religion and Reconciliation in South Africa: The Voices of Religious Leaders*. Philadelphia: Templeton Foundation Press.

Chitando, Ezra. 2010. "Equipped and Ready to Serve? Transforming Theology and Religious Studies in Africa," *Missionalia* 38(2), 187–210.

Chitando, Ezra, Tapiwa P. Mapuranga and Nisbert T. Taringa. 2014. "Zimbabwean Theology and Religious Studies During the Crisis Years (2000–2008): A Preliminary Study," *Studia Historia Ecclesiasticae* 40(1), 173–189.

Chitando, Ezra and Lovemore Togarasei. 2010. "'June 2008, Verse 27': The Church and the 2008 Zimbabwean Political Crisis," *African Identities* 8(2), 151–162.

Daas, Christopher et al. (Eds.) 2016. *Apology and Reconciliation in International Relations: The Importance of Being Sorry.* London: Routledge.

Dodo, Obediah and Gloria Dodo. 2014. "African Initiated Churches, Pivotal in Peace Building: A Case of the Johane Masowe Chishanu," *Journal of Religion and Society* 16, 1–12.

Dombo, Sylvester. 2014. "Refusing to be Co-opted? Church Organizations and Reconciliation in Zimbabwe with Special Reference to the Christian Alliance of Zimbabwe 2005–2013". *Journal for the Study of Religion* 27(2), 137–171.

Gathogo, Julius. 2012. "Reconciliation Paradigm in the Post Colonial Africa: A Critical Analysis," *Religion and Theology* 19, 74–91.

Gatwa, Tharcisse. 2005. *The Churches and Ethnic Identity in the Rwandan Crises 1900–1994.* Milton Keynes: Regnum Books International.

Gibson, James L. 2005. "The Truth About Truth and Reconciliation in South Africa," *International Political Science Review* 26(4), 341–361.

Heal Zimbabwe Trust (HZT) and Zimbabwe Civic Education Trust (ZIMCET). 2016. *Exploring Indigenous Transitional Justice Mechanisms in Zimbabwe.* Harare: Heal Zimbabwe Trust and Zimbabwe Civic Education Trust.

Hiagbe, Komi A. 2015. "The Church and Sustainable Development in Sub-Saharan Africa," *Studia Historiae Ecclesiasticae* 41(2), 164–179.

Ilo, Paul. 2014. "Faith-Based Organizations and Conflict-Resolution in Nigeria: The Case of the Christian Association of Nigeria (CAN)," *Journal of Global Initiatives* 9(2), 99–108.

Katongole, Emmanuel. 2017. *The Journey of Reconciliation: Groaning for a New Creation in Africa.* Maryknoll, NY: Orbis Books.

Kaulemu, David. 2011. *Ending Violence in Zimbabwe.* Harare: Konrad Adenauer Stiftung.

Lapsley, Michael and Stephen Karakashian. 2012. *Redeeming the Past: My Journey from Freedom Fighter to Healer.* Maryknoll, NY: Orbis Books.

Lederach, John Paul. 1997. *Building Peace: Sustainable Reconciliation in Divided Societies.* Washington, DC: United States Institute of Peace.

Longman, Timothy. 2010. *Christianity and Genocide in Rwanda.* Cambridge: Cambridge University Press.

Machakanja, Pamela. 2010. *National Healing and Reconciliation in Zimbabwe: Challenges and Opportunities.* Wynberg: Institute for Justice and Reconciliation.

Machingura, Francis. 2010. "The Reading and Interpretation of Matthew 18: 21–22 in Relation to Multiple Reconciliations: The Zimbabwean Experience," *Exchange* 39, 309–330.

Maluleke, Tinyiko S. 2001. "Can Lions and Rabbits Reconcile? The South African TRC as an Instrument of Peacebuilding," *The Ecumenical Review* 53(2).

Mangena, Fainos. 2012. *On Ubuntu and Retributive Punishment in Korekore-Nyombwe Culture: Emerging Ethical Perspectives.* Harare: Best Practices Books.

Manyonganise, Molly. 2015. "The Church, National Healing and Reconciliation in Zimbabwe: A Womanist Perspective on Churches in Manicaland (CiM)," A Thesis Submitted in Partial Fulfilment of the Requirements for the Degree of PhD in Biblical and Religious Studies in the Department of Biblical and Religious Studies, University of Pretoria.

Mbire, Moreblessing. 2011. "Seeking Reconciliation and National Healing in Zimbabwe: Case of the Organ on National Healing, Reconciliation and Integration (ONHRI)," A Research Paper Presented in Partial Fulfilment of the Requirements for Obtaining the Degree of Masters of Arts in Development Studies, Institute of International Studies, The Hague.

Metz, Thaddeus. 2018. "*Ubuntu*, Christianity, and Two Kinds of Reconciliation," in Moham-med Girma (ed.), *The Healing of Memories: African Christian Responses to Politically Induced Trauma*. Lanham: Lexington Books.

Muchena, Deprose. 2004. "The Church and Reconciliation: A Mission Impossible?" in Brian Raftopoulos and Tyrone Savage (eds.), *Zimbabwe: Injustice and Political Reconciliation*. Cape Town: Institute for Justice and Reconciliation.

Munemo, Douglas and Elinah Nciizah. 2014. "The Church in Zimbabwe's Peace and Rec-onciliation Process under the Government of National Unity," *IOSR Journal of Humanities and Social Science* 19(10), 63–70.

Olupona, Jacob K. (Ed.) 1992. *Religion and Peace in Multi-faith Nigeria*. Ile Ife, Nigeria: Obafemi Awolowo.

Onah, Nkechi G., Benjamin C. Diara and Favour C. Uroko. 2017. "Ethno-Religious Con-flicts in Nigeria: Implications on Women," *Mediterranean Journal of Social Sciences* 8(5), 61–68.

Orobator, Agbonkhianmeghe E. 2018. *Religion and Faith in Africa: Confessions of an Animist*. Maryknoll, NY: Orbis Books.

Sachikonye, Lloyd. 2011. *When a State turns on its Citizens: 60 Years of Institutionalised Violence in Zimbabwe*. Johannesburg: Jacana Media.

Schliesser, Christine. 2018. "From 'a Theology of Genocide' to a 'Theology of Reconcilia-tion'? On the Role of Christian Churches in the Nexus of Religion and Genocide in Rwanda," *Religions* 9, 34. doi:10.3390/rel9020034a.

Smock, David R. (Ed.) 2006. *Religious Contributions to Peacebuilding: When Religion Brings Peace, Not War*. Washington, DC: United States Institute of Peace.

Tarusarira, Joram and Gladys Ganiel. 2012. "Religion, Secular Democracy, and Conflict Res-olution in Zimbabwe," in Lee Marsden (ed.), *The Ashgate Research Companion to Religion and Conflict Resolution*. Farnham: Ashgate.

Toki, Tajudeen O., Muhammad A. Gambari and Muhammad A. Hadi. 2015. "Peace Building and Inter-Religious Dialogue in Nigeria," *Journal of Islam in Nigeria* 1(1), 104–116.

Tutu, Desmond. 1999. *No Future Without Forgiveness*. New York: Doubleday.

Ushe, Ushe M. 2015. "Religious Conflicts and Education in Nigeria: Implications for National Security," *Journal of Education and Practice* 6(2), 117–129.

United Nations and World Bank. 2018. *Pathways for Peace: Inclusive Approaches to Preventing Violent Conflict*. Washington, DC: World Bank.

Vaule, Lise. 2015. "Religion and Reconciliation in Rwanda: Is Religion an Obstacle or a Resource in Reconciliation?" Master's Thesis Is Submitted in Partial Fulfilment of the Requirements for the MA Degree at MF Norwegian School of Theology.

Villa-Vicencio, Charles. 2009. *Walk with Us and Listen: Political Reconciliation in Africa*. Cape Town: University of Cape Town Press.

18 Trauma and healing among children on the streets in Zimbabwe

Samson Mhizha, Tinashe Muromo, and Patrick Chiroro

Introduction

The phenomenon of children on the streets punctuating the cityscape of many urban areas is global, disquieting, and escalating (Drane, 2010; *cited in* Thomas de Benitez and Hiddlestone, 2011; Mhizha, 2010). Such children face traumatic experiences (Cummings, 2012). Though the exact numbers of street children are elusive (Thomas de Benitez and Hiddlestone, 2011), and impossible to quantify (UNICEF, 2005; Thomas de Benitez and Hiddlestone, 2011), the figure almost certainly runs into tens of millions globally (UNICEF, 2005). It is indubitable that the challenge of youth in the twenty-first century is more acute in Africa than elsewhere (Biaya, 2005; Honwana and de Boeck, 2005). The picture is strikingly grim for the street children in African towns (Biaya, 2005). The media and scholars alike decry the increase in population and menace of street children seen as "uncouth" for their antisocial tendencies in Zimbabwe (Mhizha, 2010; Muchini, 2001), with Ruparanganda (2008) warning that they are likely to emerge even in growth points and rural villages.

Most street children come from dysfunctional and disrupted families where poverty, domestic violence, divorce, criminality, and parental drug abuse are common (Buckner and Bassuk, 1997; Hagan and McCarthy, 1997). Street childhood is associated with disrupted attachment relationships with caregivers (Bowlby, 1967, 1980; Hagan and McCarthy, 1997). Most street children had faced extremely high rates of physical, sexual, emotional abuse and neglect at home and would have fled to the streets to escape from such adversity (Kidd, 2004). On the streets, the children face challenges in getting shelter and food and resort to transactional sex, survival sex, drug peddling, and stealing for survival (Hagan and McCarthy, 1997). The difficulty of surviving on the streets is compounded by the danger of sexual and physical assaults common on the streets (Kidd, 2004). Perhaps understandably, the primary goal of programmatic interventions for these street children involves reunifying these street children with their biological families (Lachman et al., 2002; Mhizha, 2010; Mhizha and Muromo, 2013; UNICEF, 2011). The current study assesses the traumatic experiences faced by the street children and their need for healing.

Causes of the increase in street children

A survey of the literature highlights that there are a number of causes that account for the increase in the number of children on the streets. A separate study is required in order to do justice to these factors. For the purposes of this chapter, we shall highlight the major sources, without undertaking an elaborate review of their content. Thus, first, the economic crisis in Zimbabwe had a major impact. Rurevo and Bourdillon, 2003; Muchini, 2001; Mhizha, 2010) are agreed that poverty is linked to street childhood. Sources such as Hanke (2008) reported inflation rates to have reached 7,96 trillion percent by November 2008. The Zimbabwe Country Analysis Working Document [ZCAWD] (2014) revealed that the Gross Domestic Product (GDP) was estimated to have fallen by 50.3%, poverty remained widespread, industrial capacity utilisation fell below 10% by January 2009, infrastructure deteriorated and skills flight in industries increased. Bratton and Masunungure (2011) observe that there were extreme shortages of staple foods. Chitando (2009) reasons that the crisis which plagued Zimbabwe was initiated by the Economic Structural Adjustment Programme (ESAP), struggles to resolve the emotive land question, political violence, and the stratospheric inflation spawned pessimism, despair, and anxiety especially among the young people. Gaidzanwa and Manyeruke (2010) plausibly wrote that that over the past decade, Zimbabwe's economy deteriorated to levels comparable to a country at war. Dodo and Dodo (2014) and Chiumia (2015) noted that unemployment rate stands at over 85%. Such a harsh economic environment pushed some children on to the streets.

Second, the HIV/AIDS crisis led to an increase in orphans, leading to some children being forced to go to the streets for survival. The HIV and AIDS challenge – with the infection rate in 2005 at 20.1% triggered a humanitarian crisis marked by orphanhood and poverty (Ministry of Health and Child Welfare [MoHCW] 2005) with life expectancy dropping to 40 years in 2006 from 60 years in 1990 due to poor nutrition and the high seroprevalence rate. The Zimbabwe National AIDS Council (NAC) (2013: 41) estimated the figures of orphans and vulnerable children (OVCs) at 1.6 million in Zimbabwe. The orphans have not been receiving grief and bereavement counseling and have lived in extreme poverty, experiencing psychosocial disorders such as depression, anxiety, social integration, self-esteem, and behaviour challenges (BRTI, 2008). Lack of school necessities, poverty, and feeling unloved have forced some to leave for the streets. Orphaned children face many adverse experiences, including abuse, exploitation, and multiple losses (Ngwenya, 2015).

Third, dropping out of school led some children on to the streets. During the peak of the crisis in Zimbabwe, some schools closed countrywide (Bratton and Masunungure, 2011), with many children dropping out of school (Mella, 2012).

Fourth, the high divorce rate contributed to the phenomenon of children on the streets. Studies have shown that family strife and divorce contribute to street childhood (Mhizha, 2010; Muchini, 2001). Divorce often results in impoverishment of the divorced mothers and their children, with the divorced mother assuming the sole responsibility of rearing the child, and providing the support and become poorer (Kendal, 2003). In some circumstances, children from divorced parents present many emotional challenges and traumas, since they view the divorce as traumatizing and betrayal by the parent (Dlamin, 2006). Some children with divorced parents end up on the streets.

Fifth, some stepchildren were so ill-treated by their stepfamilies that they ended up on the streets (Wakatama, 2007; Mansell, 2011; Beninger, 2011; Daly and Wilson, 1999). In the same vein, the sexual abuse of children also contributed to the increase in the number of children on the streets. Rumble et al. (2015) write that child sexual abuse in Zimbabwe has reached epidemic levels with serious concerns on public health and human rights. UNICEF (2011), Dube (2013), and the Research and Advocacy Unit (2015) have drawn attention to this unsettling phenomenon. Bowman and Brundige (2014), Sigworth (2009), Lalor (2004), Dube (2013), and Chitereka (2010) have reflected on the rise in child abuse in Africa and in Zimbabwe. After being sexually abused by a family member, the child feels betrayed and can drift on to the streets.

Sixth, studies have shown that street childhood in Zimbabwe is linked to certain family characteristics (Mhizha, 2010; Muchini, 2001; Rurevo and Bourdillon, 2003; Wakatama, 2007). Further, Ekpiken-Ekamen et al. (2014), Matchinda (1999), Xiang (2002), Baumrind (1967, 1991), and de Benitez, 2007 have reflected on how parenting styles contribute to children on the streets in other settings.

Experiences of children on the streets

Once on the streets, what does the literature say about the experiences of children? Arthur (2012) also writes that street children are vulnerable to streetism, which is the manner of life of street children as they live on the streets and adapt to the challenges they face on the streets. There is also substance abuse (Karabanow, 2004; Cummings, 2012; Makope, 2006; Muchini and Nyandiya-Bundy, 1991; Mhizha, 2010).

Further, street children are more likely to be sexually active, to face sexual abuse, and to have unsafe sex (Mhizha, 2010; Boakye-Boaten, 2008). Sorre and Oino (2013) report that street children are sexually precocious, they are at high risk of contracting HIV for many reasons: Peer influence; lack of information on HIV/AIDS; group sleeping; exposure to unprotected sex for pleasure or in exchange for food, protection, or money; others street children are always under the influence of drug thus putting them at a higher risk of contracting the disease. According to Sorre (2009), female street children have sex with three types of clients. The first type involved are the street boys with whom they had sex for protection and to whom they misrepresented that they were the only sexual partners. The second type involved the street-working youth for commercial reasons who were usually married and stayed at home. The final type were both municipal police and members of the uniformed police for protection.

Health, stigmatisation, and violence from the public

In the words of Ximena de la Barra (2000: 25), Senior Urban Advisor to the United Nations Children's Fund (UNICEF): "*Being poor is itself a health hazard; worse, however, is being urban and poor. Much worse is being poor, urban, and a child. But worst of all is being a street child in an urban environment.*" The previous statement clearly describes the nexus between poverty and health and sums up the magnitude of the health challenges street children go through. According to Mtonga (2011) the health condition of street children is generally poor. Many suffer from chronic diseases like TB, malaria; STDs and HIV are also common diseases among street children. Street childhood has been associated with poor physical health and mental health (Mhizha, 2010; Ndlovu, 2015).

Violence and victimisations are experiences that are common for street children. Street children are labeled a "social problem," and have found themselves at the sharp end of short-sighted policies which appear to protect wider society from "antisocial" children instead of protecting children from societal violence (De Benitez, 2007). Rurevo and Bourdillon (2003); Ruparanganda (2008); Beazley (2003), Wakatama (2007), and Ennew (1995) have explored the violence that street children are exposed to. Young people escape violent homes, only to encounter further violence on the streets (Alder, 1991; Cummings, 2012). Tudorić-Ghemo, (2005) highlighted that in Columbia street children are viewed with contempt and are often viewed as nuisances who should be murdered, and that 2,190 street youths were murdered in 1993 as social cleansing. Violence is part of the daily routine of street youth and involves peers, acquaintances, police, and strangers (Cummings, 2012).

Methodology

Design

The current study, being explorative, employed a qualitative research approach as the research design. It employed a qualitative methods approach to generate data to appreciate the lives of children on the streets. The present study combined semi-structured interviews and key informant interviews with visual methods. Interviews remain emblematic of qualitative research, affording participants the opportunity to talk more or less expansively about their lives (Ennew, 2003). This approach is qualitative and phenomenological. It involved detailed analysis of the lifeworld of the respondent; endeavours to explore personal and subjective experiences and focuses on the individual respondent's personal account and perception of a phenomenon which is different from attempts to give objective views of the phenomenon itself. The study arose from a DPhil study by the lead author.

Participants

In all, there were 14 children on the street and eight key informant interviewees. Of the 14 children on the street, seven were female, while the other seven were male. The children were aged between 12 years and 18 years. The researchers felt that they would exhaust the various categories and dimensions in the current study after interviewing the 22 participants.

The study employed purposive sampling in recruiting the participants. Purposive sampling involved choosing the sample basing on the judgement by the researchers on whether they met the inclusion criteria and this was influenced by multiple dimensions, such as time or availability (Strauss and Corbin, 1998) and at other times from the nature of the topic, the scope of the study, or the amount of useful information obtained from each participant (Morse, 1994) and the figure of 22 ensured that theoretical sampling was reached (Charmaz, 2014).

Data collection

Data for the current study were collected using semi-structured and key informant interviews. The semi-structured interviews were conducted with the children on the street. The semi-structured key informant interviews were held with the key informant interviewees.

Ethics

Consent was sought from gatekeepers of the children on the street who include the Ministry of Labour, Public Services and Social Welfare, the Harare City Council, and drop-in centre officials. Informed consent from the participants was obtained from the respondents and involved assuring them that they could terminate the interview at any time. Confidentiality and anonymity were spelt out and adhered to.

Limitations

The data collection methods in the current study being qualitative were acknowledged to have their own limitations. These limitations included not being representative of the target population from which the respondents were recruited. The 14 reunified former street children were not representative of all street children who were reunified in Harare. Again, the respondents were not recruited from all the different areas of Harare, while Harare itself cannot be representative of Zimbabwe in terms of the street children who have gone through reunification. Nonetheless, the children who were selected in the current study were clearly representative of the similar children with whom they shared characteristics.

Data analysis

Data collected in the current study were analysed using the interpretive phenomenological analysis. In this method, the researchers learnt about the respondent's psychological world in the form of constructs and beliefs that are made, given by the participants (Smith, 1996). The data analysis focused upon the generation of explanation and common themes that arose from the transcripts. Codes were assigned to the themes which reflected the shared perceptions among respondents of the investigated phenomena (in this case, the schooling challenges and experiences among the reunified former street children).

Findings

Physical and sexual abuse

It emerged from the data that children on the street drift to the streets fleeing from abuse at home. The types of abuse included both physical and sexual abuse. From the sample, two female street children got to the streets after having been raped by known members of the community. What irked one of the participants is that her grandmother accepted to be paid in a cow for that offence when she thought the perpetrator was supposed to be arrested and jailed. The 18-year old female child living on the streets said:

> *I was raped by an uncle who was close to my grandmother. I reported to the matter to the police but by grandmother then shouted at me telling me that she had already received a cow for the offence. That really incensed me. I decided to come to Harare to search for my father's relatives and got a warranty from the police after having lied to them that I knew where they were. But when I got to the city I realized that I had no chances locating them and that is how I got on to the streets.*

The other girl aged 16 years who was raped said that she reported the case to her supposed parents who later revealed to her that they were actually not her biological parents and that they had picked her from the streets where they had been living with her mother who was also a street dweller. Not only that, they told her that she was raped because she had invited the perpetrator and did not bother to report the case to the police. For that reason, she came to the streets in search of her mother and felt betrayed by her supposed parents for later disowning her.

Other children also reported leaving their families after facing physical abuse. One male 12 year old child living on the streets said that he fled home because his stepfather was always beating him while his mother did not try to protect him but was more concerned with safekeeping her marriage. Indeed stepparenting was also a strong factor why some children left home to stay in the streets. An 18-year old male child living in the streets said:

> I was staying with my father and stepmother but got into serious conflicts with my stepmother. My mother and sisters influenced me to disobey my stepmother, with whom they got into verbal and physical conflicts regularly. My father had divorced my mother. The conflicts escalated that I would steal money, food and kitchen utensils for resale while she denied me food, hid my birth certificates and stopped me from schooling. The situation became so tense with my father not resolving it that I decided to leave for the streets.

Poverty and neglect

It also emerged from the data that children on the street drifted to the streets due to poverty at home. The poverty originated from a number of factors, including orphanhood, drought, desertion by a parent, parental divorce, grand-parenting and unemployment status of the guardian. Closely related to poverty was neglect. Indeed, poverty could be buffered by parental love, but when there was neglect, the effects of poverty worsened. Some children complained that they faced neglect from guardians in the form of desertion, dropping off from school, being denied food, medical attention and clothes and sometimes being discriminated against by guardians. One 17-year old male street child revealed that after the death of his mother while staying in rural Gokwe, his father left home for his sister's place in Zhombe leaving him alone at home. Hunger forced him to leave home in search for her sister in Harare, but on reaching Harare he realized that he could not find her and ended up staying on the streets.

Family reconstitution

It also emerged from the data that street children left home for the streets as a result of family reconstitution. Indeed, the family would have been destabilized due to death or divorce. Then the family was reconstituted as the remaining parent who assumed custody of the child remarried bringing in a step-parent or the child was taken to some relative, sometimes an aunt, an uncle, a sibling, or grandparent. In one instance, a mother died, the father remained with the child, but the father left home to visit his daughter and the child stayed alone. Indeed, in most reconstituted families the majority of guardians were step-families, grandparent families, and families headed by an aunt or uncle. What seemed to bring problems was the fact that the child was traumatized by the death or divorce that was precursor to the family reconstitution. The processes of family reconstitution did not involve consulting the children who seemed either to feel alienated by the process or the new guardian, especially the step-parent. Step-parenting appeared a very sensitive family type and seemed to pre-cursor risk in children, not by mere step-parenting itself, but due to associated factors such as feelings of grief for the deceased or divorced parent, influence from the divorced parent, biological siblings and relatives of the absent parent, competition for the attention of the remaining parent with the step-parent, and the indifference of the remaining parent towards the child and their failure to rein on the step-parent.

Searching for jobs and relatives

It also emerged from the data that street children drifted to the cities or streets in search of relatives, siblings, and/or employment. Indeed, getting to the streets appeared accidental to many children after failing to locate the relatives or family members or secure the employment they were searching for. Indeed, many of the children searching for the relatives, family members, or employment were new to the city or streets and did not appreciate the lives they were going to lead. Indeed, having failed to secure employment or locate the family members or relatives, some of the children got to the streets as lost children with nowhere to go. One 17-year old male street child revealed that after the death of his mother while staying in rural Gokwe, his father left home for his sister's place in Zhombe leaving him alone at home. Hunger forced him to leave home in search for his sister in Harare, but on reaching Harare he realized that he could not find her and ended up staying on the streets.

Delinquency

Another theme that emerged from the data is that the children moved to the streets as a result of delinquency. The children reported having committed diverse acts of delinquency such as stealing, beating up parents or guardians, especially step-parents, and having engaged in premarital sex. The key informants also revealed that some of the children had committed offences such as having sex with neighbours' livestock especially goats, eating food for guests and replacing it with feaces, and illicit sexual behaviours. One 18-year old female street child who reported that she left home after some thefts and fights with her father and grandmother said:

> I think I was naughty myself. I stole my father's pornographic magazine and showed my friends the nude pictures. When my father caught me she wanted to beat me but I threw a stone at him. Months later I stole $300 from my grandmother which she was safekeeping for her *mukando*/savings club. These events made me decide to leave for the streets.

In another incident, a key informant revealed that a child left for the streets after having been caught being intimate with a goat. He said:

> The child was caught being intimate with a village head's goat. The owner for the goat suspecting magic from the incident brought the goat to the uncle who was staying with the child saying I have brought your child's wife. The guardian was not amused and feared being chased away from the village and chased away the child.

Trauma in the streets

Drug use and sexual abuse

It also emerged from the data that street children faced extreme forms of sexual abuse and drug use once in the streets. Indeed, most of the child reported having been duped into or urged to use drugs in the streets by their peers as a form of initiation. The most popular drugs they used were marijuana, glue, cough mixtures, and prescription drugs. The female street children also faced grave sexual abuse in the streets. An 18-year old female child said:

> When I got into the streets, I rejected the advances for sex that I received from my male peers. They then brewed tea for me which they had mixed with drugs. I drank the tea and slept for hours on end. I only woke up to realize that I was raped by an unknown male peer. I was still a virgin and my skirt and privates were full of blood from the abuse. It seemed they had taken turns to rape me. I had nowhere to report since I had fled from home.

In a similar incident, another 18-year old who reported having been raped again said:

> My female peers were urging me to be in love with a male peer in the streets. I refused saying I was still young but they did not relent. Finally, they gave me tea laced with marijuana that I slept unconsciously and he raped me. I started bleeding since I was still a virgin. I told them that I was going to report them to the police and they dissuaded me telling me that was the reason I had come to the streets so there was no way I was supposed to report. Ultimately I did not report and got into an affair with the guy.

Indeed, the findings revealed that the streets children faced sexual abuse in the streets with the female children at the receiving end. Most of the female children end up being "married" to fellow street children in the streets.

Physical abuse

Apart from sexual abuse, street children faced physical abuse from fellow street children and also members of the public. The street children decried that they faced *chitororo* (banditry) from older and bigger street dwellers who snatched their food, money, clothes, and blankets from them. The children reported that they had nothing to do to save themselves from that *chitororo* (banditry). Other children reported that on becoming bigger and older, they also used the same *chitororo* (banditry) to younger and weaker street children. It should be echoed that the violence was mainly a way of eking a living since the younger children earned more money through begging than the older ones. The other challenges alongside the physical abuse was fighting as rival groups faced off in fights for blankets, food, territory, and girls. The weaker children were also forced to work for the bigger and older street children in begging and submitting the earnings to the older children.

Ill-health

The children on the street also indicated that they face health challenges. Indeed, the children faced different illnesses such as bronchitis, skin problems,

HIV, sexually transmitted infections such as syphilis, and wounds from fights and vehicle accidents. Regarding HIV, five participants had been tested and found seropositive. Three (two male and one female) of these five children on the streets were born with the disease while the other two female children contracted the disease in the streets. All the five children were on anti-retroviral therapy (ARVs). The children on ARV medication moved around with their ARVs, but also reported losing their bags where they had put the drugs or sometimes their peers took away the drugs believing that they were psychoactive drugs.

Worry and suicidal tendencies

Negative emotional experiences were predominant among the children on the street, with worry ranking the most prevalent. The children reported worrying over what they were going to eat, wear, and do in the future. The children resorted to drugs which ameliorated the worries, at least temporarily. Most children revealed after taking the drugs "*tinosticka*" (maintained "sticking" or "freezing" stance) that they could sleep as if dead for hours on ends. The drug-induced freezing stance was also beneficial to handle the cold and cold weather, hunger, and stresses the children encountered in the streets. Related to worry were the suicidal tendencies in some of the children on the street. Indeed, there were reports of some children who had committed suicide in the streets. One 18-year old female child on the street confessed to having wanted to commit suicide when her boyfriend died by throwing herself into moving cars and was saved by her alert friends. Similarly, another 17-year old female child revealed having tried to kill herself using insecticides but was saved by her colleagues and in one incident she woke up at Parirenyatwa Hospital.

Interventions and need for rehabilitation and family healing

Family reunification

It also emerged from the data that some children on the street reunified with their parents through diverse means. Some of the children returned home on their own, with some staying for good at home but most returning to the streets after due to the failure to resolve the problems that had forced them into the streets. Other children were reunified by non-governmental organisations (NGOs) providing services for the children with or without the government. It also came out that the reunification was also fraught, with poor family tracing and lack of reunification kits. Poor family tracing involving returning the child without having established if the family was going to accept the child. The reunification kits are the financial and material resources children are supposed to be given when they are being reunited to help them deal with financial and economic challenges at home. The reunification ideally should include money for household needs, certain foodstuffs, and school requirements such as money for fees, stationery, and uniforms.

Schooling

It also emerged from the data that the interventions also involved and included schooling. The schooling was either academic or vocational training. In terms of academic schooling, the children were offered informal and/or formal schooling to resume studies at both primary and secondary levels. Some of the children proceeded to Advanced Level, with some even proceeding to college or university education. Regarding vocational training, the children were offered places in different fields such as welding, mechanics, carpentry, bakery, dressmaking, sewing, hairdressing, and cosmetics. A worrying finding was that some of the children did not complete the schooling due to funding challenges and behaviour problems related to streetism. It occurred that some of the children returned to the streets to hook up with their husbands, some regressed to drug abuse and prostitution.

Clear need for healing (rehabilitation and family therapy)

The data also showed that the children clearly needed healing to really adjust in the society to make optimal use of their potential and the different interventions provided to them. The children developed addictions while on the streets which made integration very difficult. The behaviours related to addictions included prostitution, use of vulgar language, drug use, thieving, and stealing. This means that the children needed rehabilitation. It was also apparent that even the families of origin required therapy as the behaviours that drove the children continued. The families seemed to have challenges such as dysfunctional parenting styles related to abuse and neglect. The need for healing was underscored by the finding that some of the children on the street failure to manage their emotions and also to failure to stop behaviours such as substance use, permissive sexuality, and stealing. Indeed, the children revealed a motivation to stop such behaviours but failure to manage the behaviour change; something that can be made possible of rehabilitation is undertaken. An 18–year old female child said:

> In the streets I started behaviours such as use of drugs and prostitution and failed to stop such behaviours. I remember when I tried to stop smoking, I almost cried when I saw some man smoking a cigar. I think I need professional help in stopping the smoking. I cannot stop smoking cigarettes and marijuana on my own. I have been to South Africa, there they have better systems they can help their children go through that.

Echoing the same sentiments, an 18-year old male child said:

> When I start worrying, I cannot deal with the worry myself. I need drugs
> to thwart the depressive feelings as I ponder about what I will eat, what my
> life will be like, thinking about why my guardians abused me and a lot of
> other issues. I sometimes ponder suicide. My life is a tragedy.

Similarly, speaking about the need for resolution of family problems that cata-
pulted them into the streets, an 18-year old male child said:

> When I was taken home for family reunification, the reunifying officer
> talked with my aunt in my absence. I do not know what they discussed and
> what was said about me. I would have wanted them to discuss my issues in
> my presence. What irked me is that the problems that drove me into the
> streets were not resolved as my stepmother resumed accusing me of stealing
> her money and food, denied me food while I also began stealing her uten-
> sils and money. I think our family needed to be talked with by professionals
> so that each of us would stop their problematic behaviours.

Thus, the previous findings highlight that it is imperative to provide healing or
rehabilitation to the street children and their families to resolve the challenges
related to the trauma they faced at home and in the streets.

Discussion

The data revealed that the street children really face traumatic experiences at
home, including physical abuse, sexual abuse, family separation, and reconstitution in the form of orphanhood, parental divorce and step-parenting, poverty,
and HIV stigma. Sometimes the children respond to the family crisis through
delinquency which further worsens their situations at home. These traumatic
experiences at home force the children to decide to leave home either in search
for jobs or relatives in the city.

On the streets, the children face further traumatic experiences as they are
further sexually and physically abused by peers and other adults on the streets,
rounded-up by the police and dumped in far-away places. The data suggest
that the trauma faced by the children seems to worsen once on the streets. The
victimization worsens. Violence is part of the daily routine of street youth and
involves peers, acquaintances, police, and strangers (Alder, 1991; Cummings,
2012). Young people escape violent homes only to encounter further violence
on the streets (Cummings, 2012).

In terms of interventions, the children are normally reunified with their families, though the reunifications seem hurriedly done, with poor family tracing,
limited resources, and poor coordination as the major disabling factors. Indeed,
the children note that the children are just dumped home without even sufficient

resolution of the factors that drove them into the streets. Feeny (2005) decried the poorly resourced and implemented reunification programmes in Africa.

Schrader, McMillan, and Herrera (2014) described the Juconi theoretical framework which incorporates both attachment and trauma theories. The model holds that for family reunification gains, especially with regards to schooling, to be sustained, it is essential first to heal the effects of trauma. Yet, in Zimbabwe, there are no efforts to offer therapeutic interventions. Risky behaviours such as substance use, poor relationships, and streetism can only be addressed through therapy according to the model. The model assumed without sufficient rehabilitation on the children, there were schooling and reunification challenges.

Recommendations

The following recommendations are suggested. It is herein suggested that families, parents, and guardians are trained on parenting children in ways that do not abuse the children. They should strengthen the attachment bonds with the children. Children find it hard to stay with abusive parents and guardians. School authorities should be trained to provide unique and specific education that meets their background and circumstances of children on the street.

For the children who are on the streets, the government should provide health and education services. When it comes to family reunification, it is pertinent that the programmes should be well-funded and well-coordinated. They should include reunification kits, thorough family tracing, and flexibility.

Such education should include training in life skills and vocational training and should include facets such as decision-making, interpersonal skills, stress and coping with it, health literacy, and emotional intelligence. Regarding vocational skills, the individual children on the street and former street children should be free to select courses they want from an array, including mechanics, welding, farming, sewing, embroidery, brickwork, carpentry, computer literacy, and programming among many others. The government should avail funding for such education.

Perhaps more importantly, the government should provide rehabilitation and therapeutic services to children on the street to help them deal with the adverse psychological and emotional experiences both at home and in the streets. There should be advocacy to deal with stigma, labelling, and stereotypes the street children face in schools and communities.

Conclusion

The current study has shown that street children face many traumatic experiences at home which drive them into the streets. These include physical and sexual abuse, family separation and reconstitution in the form of orphanhood, parental divorce and step-parenting, poverty and HIV stigma. Once in the streets, the traumatic experiences worsen as the children are subjected to further abuse by their peers, adult street dwellers, and the police. In terms of interventions, it is deplorable that street children are provided with poorly resourced and funded interventions like family reunification without therapeutic support. The majority failed to properly integrate in society evidently showing a need for thorough family reunification grounded in rehabilitation and ensuring restoration of attachment relationships with caregivers. Healing the children on the street is a major investment in the process of healing Zimbabwe.

References

Alder, C. 1991, 'Victims of violence: The case of homeless youth', Australian and New Zealand *Journal of Criminology, 24*, 1–14.

Arthur, I. S. II. 2012. "Streetism: A socio-cultural and pastoral theological study of a youth problem in Ghana," Unpublished Doctoral Thesis, Emory University, Atlanta, Georgia.

Baumrind, D. 1967. "Child Care Practices Anteceding Three Patterns of Preschool Behaviour," *Genetic Psychology Monographs* 75, 43–88.

Baumrind, D. 1991. "The Influence of Parenting Style on Adolescent Competence and Substance Use," *Journal of Early Adolescence* 11, 56–95.

Beazley, H. (2003). The construction and protection of individual and collective identities by street children and youth in Indonesia. *Children, Youth and Environments, 13* (1), 899–902.

Beninger, C. 2011. *Stepfamilies in Namibia: A Study of the Situation of Stepparents and Stepchildren and Recommendations for Law Reform.* Windhoek: Legal Assistance Centre.

Biaya, T. K. 2005. "Youth and Street Culture in Urban Africa," in A. Honwana and F. de Boeck (eds.), *Makers and Breakers: Children and Youth in Postcolonial Africa.* Oxford: James Currey.

Biomedical Research and Training Institute. 2008. *Situational Analysis of Orphaned and Vulnerable Children in Eight Zimbabwean Districts.* Cape Town: Human Sciences Research Council.

Boakye-Boaten, A. 2008. Street children: experiences from the streets of Accra. Research Journal of International Studies, 8, 76–84.

Bowman, C. and E. Brundige. 2014. "Child Sex Abuse Within the Family in Sub-Saharan Africa: Challenges and Change in Current Legal and Mental Health Responses," *Cornell International Law Journal* 47(2), 232–297..

Bowlby, J. 1969. *Attachment and Loss, Vol. 1: Attachment.* New York: Basic Books.

Bowlby, J. 1980. *"Attachment and Loss" vol. 2. Separation, Anxiety and Anger.* New York: Basic Books.

Bratton, M. and E. Masunungure. 2011. "The Anatomy of Political Predation: Leaders, Elites and Coalitions in Zimbabwe 1980–2010," *Developmental Leadership Program,* Research Paper 09.

Buckner, J. C. and E. L. Bassuk. 1997. "Mental Disorders and Service Utilization Among Youths from Homeless and Low-Income Household Families," *Journal of the American Academy of Child and Adolescent Psychiatry* 36, 890–900.

Charmaz, K. C. 2014. *Constructing grounded theory,* 2nd ed. Thousand Oaks, CA: Sage.

Chitando, E. 2009. "Deliverance and Sanctified Passports: Prophetic Activities Amidst Uncertainty in Harare," in Liv Haram and C. Bawayamba (eds.), *Dealing with Uncertainty in Contemporary African Lives.* Uppsala: Nordiska AfrikaInstitutet.

Chitereka, C. 2010. "Child Sexual Abuse in Zimbabwe: The Agenda for Social Workers, 20," *Asia Pacific Journal of Social WORK and Development* 29, 32.

Chiumia, S. 2015. "Is Zimbabwe's Unemployment Rate 4%, 60% or 95%? Why the Data Is Unreliable," *Africacheck,* 30 October. https://africacheck.org/reports/is-zimbabwes-unemployment-rate-4-60-or-95-why-the-data-is-unreliable/ (accessed on 20 February 2017).

Cummings, P. 2012. "Factors Related to the Street Children Phenomenon in Major Towns in Sierra Leone: A Comparative Study of the City's Street Children and Children in Normal Family Homes," A Dissertation Submitted to St. Clements University.

Daly, M. and M. Wilson. 1999. *The Truth About Cinderella: A Darwinian View of Parental Love.* New Haven: Yale University Press.

De Benitez, T. S. 2007. *State of the World's Street Children: Violence.* London: Consortium for Street Children.

De la Barra, X. 2000. *United Nations Commission on Economic, Social and Cultural Rights* (UNESCO) General Comment No. 14, August. New York: UNESCO.

Dlamini, N. 2006. "Measurement and Characteristics of Single Mother in South Africa: An Analysis Using 2002 General Household Survey," Unpublished Thesis, University of Kwazulu-Natal, South Africa.

Dodo, O. and Dodo, T. 2014. *"Unemployment and Conflict in Zimbabwe: An Analysis and Resolution" in Development Policy and Practice: Making Use of Population Census Data in Zimbabwe.* Harare: IDA.

Dube, R. 2013. *"She Probably Asked for It!" A Preliminary Study into Zimbabwean Societal Perceptions of Rape.* April. Harare: Research & Advocacy Unit.

Ekpiken-Ekamen, R., A. E. Ayuk and R. A. Adadu. 2014. *Causal Effects of Street Children in Nigeria: Implications for Counselling* 5(8), 154–158.

Ennew, J. 1995. "Outside Childhood: Street Children," in B. Franklin (ed.), *The Handbook of Children's Rights-Comparative Policy and Practice.* London: Routledge.

Ennew, J. 2003. "Difficult Circumstances: Some Reflections on 'Street Children' in Africa," *Children, Youth and Environments* 13(1), 128–146.

Feeny, T. 2005. *In Best or Vested Interests? An Exploration of the Concept and Practice of Family Reunification for Street Children.* London: The Consortium for Street Children.

Gaidzanwa, R. B. and C. Manyeruke. 2010. *Livelihoods Situational Analysis of University of Zimbabwe Female Students.* Harare: Students Solidarity Trust.

Hagan, J. and B. McCarthy. 1997. *Mean Streets: Youth Crime and Homelessness.* New York: Cambridge University Press.

Hanke, S. T. 2008. *From Hyperinflation to Growth, Centre for Global Liberty and Prosperity, Development Policy Analysis:* Washington, DC: CATO.

Honwana, A. and F. de Boeck. 2005. *Makers and Breakers: Children and Youth in Post-Colonial Africa.* Oxford: James Currey.

Karabanow, J. 2004. *Being Young and Homeless: Understanding How Youth Enter and Exit Street Life.* New York: Peter Lang.

Kendall, D. 2003. *Sociology in Our Times,* 4th ed. Belmont: Wadsworth and Thomson Learning.

Kidd, S. A. 2004. "The Walls Were Closing in and We Were Trapped: A Qualitative Analysis of Street Youth Suicide," *Youth and Society* 36, 30–55.

Lachman, P., X. Poblete, P. O. Ebigbo, S. Nyandiya-Bundy, R. P. Bundy, B. Killian and J. Doek. 2002. "Challenges Facing Child Protection," *Child Abuse & Neglect* 26, 587–617.

Lalor, K. 2004. "Child Sexual Abuse in Sub-Saharan Africa: A Literature Review," *Child Abuse & Neglect* 28, 439–460.

Makope, V. 2006. *A Zimbabwean Street Story.* Harare: German Agro Action.

Mansell, P. 2011. "Young Adult Stepchildren's Experiences of Relationship with Stepmothers," Unpublished Doctoral Thesis Clinical Psychology, The University of Auckland.

Matchinda, B. 1999. "The Impact of Home Background on the Decision of Children to Run Away: The Case of Yaounde City Street Children in Cameroon," *Child Abuse and Neglect* 23(3), 245–255.

Mella, M. 2012. "An Investigation into the Nature and Extent of the Economic Exploitation of Street Children in Zimbabwe: A Case Study of Harare Central Business District," Unpublished Master's Thesis, University of Zimbabwe, Harare, Zimbabwe.

Mhizha, S. 2010. "The Self-image of Adolescent Street Children in Harare," Unpublished Master's Thesis, University of Zimbabwe, Harare, Zimbabwe.

Mhizha, S. and T. Muromo. 2013. "An Exploratory Study on Challenges Faced by Street Children in Harare Regarding Schooling," *Zimbabwe Journal of Educational Research* 25(3), 350–368.

Ministry of Health and Child Welfare. 2005. *National Health Profile: Zimbabwe National HIV and AIDS Estimates, 2005 Preliminary Report.* www.mohcw.gov.zw (accessed on 15 February 2007).

Morse, J. M. 1994. "Designing Funded Qualitative Research," in N. K. Denzin and Y. S. Lincoln (eds.), *Handbook of Qualitative Research.* Thousand Oaks, CA: Sage, 220–235.

Mtonga, J. 2011. "On and Off the Streets: Children Moving Between Institutional Care and Survival on the Streets," Unpublished Master's Thesis, Norwegian University of Science and Technology.

Muchini, B. 2001. *A Study on Street Children in Zimbabwe.* www.unicef.org/evaldatabase/index_23256.html (accessed on 6 February 2007).

Muchini, B. and S. Nyandiya-Bundy. 1991. *Struggling to Survive: A Study of Street Children in Zimbabwe.* Harare: UNICEF-Zimbabwe.

National Aids Council. 2013. *Zimbabwe HIV/AIDS Situation: HIV/AIDS Numbers.* Harare: National AIDS Council.

Ndlovu, I. 2015. "Life Experiences of Street Children in Bulawayo: Implications for Policy and Practice," PhD thesis, The Open University.

Ngwenya, M. 2015. "An Investigation into Challenges Faced by Communities-Based Interventions for Orphans and Vulnerable Children in Mutare, Zimbabwe," Unpublished Master's Thesis UNISA South Africa.

Research Advocacy Unit (RAU). 2015. *What Happens to Perpetrators of Sexual Abuse in Zimbabwe: Examining the Outcome of Cases Heard at the Magistrate's Court in Harare, Zimbabwe from 2013 to 2015?* Harare: RAU.

Rumble, L., Mungate, T., Chigiji, H., Salama, P., Nolan, A., Sammon, E., and Muwoni, L. 2015. Childhood Sexual Violence in Zimbabwe: Evidence for the Epidemic against Girls *Child Abuse and Neglect International Journal, 46,* 60–66

Ruparanganda, W. 2008. "The Tragedy of Procrastinating? A Case Study of Sexual Behaviour Patterns of Street Youth of Harare, Zimbabwe in the Era of HIV and AIDS Pandemic," Unpublished Doctoral Thesis, University of Zimbabwe, Harare, Zimbabwe.

Rurevo, R. and M. F. C. Bourdillon. 2003. *Girls on the Streets.* Harare: Weaver Press.

Schrader McMillan, A. and E. Herrera. 2014. *Strategies to Ensure the Sustainable Reintegration of Children Without Parental Care: JUCONI.* Mexico: Family for Every Child and Juconi. www.familyforeverychild.org/wp-content/uploads/2014/01/Children-s_Reintegration_in_Mexico.pdf.

Sigworth, R. 2009. *"Anyone Can Be a Rapist": An Overview of Sexual Violence in South Africa.* Johannesburg: Centre for the Study of Violence and Reconciliation.

Smith, J. A. 1996. "Beyond the Divide Between Cognition and Discourse: Using Interpretative Phenomenological Analysis in Health Psychology," *Psychology and Health* 11, 261–271.

Sorre, B. 2009. *Patterns of Migrations Among Street Children in Kenya: An Ethnographic Account of Street Children in Kisumu Municipality.* Saarbrücken, Germany: Lambert Academic Publishing.

Sorre, B. and P. Oino. 2013. "Family Based Factors Leading to Street Children Phenomenon in Kenya," *IJRS, India* 2(3), 148–155.

Strauss, A. and J. Corbin. 1998. *Basics of Qualitative Research: Techniques and Procedures for Developing Grounded Theory.* Thousand Oaks, CA: Sage.

Thomas de Benitez, S and Hiddleston, T. (2011). Promotion and Protection of the rights of children working and/or living on the street OHCHR Global Study. Genava: The Office of the United Nations High Commissioner for Human Rights (OHCHR)

Tudorić-Ghemo, A. 2005. "Life on the Street and the Mental Health of Street Children – A Developmental Perspective," Unpublished Master's Thesis, University of Johannesburg, Johannesburg, South Africa.

United Nations Children's Fund. 2005. *State of the World's Children 2006: Excluded and Invisible.* New York: UNICEF.

United Nations Children's Fund. 2011. *National Baseline Survey on the Life Experiences of Adolescents.* Harare: UNICEF.

Wakatama, M. 2007. "The Situation of Street Children in Zimbabwe? A Violation of the United Nations Convention on the Rights of the Child (1989)," Thesis Submitted for the degree of Doctor of Philosophy at the University of Leicester.

Xiang, R. 2002. "A Study of Street Children," in H. Q. Zhang, R. Xiang and W. H. Gao (eds.), *Voices of the Disadvantaged Group and the Interventions of Social Work.* Beijing: Chinese Financial and Economic Publishing House.

Zimbabwe Country Analysis. Working Document (ZCAWD). 2014. "United Nations Country Team (UNCT) and the Government of Zimbabwe (GoZ): Harare," www.zw.one.un.org/sites/default/files/Publications/UNZimbabwe/Country%20Analysis_FinalReview_3Oct2014.pdf (accessed on 18 March 2017).

19 The environmental healing promises of a Zimbabwean traditional religio-mythical paradise

Nisbert Taisekwa Taringa

"For when we see with spiritual eyes, we remain in service to nature; we see nature as the originator of our tools, and we know that our tools or our technology must be used in harmony with nature's design and purposes, which are to maintain and serve the individual and the community."

(Some, 1998: 65)

Introduction

There is a global recognition for a need for a new, more environmentally healing imagination of nature. This is a healing imagination that sees nature as active, meaningful, subjective and spiritual, re-evaluates it, while recognizing humanity as part of nature, encouraging caring human action towards it. In this recognition, there is need to consider religio-cultural resources as a possible influential source of such a new recognition of nature, linking humanity to a wider environmental reality and providing the existential support, moral authority, and institutional organization able to heal the environment (Watling, 2009). This chapter therefore explores potential mythical paradise visions in Shona traditional religio-cultural mythical thought, with reference to the *Mwedzi* myth of creation, that can cultivate attitudes to the natural environment that can act as a basis for orienting people toward overcoming and healing the environmental crisis in Zimbabwe, in order to ensure a balance between sustainable economic activities and ecological justice. I assume that there is need for something more than environmental policies, something which African (Shona) traditional religio-cultural mythical paradise visions can provide. The central question is: To what extent can African (Shona) traditional religio-cultural mythical thought be seen as a legitimate, meaningful, powerful, way of inculcating environmental healing consciousness and imagination? I begin by a brief summary of the global complexity of issues at the heart of the environmental crisis. After this I consider environmental damage in Zimbabwe. This is followed by a critique regarding the limits of the modern view of nature that I intend to pit against the healing potential of African (Shona) traditional religio-cultural mythical thought. The section follows my critique deals with presentation and interpretation of the Mwedzi myth of creation.

The global complexity and scope of the environmental crisis

The formidable challenges relating to the environmental crisis have been well acknowledged and documented. Mary Tucker and John Grim, for example, note the extent of the issues and acknowledge that it is wide ranging. Their observation is captured as follows:

> From resource depletion and species extinction to pollution overload and toxic surplus, the planet is struggling against unprecedented assaults. This is aggravated by population explosion, industrial growth, technological manipulation, and military proliferation heretofore unknown by the human community. From many accounts the basic elements that sustain life – sufficient water, clean air and arable land – are at risk. The challenges are formidable and well documented.
>
> (Tucker and Grim, 2001: xiii)

Young (2005: 281) is more elaborate and unpacks the complexity and scope of the environmental crisis. He enumerates the following challenges:

1   Ozone depletion, releasing ultraviolet radiation that threatens to severely damage humans, other animals, and plants.
2   Emissions resulting in the "greenhouse effect" and the dangerous elevation of the earth's temperature, with a host of negative consequences.
3   Deforestation, including, but not limited to, the important tropical rain forests.
4   Pollution of the air, earth, and water.
5   Desertification, caused by depletion of the earth's soils through current agricultural practices.
6   Population growth that threatens to exceed the carrying capacity of the earth, unless we learn to distribute resources more equitably.
7   Extinction of species, which threatens the planet's biodiversity.
8   Consumption of natural resources faster than they can be replenished.
9   Proliferation of nuclear, biological, and chemical weapons of mass destruction.

In light of this crisis, Tucker and Grim (2001: xiv) aptly draw our attention to the fact that the causes cannot be explained exclusively in terms of economic, political, and social factors. For Tucker and Grim (2001: xiv) the environmental crisis is also a moral and spiritual crisis. They, therefore, call for the re-examination of religions in the light of the current environmental crisis.

Further, they argue, "Religious traditions may indeed be critical in helping to reimagine the viable conditions and long range strategies for fostering mutually enhancing human–earth relations" (Tucker and Grim, 2001: xiii). "They may help to supply both creative resources of symbols, rituals, and texts as well as inspiring visions for reimagining ourselves as part of, not apart from, the natural world" (Tucker and Grim, 2001: xiii). Young (2005: 281) shares the same view when he states, "Many today are saying that since the roots of the present environmental crisis are spiritual, the solution must come from religious resources as well. At the least, it is clear that any analysis of the ecological crisis must include attention to the possible role religions have played in creating it, and their potential for resolving it." This ties in very well with the assumption that environmental degradation is a problem to which religions are prepared to respond constructively. In the light of this assumption, religious people may follow three possible approaches, namely (1) recovering wisdom in the traditions they have inherited, (2) reforming these traditions in light of the new situation, or (3) replacing traditional religion in favour of something new and more suited to the current crisis (Bauman et al., 2011: 59).

In this chapter, I incline myself to recovering wisdom from inherited religio-cultural traditions. I believe in the validity of core African (Shona) traditional religio-cultural mythical thought in addressing anthropocentric environmental attitudes. I therefore argue that the Shona Mwedzi myth of creation has resources for constructively responding to carelessness and inattention that that have led to ecological devastation. It is my strong contention that the myth contains wisdom about the relationship of humanity and nature, and that we pay attention to the urgent need to heal the environment.

I therefore focus on the power of one traditional Shona myth of creation to foster environmental healing mythical paradise visions. My idea that a solution should come from African religio-cultural tradition tends to express concern about the limits of the modern Western view of nature regarding the need for healing the environment in Zimbabwe.

Ecological damage: the wounded natural environment in Zimbabwe

The destruction of the natural environment in Zimbabwe is caused primarily by two seemingly unsustainable economic activities. These are the Fast Track Land Reform programme, which started in the year 2000, and persistent artisanal small-scale mining activities. The natural environment is put under pressure by these activities. One of the effects of the Fast Track Land Reform Programme is the massive cutting down of trees. Following are a few examples.

We have been allocated land in the area . . .

> The chief was also engaged in a wrangle with farmers. One of the most worrying environmental disasters was the massive destruction of trees in the area adjacent to the Great Dyke around Kildonia area, near Mutoroshanga. Several vehicles and trucks were seen loaded with firewood going from the area to Harare. They bought large stocks of firewood for resale, which was big business in Harare. Most of the farmers said they had been allocated the land and that is why were cutting down trees so haphazardly. "We have been allocated land in the area".

Deforestation was controlled by well-organized cartels that included politicians, businessmen and farmers. The chief was facing resistance. The chief's lamentation is captured in the following words: "The farmers are now blatantly defying my orders to vacate the area, despite the promise to have land reallocated to them elsewhere. We are fighting running battles with these farmers almost every day, but some of them are seeking protection from political leaders and this is very sad for our environment. I gave them a three day eviction notice but they resisted eviction order." There was also rampant cutting down of trees near a sacred shrine called Maringambizi, which had traditionally been a place reserved for ancestral worship and performing traditional rituals. Chief Zvimba has made an arrangement with ministry of lands to take over all the places that are considered sacred in the area.

(Bwititi in Taringa and Sipeyiye, 2013: 59)

"Clear most of the trees to farm! This section has not been used for crops . . ."

When Phides Mazhawidza was shown her newly allocated A2 farm in Goromonzi, she was dismayed to find that it was covered with trees. While she admired the miombo woodlands with its beautiful musasa and munondo trees, her heart sank when she realized that she would have to clear much of it to farm. Phides' farm was a subdivision of a large commercial farm in a region of high agricultural potential and her section had not been used for crops.

(Hanlon et al., 2013: 175)

Land reform means unused land is being cleared and land is being used intensively, which makes trees a key issue. There is an increased demand for wood for fuel, in particular for curing tobacco and to sell to urban dwellers. So far land-reform farmers seem to be managing their trees, but they will need to be monitored. Fast track land reform and economic crisis caused by hyperinflation have created two serious environmental problems that will not be solved by simple enforcement.

(Hanlon et al., 2013: 187)

Cutting down trees and veld fires

Maposa et al. (2011: 160) decry the impact of the land reform on the environment:

In spite of the fact that the Land Reform program has posited some apparent successes in the particular provision of land as a source of livelihood for thousands of peasants who were landless, it is causing almost unmitigated environmental disaster. It is a hard reality to note that varimi vatsva (new farmers) are involved in wanton tree cutting in resettled farmlands. Trees are disappearing at catastrophic rapidity. This is causing deforestation, an issue that is intrinsically linked to environmental degradation. Kwekwe Town is fast turning into a desert. The reasons are not far to seek. The new farmers have occupied the adjacent former white commercial farming properties such as Congela, Dunlop Extension, Milsonia Ranch and Maivalle Ranch.

Apart from the indiscriminate cutting down of trees, varimi vatsva have been widely accused of causing veld fires in the former white farmlands across the country. However from the onset, it must be stated that the issue of who causes the fire is a contentious one. Firstly, it is alleged that communal peasants cause veld fires. Fire outbreaks commonly occur during the dry season when conditions favor the spread of the fire from one point to the other. The communal peasants move around and smoke out bees in search of honey from the veld. Secondly some varimi vatsva incidentally cause veld fire during land preparation. Despite being motivated by the practical need to survive, varimi vatsva are the chief culprits in the sense that they are also involved in hunting animals for game meat in their new found domains.

Maposa et al. (2011: 161)

Small-scale artisanal mining activities

Gwenero (2016: v) decries how small-scale artisanal mining activities have ravaged the environment. There is rampant land degradation, siltation, deforestation, water pollution, and loss of aquatic life and loss of biodiversity. One need not wonder why as early as 2007 the then deputy minister of environment made the following remarks when he visited the Marange Diamond fields:

The environment has been ruined. If we allow panning to continue the country cannot afford its reclamation . . . What I have seen is land destruction at its worst. Who will be responsible for filling these shafts? The extent of the plunder is shocking. It is as if these people were using motorized machinery like graders when they were using picks and shovels.

(Manica Post 16 March 2007)

The two economic activities, namely agriculture and mining, which I have presented previously show that there is an urgent need to focus on healing the environment. Currently, in Zimbabwe, the focus of healing and reconciliation seems to be mainly on human relationships. In the previous scenarios, there is a concern that land reform and economic crisis have created serious environmental problems that will not be solved, as Hanlon et al. (2013: 187) correctly state, by simple enforcement. There is need for a change of attitude. It is in this light that I call for a crucial reconsideration of the role of African (Shona) religio-cultural tradition as a healing resource that has the potential of reinstating green spirituality. This entails a critique of modern Western views of nature.

The limits of the modern Western views of nature

The modern worldview has a tendency to view nature as disenchanted. It also inclines itself to assert the mastery of human beings over other aspects of nature. The modern view of nature revolves around: The pre-eminence and natural superiority of humans. This advocates, first of all, the view that people are like God in their wisdom, inventiveness, creativity, and intelligence. So it is human destiny and nature to master creation (Kinsley, 1995: 126). Secondly, there is the issue of the disenchantment of nature. Here the view is that nature is not sacred. God created it, but it is not divine. It is only human beings who are endowed with souls and made in the image of God. So creation is not animate in the sense of containing souls (Kinsley, 1995: 127). Thirdly, we have the investigation and domination of nature. The spirit of this orientation is captured in the following words "The new man (sic) of science must not think that the inquisition of nature is in any way forbidden. Nature must be bound into service and made a slave, put in constraint and moulded by mechanical arts. The searchers and spies of nature are to discover her plots and secrets" (Kinsley, 1995: 129). The scientific analysis and experimentation implied in the previous quotation is related to a fourth idea. This is the idea of objectivity and aloofness. This position emphasises that human beings are different and stand apart from the rest of the natural world. So it is not possible to think of nature as consisting of beings with which one could establish rapport (Kinsley, 1995: 130). Fifthly, there is the notion of infinity. This fosters the idea that reality consists of an open universe infinite in size. (Kinsley, 1995: 131). The mastery of nature implied in the notions that we have mentioned so far presupposes a certain notion of progress. In the modern worldview, progress means moving "from a condition in which nature overwhelms, dominates, humbles, or confines human beings to a condition in which human beings conquer, control, and manipulate nature for their own purposes or for the well-being of the human race" (Kinsley, 1995: 132) As a result, nature is viewed primarily as a resource to be exploited in the human quest for progress.

This way of viewing nature squares very well with dualistic attitudes. Thus, "Dualism is the tendency to divide reality into polar opposites, one pole superior and the other inferior (hierarchy). The great dualisms of the Western tradition are familiar: God and world, heaven and earth, spirit-soul-mind and nature-body-matter, men and women, good and evil, winners and losers, and culture and nature" (Martin-Schramm and Stivers, 2003: 20). Some dualisms simplify what is often a complex reality. A dualistic frame of mind may be deeply troubling, when polar opposites are disconnected, value judgement places one pole above the other, and social custom and attitudes toward nature are formed according to these judgements. The oppression of people and the degradation of nature may be fostered under these circumstances (Martin-Schramm and Stivers, 2003: 20).

In the light of the limitations of dualistic in fostering environmentally friendly attitudes I argue for counter imaginations of nature and humanity that are based on African understandings of: (1) relational personhood, (2) relational ontology, and (3) relational epistemology. My argument is consistent with observations of the global recognition of the need for a new, more environmentally friendly/benign imagination of nature, seeing it as active, meaningful, subjective, and spiritual, re-evaluating it, recognizing humanity as part of nature, and encouraging caring human action towards nature. In this context religion is regarded as a possible influential source of new recognition of nature, linking humanity to a wider environmental reality and providing the existential support, moral authority, and institutional organization able to address environmental issues (Watling, 2009: 2–3).

We may also speak of idealized religious imaginations of nature and humanity's place in it, envisaging a more environmentally oriented humanity in a cooperative, harmonic, interdependent, sacred relationship with nature (Watling, 2009: 2–3). We may imagine a more environmentally friendly, cooperative, humble, and spiritual humanity in tune with nature. The way nature is imagined leads to the way humanity interacts with it, dominating or liberating, degrading or protecting it (Watling, 2009: 2–3).

In this chapter, I therefore explore the possibility of such ideal imaginations in African traditional religion. The exploration is based on analysing a Shona myth of creation. This creation myth is popularly known as the *Mwedzi* myth of creation. My rationale for choosing myth is well captured in the following words:

> Myth, perhaps most appropriately described as sacred wisdom, is critical to understanding religions. Myths contain a people's worldview; they encapsulate and condense . . . views of the world, of ultimate reality, and of the relationship between the creator, the universe, and humanity. Mythology answers questions of meaning and value about a people's place, and relations with the larger world. Myths contain a people's worldview and spiritual vision. Myth teaches humanity to find the sacred in and through all aspects of the natural world and expose humanity as just one part of an on-going sacred life that includes the entire cosmos.
>
> (Kemerer, 2012: 21)

This conception of myth is crucial in the sense that it does not necessarily relegate mythical thinking to fiction or fairy tale. We follow a phenomenological interpretation of myth that emphasises the meaning and significance of myths. In fact, the previous definition implies phenomenology's understanding of myth as sacred stories. So, next we explore the *Mwedzi* myth of creation in the light of the earlier understanding of myth.

The *Mwedzi* myth of creation

> In the beginning, Mwari (God) created the first man, *Mwedzi*, (moon) whom he placed in a pool. He asked to be released into the world for the pool of life was boring. He was given a go ahead after a bitter debate with Mwari. Mwari had insisted that *Mwedzi* would regret it, since the earth was a lonely and desolate place.
>
> After a few days pondering, *Mwedzi* came back to Mwari and complained that he wanted a partner. He was given *Massasi* (*Nyamasase*, the evening star). The two departed to the earth. In the evening, they made fire to warm their bodies. *Mwedzi* had a medicine horn. He grabbed it and rubbed its oil on his index finger. Suddenly he jumped to the side where *Massasi* was after having remarked that he was capable of jumping to the other side of the furnace. He touched *Massasi*. She became pregnant. *Massasi* bore trees, grass, cattle and goats and also the herbivores of the forest

After two years, Mwari took *Massasi* back to the pool leaving *Mwedzi* lonely. *Mwedzi* petitioned for another wife. He was given *Morongo*, the morning star. Mwedzi repeated the same act and *Murongo* conceived. She gave birth to the first boys and girls, wild carnivores such as the lion and its kind, the civet cat and the snake. Morongo later copulated with the snake. *Murongo*, like *Mwedzi*, had committed incest. The snake bit Mwedzi, who had now assumed the place of sovereign (*Mambo*). He became ill. There was drought, starvation, and death. Many people died and *Mwedzi*'s sons consulted *hakata* (divination bones). They were instructed to perform a ritual. Things were brought to normal when they chose a king.

(Banana, 1991: 45)

Visions of the paradise based on the myth

Overall, the myth implies that the Shona people do not generally hold an idea of "nature" separate and apart from humanity or from the spirit world. Instead, they most often view the supernatural world as here, among us, and they tend to view humans as just one part of a perpetual sacred life that encompasses the entire cosmos. For the Shona people, the environment and the supernatural realm are interconnected. This stems from the observation that elements of nature are children of human beings. So the Shona this means that they are all surrounded with creative energies flowing through trees, grasses, streams and rivers, mountains, rivers, sea, sky, and all galaxies, animals, birds, and humans. The ecosystem is viewed with awe. As a result, the Shona people also tend to understand their expansive community as interdependent. The myth generally illustrates the fact that all living things and natural entities have a role to play in maintaining the web of life. In light of this general analysis, later I discuss Shona visions of the paradise implied in the myth, particularly ecological imaginations that imply relational ontology, relational personhood and relational epistemology. These visions have a potential for forming the bedrock of a healing attitude towards the environment.

Relational ontology

At the heart of Shona myth is a relational ontology based on kinship with nature. From the myth we note that "*Massasi* bore trees, grass, cattle and goats and also the herbivores of the forest (abyss). *Mwedzi* repeated the same act and *Murongo* conceived. She gave birth to the first boys and girls, wild carnivores such as the lion and its kind, the civet cat and the snake." This implies that human beings and nature are related. This kinship is consistent with Mbiti's (1969: 135) observation about kinship among Africans in general. He notes that

Indeed this sense of kinship binds together the entire life of the tribe and is even extended to cover animals, plants, and non-living objects through the totemic system. Almost all the concepts connected with human relationships can be understood and interpreted through the kinship system. This it is which largely governs the behavior, thinking, and whole life of the individual in the society of which he is a member.

The idea of kinship is based on the belief that all people are descended from a common ancestor who long ago lived in their territory (Paris, 1995: 77). In the myth, nature and human beings originate from a common ancestor, *Mwedzi*. The status of nature vis-à-vis humans in Shona society must therefore be imagined, and primarily be considered in the context of kinship. In this context the key word is "relationship." In fact, we may speak of ontological relationship. The Shona view the world in such a way that everything in the universe is due to relationships. Everything is interconnected, interwoven, one, everything can relate to us and we can relate to every "thing" as one.

This relational ontology is a complete unity or solidarity, which nothing can break or destroy. To destroy or remove one of the categories is to destroy the whole of existence including the destruction of the creation, which is impossible. One mode of existence presupposes all the others, and a balance must be maintained so that these modes neither drift too far apart from one another nor get too close to one another. From the myth we note that "Morongo later copulated with the snake. *Murongo* like Mwedzi had committed incest. The snake bit Mwedzi, who had now assumed the place of sovereign (*Mambo*). He became ill. There was drought, starvation, and death. Many people died and *Mwedzi's* sons consulted *hakata* (divination bones). They were instructed to perform a ritual. Things were brought to normal when they chose a king." (Banana, 1991: 45). Generally, the relational ontology drawn from the myth is one based on a kinship model that sees, as Johnson (1993: 30) observes;

> Human beings and the earth with all its creatures are intrinsically related as companions in a community of life. Because we are all mutually interconnected, the flourishing or damaging of one ultimately affects all. This kinship attitude does not measure on a scale of higher or lower ontological dignity but appreciates them as integral elements in the robust thriving of the whole.

Relational personhood

The relational ontology discussed earlier rests on a kind of relational personhood. The relationship between animals such as the snake and figures such as the morning star Morongo in the myth imply that there is no total alienation between human and nonhuman. This points to the view that the Shona person is a composite of relationships. In fact, the person is "dividual," not individual. A person constitutes relationships. They relate to others. The "other" is nature. A person does not individuate, but "dividuates" other beings in their environment. The "I" is not the primary axis of Shona culture.

From the myth we can infer a Shona worldview characterized by seamless interconnection between the divine, human, and natural worlds. Nature is not unimportant. Divine-human relations do not exclude relationships between humans and nature. This leads us to imagine a "we-ness" as opposed to a materialistic framing of the environment as alien to us and develops an awareness and sense of self and others. This means developing a sense of belonging and coming to know our responsibilities and ways to relate to the self and others. This breeds a vision based on focusing our attention on our interrelatedness and our interdependence with each other and our greater surroundings.

The Shona environmental vision entails imagining the *nyika* (country) not only as the land and the people, but also including entities such as water bodies, animals, plants, the climate, skies, and spirits. Are entities live in close relationship with one another. All things are recognised with their place in the overall system. Relationships are not oppositional, nor binary. Relations serve to define and unite, not to oppose or alienate. Both this relational personhood and this relational ontology should be undergirded by an implied relational epistemology.

Relational epistemology

From the Shona creation myth, it can be noted that nature is not unimportant. At the heart of the myth is an implied relational epistemology. This is based on the assumption that divine-human relations do not exclude relationship between humans and the natural. There is no materialistic framing of the environment as alien to humanity. The myth fosters a relationality which frames the environment as "nested relatedness." It is not premised on the dichotomous opposition of culture and nature as good or evil. This relational epistemology privileges knowing how to behave within relationships in order to nourish these relationships over knowing things in and for themselves as objects separate from the human community.

Conclusion

In light of the global recognition of the need for a new, more environmentally imagination of nature, in this paper I have explored such ideas in Shona traditional religion, by analysing the Mwedzi myth of creation. I have acknowledged the environmental challenges and took heed of the call to explore possibilities of religious environmental visions and in particular I explored what could be termed African traditional religious environmental visions. In light of the ideal of a more environmentally friendly, cooperative, humble, and spiritual humanity in tune with nature, I have demonstrated the possibility of new ways of imagining the relationship of humanity and nature that foster a relational perception of the environment based on relational ontology, relational personhood, and relational epistemology inferred from the African (Shona) traditional religio-cultural myth of creation. As a result, my main argument in this chapter is that African (Shona) traditional religio-cultural mythical thought must be seen as a legitimate, meaningful, powerful, way of inculcating environmental healing consciousness, a view able to rekindle traditional African (Shona) green spirituality. Whereas most scholars have approached the theme of national healing, reconciliation, and integration in terms of uniting different ethnic and political groups, in this chapter I have demonstrated the urgency of healing the land. It is only the land that is healed that can carry healed individuals, communities, and the nation. The healing of the land of Zimbabwe from environmental degradation caused by the land reform exercise and unmonitored mining activities is, therefore, an extremely urgent undertaking. The healing of the land of Zimbabwe constitutes the primary and most pressing theme in the discourse on national healing, integration, and reconciliation. The politics of land reform must now be replaced by the politics of healing the land, promoting care for the environment and giving rise to prosperity.

References

Banana, C. 1991. *Come and Share: An Introduction to Christian Theology*. Gweru: Mambo Press.

Bauman, W. A., R. R. Bohannon II and K. J. O'Brien. 2011. "Ecology: What Is It, Who Gets to Decide, and Why Does It Matter?" In W. A. Bauman, R. R. Bohannon II, K. J. O'Brien (eds.), *Grounding Religion: A Field Guide to the Study of Religion and Ecology*. New York: Routledge, 49–63.

Bwiti, K. 2000. "Chief Zvimba's Bold Stand for Nature," *The Sunday Mail*, 20–26 December.

Gwenero, L. H. 2016. "Effects of Artisanal Small Scale Gold Mining Activities on the Environment and Livelihoods: A Case Study of Shurugwi," Dissertation Submitted in Partial Fulfilment of the Requirements of the Bachelor of Arts in Development Studies Honour's Degree, Faculty of Arts, Department of Development Studies, Midlands State University, Gweru.

Hanlon, J., J. Manjengwa and T. Smart. 2013. *Zimbabwe Takes Back Its Land*. Cape Town: Jacana Media.

Johnson Elizabeth, A. 1993. *Women Earth and Creator Spirit*. New York: Paulist Press.

Kemerer, Lisa. 2012. *Animals and World Religions*. Oxford: Oxford University Press.

Kinsley, D. 1995. *Ecology and Religions: Ecological Spirituality in Cross-Cultural Perspective*. Englewood Cliffs, NJ: Prentice Hall.

Some, Malidoma Patrice. 1998. *The Healing Wisdom of Africa: Finding Life, Purpose Through Nature, Ritual and Community*. New York: Tarcher/Putnum.

Maposa, R. S., J. Hlongwana and T. Muguti. 2011. "Liberation Theology and the Depletion of Natural Resources, A Smart Partnership? An Appraisal on Varimi Vatsva in the Former Commercial White Farms in Zimbabwe," *Journal of Sustainable Development in Africa* 13(2), 155–167.

Martin-Schramm, J. B. and R. L. Stivers. 2003. *Christian Environmental Ethics: A Case Method Approach*. New York: Orbis Books.

Mbiti, John S. 1969. *African Religions and Philosophy*. London, Ibadan and Nairobi: Heinemann.

Paris, Peter J. 1995. *The Spirituality of African People: The Search for a Common Moral Discourse*. Minneapolis: Fortress Press.

Taringa, N. T. and M. Sipeyiye. 2013. "Zimbabwean Indigenous Religions and Political Drama: The Fast-Track Land Reform and Fast-Track Change to Attitudes to Nature,

2000–2008," in Chitando Ezra (ed.), *Prayers and Players: Religion and Politics in Zimbabwe*. Harare: SAPES Books, 51–61.

Tucker, Mary Evelyn and Grim, John. 2001. *Daoism and Ecology*. Cambridge: Publications of the Center for the Study of World Religions, Harvard Divinity School.

Watling, Tony. 2009. *Ecological Imaginations in the World Religions: An Ethnographic Analysis*. London: Continuum.

Young, William. 2005. *The World's Religions: Worldviews and Contemporary Issues* (2nd ed). Upper Saddle River, NJ: Pearson Prentice Hall.

Index

Note: Page numbers in **bold** indicate a table on the corresponding page.

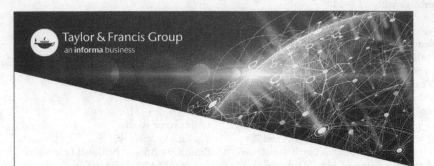

Printed in the United States
by Baker & Taylor Publisher Services